Ethical Questions in Dentistry. Second Edition

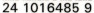

Ethical Questions in Dentistry

Second Edition

James T. Rule, DDS, MS

Professor Emeritus
Department of Pediatric Dentistry
Dental School
University of Maryland
Baltimore, Maryland

Robert M. Veatch, PhD

Professor of Medical Ethics
The Kennedy Institute of Ethics
Georgetown University
Washington, DC

Quintessence Publishing Co, Inc

Chicago, Berlin, Tokyo, Copenhagen, London, Paris, Milan, Barcelona,
Istanbul, São Paulo, New Delhi, Moscow, Prague, and Warsaw

To My Son

Timothy Cornwall Rule

—JTR

To My Father

Cecil Ross Veatch
September 19, 1905–May 6, 1977

—RMV

Library of Congress Cataloging-In-Publication Data

Rule, James T.
  Ethical questions in dentistry / James T. Rule, Robert M. Veatch.-- 2nd ed.
      p. ; cm.
  Includes bibliographical references and index.
  ISBN 0-86715-443-8 (softcover)
  1. Dental ethics. 2. Dental ethics--Case studies.
  [DNLM: 1. Ethics, Dental--Case Reports. WU 50 R935e 2004] I. Veatch,
Robert M. II. Title.

  RK52.7.R85 2004
  174.2'976--dc22

                                        2004007423

quintessence
books

©2004 Quintessence Publishing Co, Inc

Quintessence Publishing Co, Inc
551 Kimberly Drive
Carol Stream, IL 60188
www.quintpub.com

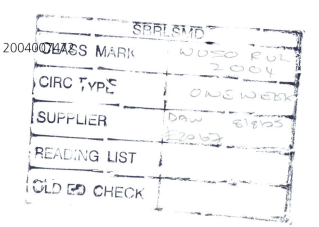

Editors: Lisa C. Bywaters and Lindsay Harmon
Cover and internal design: Dawn Hartman
Production: Susan Robinson

Printed in the USA

Table of Contents

Cases

Preface to the Second Edition

In the 11 years since the first edition of this book was published, much has happened in the field of dental ethics. An ethics curriculum is now required in all US dental schools. New books on dental ethics have been published, including several from other countries, and two in this country are now in their second editions. The American College of Dentists has published an ethics handbook for dentists and now includes a section on dental ethics in each issue of its journal. The membership of the US-based Professional Ethics in Dentistry Network has increased significantly, and an international dental ethics association has been formed called IDEALS—the International Dental Ethics and Law Society.

Even as recognition of the importance of dental ethics has grown, concerns about the ethical foundations of the profession may also have increased. There is some unease within the profession—possibly also reflected in public attitudes—about a tendency for increasing numbers of dentists to put their own interests above those of their patients.

The second edition of this book is designed to deal directly with issues such as this. Its goals are the same as those of the first edition: to help sensitize dental professionals to the important role of ethics in dentistry and to provide a general approach to ethical reasoning in dental-related problem solving. However, in order to better implement these goals, we have made several important changes, some of which were shaped by constructive criticism of the first edition.

As a frame of reference for the rest of the book, we have included an entirely new chapter on professions. Using frequent references to dentistry, it begins with a brief history of the development of professions that is essential to understanding their structure and function today. It presents both the traditional idealized perspective of professions and the views of their critics. For professionals, both outlooks are required reading.

Of special significance for newcomers to the discipline of ethics is the expansion and modification of the format of the case discussions. The discussions now contain an increased amount of relevant background material and additional guidance in the techniques of ethical problem solving.

To find space for these innovations, two adjustments were made. One was to eliminate the chapter on research. (A few of its cases were retained and moved to other chapters.) We also eliminated cases that we had reason to believe were not widely used for discussion by students and others. The first edition contained 111 cases; the second contains 88.

The final important change was the introduction of new and timely cases—12 of the 88 did not appear in the first edition. Unlike the cases in the first edition, which were presented from the perspective of the individual practitioner, many of the new cases invite discussion on ethical issues faced by the entire profession of dentistry—for example, access to care, licensure, and the corporate sponsorship of graduate education.

Preface to the First Edition

Every day of their professional lives, dentists face decisions that have ethical content. Most often the issues involve the utilization of complicated diagnostic or technical skills in the delivery of patient care. The way these skills are used is based on the values of both the dentist and the patient. Every recommendation by a dentist and acceptance by a patient has ethical substance, in its potential for patients to be helped or harmed or their wishes and values to be respected or ignored. Sometimes a practitioner's recommendation may conflict with what the patient wants. Sometimes what the patient wants may sound foolish to the dentist. How the dentist responds to these problems and many others determines the character of a dentist's practice.

Some situations occur so often that they may not even be recognized as having ethical content. Other times the circumstances are complex, and the answers are not readily apparent. However, in both situations a background in philosophical ethics can be helpful as support for making sound decisions. Unfortunately, while technological advances and changes in societal perspectives over the last 20 years have increased the ethical challenges inherent within dentistry, the response of dental schools has been relatively recent. Further, although at present 80% of all dental schools offer courses in ethics, the emphasis in many is on jurisprudence.

This does not mean that dentists are not interested in or disturbed about ethical issues. In recent years, published reports have shown concerns about poor quality of care, violations of public trust, flagrant advertising, self-regulation, informed consent, interactions with impaired or incompetent colleagues, financial interactions with patients and insurance companies, and several others. Dental practitioners have developed a variety of approaches, including the reliance on values instilled during dental school, discussions with colleagues and consideration of the ADA Code of Ethics, and their own personal standards, to resolve these problems. However, a general approach to ethical reasoning in dental-related problem solving has not been available to either the dental practitioner or the dental student. This book is intended to address that deficiency.

Acknowledgments

Of great importance in facilitating the completion of the second edition was James Rule's opportunity to serve as a Senior Visiting Fellow at Creighton University's Center for Health Policy and Ethics in Omaha, Nebraska in the autumn of 2003. The support of Center Director Ruth Purtilo, PhD, and each of the Center faculty, as well as the facilities of Creighton University were extremely valuable. Especially important was the generosity of Jos Welie, PhD, who freely offered his time and his perspectives in many discussions of ideas and issues related to this book. These discussions, among other benefits, contributed to the formulation of some of the new cases that appear in this edition. Dr Welie, along with Dr Ruth Purtilo and Dr Amy Haddad, also reviewed the chapter on professions and made valuable suggestions for its improvement.

As with the first edition of this book, Dr Rule also remains indebted to the University of Maryland for its sabbatical policies and its Department of Pediatric Dentistry for its many years of support. Both were essential contributions to this publication.

We are also grateful for discussions about ethical issues facing dentistry that were held with Dr Wayne Barkmeier, dean of Creighton University School of Dentistry and especially with Dr Richard R. Ranney, former dean of the University of Maryland, who made many important contributions to several of the cases. Once the decision was made to create space in the second edition for new material by eliminating some of the cases from the first edition, Dr Muriel Bebeau provided invaluable information in deciding which cases might be excluded. Dr Andrew E. Allen, Dr Margaret E. Wilson, and Dr Louis DePaola were helpful in updating clinical and scientific information or reviewing issues about old and new cases. Finally, Dr Richard Manski reviewed the chapter on ethical issues in third-party financing and made helpful contributions to the revision. John F. Rule's editorial reviews were once again helpful, and Joanne Rule's support was indispensable.

Introduction

Working through this text, you will find your own answers to ethical questions that dentists face every day. The following case is just one example of the issues to be discussed.

A third-year dental student who worked evenings as a dental assistant described to one of her professors this prototypical example of the kinds of ethical problems encountered in dentistry:

Case 1: Which Patient Benefits?

Ms Andrea Armstrong, aged 37, has been a patient in the practice of Dr Ted Davis for 4 years. She entered his practice seeking treatment for several missing teeth and significant periodontal disease. With unusual candor, she told Dr Davis that she had been an intravenous drug user several years prior to entering his practice. She attributed her deteriorated oral condition to the personal neglect that accompanied her active addiction. During that period she had lived with a man with whom she shared her habit. The relationship ended, and she subsequently received treatment for her addiction.

She is now drug free and involved in a healthy relationship with a man named John Ariana. They live together and plan to be married. But a serious problem has arisen as of her current recall visit: She has become HIV positive and believes she was infected by her former lover.

Dr Davis plans to continue to treat Ms Armstrong. However, he now faces a problem in relation to her fiancé, who recently entered Dr Davis's practice at the suggestion of Ms Armstrong. Based on indirect and separate conversations with each patient, Dr Davis has become convinced that Ms Armstrong has not told her partner of her HIV status, and the idea gnaws at him. He feels that Ms Armstrong is clearly obligated to disclose her HIV conversion to her fiancé. He also feels that he has a duty to tell Mr Ariana. Compounding this dilemma is Dr Davis' commitment to keep his patient's confidences. He fears litigation should he fail to do so.

DISCUSSION:

How should Dr Davis handle these conflicting obligations? Does confidentiality for Ms Armstrong override the need to inform Mr Ariana? How does one approach this ethical dilemma, in which both disclosure and nondisclosure could possibly be justified? These questions will be explored in chapter 7 when we examine the ethics of confidentiality. But first, we must clarify exactly what ethics is and how ethical problems can be examined. Only then will we be in a position to provide a more detailed analysis of Dr Davis' problem.

Like all professions, dentistry faces ethical situations on a daily basis. Some, such as the previous case, are similar to those encountered in medicine. Many, however, are unique to the practice of dentistry. A few are encountered so often they may not even be recognized as having ethical content. Other cases, like that of Dr Davis, require some background in the discipline of ethics as support for making sound decisions.

Technological advances and a shift in attitudes within society have created more clinical situations that require ethical analysis. Texts such as this one and professional ethics programs in dental schools throughout the country have only begun to prepare their students to handle those situations.

Goals and Format

The primary goal of this book is to comprehensively present the ethical problems in dentistry and to suggest approaches to their resolution. The text is organized into three parts. Part I introduces the major ethical theories and principles and gives examples that encapsulate their application to dental practice. It also introduces a format for ethical case analysis that is illustrated using the case of a troublesome patient's request for mood-altering drugs. Parts II and III consist exclusively of ethical analyses of cases. Most of the cases are based on actual events associated with patient care and were solicited from generalists and specialists in various parts of the country, thus providing a national picture of ethical issues in dentistry. Names and details have been modified to provide anonymity and clarity of the issues. A few cases were taken from published reports in dental literature and the public press, in which instances real names and details are provided. In addition, certain cases were written as ethical issues facing the profession at large, rather than an individual practitioner.

Part II discusses ethical principles by using case histories to illustrate the following: beneficence (acting to benefit the patient), nonmaleficence (avoiding harm), fidelity (obligations related to trust and confidentiality), autonomy (including problems of informed consent), veracity (truth-telling), and justice in the allocation of dental resources.

Part III rounds out the discussion with cases representing special topics such as ethical issues in dental schools; third-party financing; HIV-infected patients and dentists; and incompetent, dishonest, and impaired dentists.

Altogether, the organization and contents of this book give the reader both the basic fundamentals of ethics and a broad perspective of the types of ethical issues that dentists encounter. In addition, the examples of ethical reasoning illustrated in the case and analysis sections provide useful guidelines for the resolution of ethical problems encountered in professional life.

Part I
Ethical Questions:
Theory and Principles

chapter 1

An Overview of Ethics in Dentistry

In this chapter

The Influence of Society and Medicine

Society's Increasing Concern

Ethical standards in modern society are in a time of rapid flux and show the contradictions that characteristically attend such changes. This period of ethical re-evaluation received an abrupt stimulus in the 1960s from the great upheavals over civil rights and the Vietnam War. Contrasted with this is the current widespread concern about the behavior of public persons. A president has been impeached. Congressional ethics committees have taken aggressive action against colleagues. Distrust between political parties is increasingly problematic. Business leaders have been put on trial for deception and dishonesty. Public trust in institutions of all sorts, including most professions, has diminished.[1] Consumers are better informed and demand more and better services, including those related to health care. On the other hand, strains of contradictory value systems run throughout society. Large segments of society are becoming more materialistic, more self-serving, less reflective, and less concerned for the welfare of the community.[2]

Despite these views, there is a growing advocacy for limiting what has been almost a century-long endorsement of unchecked "progress." Significant portions of the population now feel that the world ecology is at risk, that resources are finite and must be guarded, that technology has created important ethical issues not previously recognized, and that there is something seriously wrong with our health care system, both its cost and its benefits.[2]

Upheaval in Medicine

Thirty years ago, there was little formal intellectual work that considered ethical questions in the health care professions. What ethical discussion existed was more or less limited to questions about physicians' practices and how they were interrelated: Should physicians extend professional courtesy? Should they conceal from a patient their disagreement with a colleague's diagnosis?

During the three intervening decades, medicine's increased preoccupation with ethics has been phenomenal. The output of ethics literature was minimal in 1970. By 1980 the number of MEDLINE ethics references cited was 313. The number grew to 780 by 1989 and has continued to grow even more rapidly since then. Ethics consultants in hospitals are now commonplace, and most larger hospitals have ethics committees that offer a formal review of problems with ethical overtones.[3] In addition, newspapers regularly feature stories illustrating ethical issues involving difficult decisions to be made at the end or the beginning of life.

One of the most important reasons for the growth in concerns over ethics is rooted in the tremendous technological advances that, at great cost, offer prolonged or improved life quality. With high-tech enhancements come questions about who gets the care, who pays for it, and how those decisions are made. Especially important are concerns over genetic engineering, reproduction, and termination of care.[4,5]

The huge increase in the cost of care is also of special concern. In 1960 the dollars spent on medical care were 5.9% of the gross national product. By 1990 the amount had risen to 12.2%[6] and by 2001 to 14.1%.[7] Considering the extent of the increase, it is natural to expect citizens to be concerned about ethics. This is especially true when the impact of the dollars spent is questionable. For example, the United States spends two and a half times as much money per capita on health care as does Britain, but life expectancy and other health parameters are quite similar.[8]

Consider, too, that most medical care is now covered, at least in part, by some form of health insurance. Health insurance in itself generates its own ethical issues. Traditional third-party payment systems encourage overtreatment and overutilization. Health maintenance organizations (HMOs) encourage undertreatment and underutilization.[8]

Several other factors have contributed to the increased attention or concern about ethical issues. Ethicists have branched out beyond their traditional roles in philosophy departments to enter the health care arena. Undergraduate courses in bioethics and concerns for the ability of future physicians to deal with the increasing complex ethical issues in medicine have set up demands for ethics courses in medical schools that previously had none. Practicing physicians, because of their lack of training in ethics, are often poorly prepared to deal with the ethical issues encountered in daily practice.[4]

Physicians also have nagging concerns about the desirability of medicine as a profession. Increasing controls by the federal government and by the insurance industry have decreased the time that physicians have available for patient contact. Public trust in physicians is of concern. The nature of medical practice is changing in that more doctors are being employed by organizations. Although physicians continue to control policies in these organizations, they perceive the trend toward "captive" physicians as being undesirable.[1] Finally, since 1983, physicians' incomes, while still very high, have started to decline for the first time.[8] These factors, coupled with the decline in the college-age population and the increased attractiveness of other scientific, professional, and business occupations, have led to a decrease in the number of applicants to medical school. All of these factors form a context for the ethical issues that must be faced in today's society.

Dentistry as a Reflection of Medicine

The recent growth of ethics literature in dentistry has been significant but is nearly 15 years behind medicine in terms of its analysis of dental-related ethical problems. Additionally, although a few books on dental ethics are available, the literature is almost exclusively limited to journal articles, whereas hundreds of books have been written on themes of medical ethics. Until 1993, when the first comprehensive books on dental ethics were published, the only applicable book available was limited to issues of informed consent.[9]

Still, there is a rising interest in ethics in dental education. The American Dental Association's (ADA's) Commission on Dental Education has set standards for ethics education and has made it a requirement for accreditation. In addition, all dental hygiene schools[10] now have courses in professional ethics. However, the ability of these courses to stimulate valid ethical reasoning may be of concern because few of the faculty have formal training in ethics.

In clinical dentistry, the interest in ethics is considerably different from that of medicine. For example, there is nothing comparable to the ethics consultants or ethics committees that are becoming routine in the hospital practice of medicine. The main consideration in dentistry has not been about specific clinical issues such as that of the termination of care. Rather, it has focused on the ethical standards of the profession in the sense of concerns for excellence in the quality of care and the need to maintain public trust. The leadership in this regard has come from the American College of Dentists. The growing number of ethics-oriented continuing education courses is a reflection of those concerns.

Some of the ethical issues in clinical dentistry derive from technological advances that have somewhat paralleled those in medicine, although with fewer dollars at stake and less involvement in life-sustaining issues. Nevertheless, costly innovations such as computer-generated restorative procedures (ie, CAD/CAM), along with the increasing use of implants and lasers, not only serve to improve the quality of care but also make care more inaccessible to less affluent people.

The increases in costs of care in dentistry have been substantially less than those in medicine, but they still present ethical concerns in terms of the resulting benefits. In medicine the huge increase in costs has not improved morbidity or mortality statistics. In dentistry there has been a steady decline in caries rates in children and young adults over the last 40 years and a decline in periodontal disease as well. However, these improvements appear to be related less to patient care provided by dentists than to water fluoridation and the increased use of improved oral home care products, especially fluoride dentifrices and therapeutic mouthrinses.

In another parallel with medicine, the growth of dental health insurance has been significant. However, it has not reached the high level of coverage experienced for medical insurance. Statistics from 2000 show that 85.4% of the population had some form of general health insurance, whereas only 57.4% had some form of dental insurance coverage.[11] Nevertheless, the entrance of insurance into dental practice has fostered significant ethical concerns about overtreatment and undertreatment, just as it has in medicine.

Medicine is becoming more concerned over its public image and its desirability as a profession. Dentistry, always sensitive to issues of public opinion and professional status, has also experienced some recent decline in that regard. The 2001 Gallup Poll on honesty and ethics in American professions placed dentistry eighth from the top, below nurses, pharmacists, veterinarians, physicians, grade-school and high-school teachers, and clergy, and immediately below college teachers.[12] While eighth is not bad, it is several steps down from the top two or three rankings, where dentistry stood for decades. In one of his monthly commentaries in the *Journal of the American Dental Association*, Gordon Christensen offered five reasons why the public's attitude toward dentistry may be changing. They include: "having a commercial, self-promotional orientation; planning and carrying out excessive treatment; charging high fees without justification; providing service only when it is convenient; refusing to accept responsibility when treatment fails prematurely."[13] Incomes of dentists, having declined over most of the 1980s, are now increasing once again. And although there is concern within dentistry about the trend for dentists to be employed by organizations rather than to be self-employed, the view of dentistry by dentists is improving.

How Dentists Perceive Ethical Problems

The Nature of Ethical Problems

What constitutes an ethical problem in contrast with a clinical, scientific, or legal problem? It might appear that some problems are purely clinical or scientific. However, such a view is illusory if by that we mean that clinical or scientific decisions can ever be made without some value judgment. Every clinical, scientific, or legal problem involves an evaluative component. Evaluations can often be identified when words of appraisal appear, such as good or bad, right or wrong, should, ought, or must. Sometimes the evaluative words are not as conspicuously evaluative, but they convey value judgments nonetheless. Claiming that an effect is a "benefit" or that a treatment is "indicated" conveys such a judgment, as does identifying an effect as a "harm" or a "side effect."

Of course, not all evaluations are moral evaluations. Some value judgments are esthetic, cultural, or merely matters of personal taste. Certain evaluations, however, are indeed ethical. Most of us can rely on common sense to tell the difference between ethical and other kinds of evaluations. The formal criteria of ethical evaluations will be discussed in chapter 3. What is critical to know at this point is that all clinical or scientific decisions require evaluations. Decisions are easy when the difference between good and bad is clear-cut. In other situations, decisions are more difficult, and choices must be made between good and good or between two evils.

The use of local anesthetics for cavity preparation offers a good example of the role of values in decision making. Dentists are taught to use local anesthetics almost routinely in cavity preparations to maximize patient comfort. The use of local anesthetics may also reduce the stress felt by the dentist who then does not have to worry about hurting the patient. It can also result in better treatment because, for example, more thorough caries removal is possible under good local anesthesia. In general, dentists value these consequences of local anesthesia to the extent that they often use it routinely even though procedures may be possible without it. Sometimes dentists may value the benefits of local anesthesia so much that they may refuse to treat a patient who requests that no local anesthesia be given or may try to pressure a reluctant patient to accept it. The frequent use of local anesthesia is not a major value issue in dentistry, but it does show the value dentists place on their ability and desire to relieve pain. Patients may hold values that differ from the dentist's and lead to rejecting local anesthesia. They may find the discomfort of the injection worse than that of the drilling or they may not want to experience the posttreatment feeling of anesthesia. There is nothing incorrect about these judgments; they are simply different from those that dentists often make. Failing to ask patients about their judgments may lead to treatment without adequate consent.

Evaluation may become an ethical issue when the dentist realizes that the evaluation involves a trade-off between the value of reducing pain and other values that the patient may affirm. For example, the patient may fear the side effects of the anesthetic, may object to its duration, or may simply have a psychological constitution that tolerates dental pain. It is clear that there is no definitively correct value judgment here. The value judgment of the dentist and the patient may conflict. The dentist who does what he or she thinks is best for the patient could end up violating the autonomy of the patient.

Ethical Versus Legal

People sometimes confuse ethical and legal problems. Both the ethical and the legal involve evaluations. Ethical evaluations, however, appeal to what is believed to be an ultimate standard of right and wrong. Legal evaluations appeal to the evaluations of a particular society. Moreover, they merely express the society's minimal standards of behavior that can be enforced. Hence, it is possible that some behaviors could be legal, but still unethical. Alternatively, some behaviors that are illegal might nevertheless be ethical. This could occur if a society makes a value judgment that ultimately turns out to be wrong. Laws enforcing slavery are an extreme example where the legal and the ethical are not identical.

Changing attitudes within society about health care and the growing tendency toward initiating malpractice suits has stimulated attitudinal changes within the profession. Thus, instead of viewing the law as a guide for providing treatment that is in the interests of their patients, dentists often view the law as specifying the behavior necessary to avoid malpractice.[14]

As a result, differences between law and ethics must be noted as well as similarities. It may be legal for a general dentist to provide comprehensive orthodontic care without adequate training but unethical to do so. Conversely, a dentist may consider it ethically justifiable to correct a cross-bite for a patient on a state medical assistance program with a relatively expensive treatment not covered under the program and charge the program for a relatively less expensive but insurance-covered space maintainer. This action, however, is illegal because, in actuality, no space maintainer is required or placed.

In a 1988 study, Hasegawa et al[15] presented a group of practitioners with a series of perplexing clinical ethical situations and asked them to identify whether they represented ethical or legal problems. Although the dentists generally tended to identify the problems as being primarily ethical in nature, younger dentists tended to view them as legal and older dentists tended to view them as neither ethical nor legal. In addition, issues of informed consent were identified by all groups predominantly as being legal rather than having to do with the ethical issue of patient autonomy. It is apparent that some confusion exists within the profession over the very nature of, and foundation for, the relationships between patient and dentist.

Ethical Issues Faced by Dentists

The clinical ethical situations referred to already were predominantly derived from work done by Bebeau and Speidel[16] with a group of Minnesota dentists. Some of the situations came from cases gathered by Hasegawa himself.[15] These examples, coupled with examples reported in a survey of Florida dentists by Holloway et al,[17] form the main part of a compilation presented here of ethical problems as seen by practicing dentists. To these are added other individual contributions appearing in the published literature, along with a survey of issues presented by Dummett in the *Encyclopedia of Bioethics*.[18]

Quality of Care

One of the most frequent expressions of concern is for quality of care.[19] Care might be deemed inadequate if it involves the delivery of substandard care without the patient's knowledge, without consideration of the patient's wishes, without justification by virtue of special circumstances, and motivated by financial gain. No data are available to show the prevalence of this sort of treatment, but it nevertheless has been a recurrent concern in dentistry. Quality of care issues are often linked with other factors.

Advertising

Advertising is one such factor linked with quality of care.[17,18,20] Although in the past some dentists considered all advertising unprofessional, now the primary concern is dentists whose marketing and advertising activities are considered false or misleading. The ADA code of ethics states that "no dentists shall advertise or solicit patients in any form of communication in a manner that is false or misleading in any material respect."[21] Nevertheless, there is a widespread opinion among dentists that misrepresentation is only part of the problem. Many dentists believe that aggressive marketing practices such as discount ploys are not only in bad taste but also diminish the profession in the public eye and probably represent the activities of those who are more interested in profit than in the quality of service.

Self-regulation Practices/"Denturism"

Two other factors that concern dentists deal with the quality of care issue. One is the need to have adequate *self-regulation* and *quality assurance* practices, both to protect the public and to preserve the profession's autonomy.[18,22,23] The other is the movement toward "denturism," which permits laboratory technicians to provide complete prosthetic services, including their clinical components. Dentists are widely opposed to this movement on the basis of concern for an increased risk of substandard and potentially harmful services to patients.[18]

Patient Autonomy

Another set of important issues involves patient autonomy. Issues of *informed consent*[15,17,18,24,25] and the need to put the *patient's interest first*[17] are considered very important. Informed consent is a significant ethical challenge to the dentist because of the large number of different materials and different techniques available for the same or similar problems. Under such circumstances, how much information does the patient need to know to make an informed decision?

Conflicts with Patients

Considerable concern is expressed regarding dentist-patient conflicts and resolutions to such conflicts. One category of conflicts deals with those *precipitated by the dentist.* For example, consider the patient who is unable or unwilling to comply with the home care expectations of the dentist while the dentist wonders whether continuation of the treatment is justifiable.[15] Another example is the management of the questionable child abuse case where the dentist's actions could help the patient but harm the parent.[26] Problems involving the use of potential aversive behavior control techniques in uncooperative children who require dental treatment are also sources of ethical conflict. A final example involves the question of how much training is necessary in a new technique such as implant placement prior to performing it on patients.[15,19]

Another category of conflicts with patients includes those *precipitated by the patient.* The most frequent situation is the patient who requests a procedure that is contrary to the training and standards of the dentist.[15,17] An example is the request for complete-mouth extraction by a patient who has an essentially intact dentition that can easily be saved. Another example is the patient who requests sedatives or pain medication when the dentist is not sure of the necessity.

Justice

Several concerns are over issues of justice. What are the *obligations regarding treatment* for patients not of record who are in pain, for patients with AIDS,[27] or for patients whose prior treatment has failed?[15] Should the dentist *discontinue treatment* when the patient's payment schedule is behind or has stopped altogether?[15] Should the dentist become involved in *treating special patients*, including the handicapped, the aged, and those in nursing homes[18,28,29] or other community programs when that involvement would intrude on a busy and prosperous practice?[18] Is the dentist obligated to provide any free services? If so, for whom and to what extent?

Intraprofessional Relationships

The management of intraprofessional relationships is a major concern among dentists.[15,17,18,28] Examples include the discovery of pathoses overlooked by a colleague when temporarily covering a colleague's practice[28] and other situations where communication with patients without criticizing colleagues is the norm. Referral practices that are based on factors other than the patient's interest are also sources of concern. Among the most difficult problems are those where colleagues should be confronted with their incompetence or when incompetence should be reported.[17]

Financial Transactions

A final series of ethical issues concerns financial transactions pertaining to patients. Some of these issues involve *direct transactions* such as requests by patients to falsify billing (as in the predating of insurance claims),[15,28] decisions on who pays when treatment fails,[15] the charging of different fees for the same service under varying circumstances, charging but not providing services, and fee splitting.[17]

A more troublesome set of issues exists with respect to *dental benefit plans*.[15–17,20,30,31] Dentists perceive these problems as involving issues of the waiving of co-payments and the temptation to tailor the treatment plans of patients to the type of coverage existing in the insurance plan. The latter category contains threats both to the autonomy of the profession (in terms of who controls the treatment) and to the appropriateness of care given to patients.

The types of problems cited have appeared in the literature but the ethical considerations involved in approaching these problems are not clearly defined. However, a report has been published that proposed and described values that are held by the profession of dentistry and are important foundations for ethical decision making. These will be discussed in the next section. Ethical decision making related to problems such as those previously mentioned can be assisted by considering the care-related values that are important to the profession. The next section will present a hierarchy of such values that has been proposed for dentistry.

Values in Clinical Dental Ethics

Ozar and Sokol's Proposal for Six Values in Dentistry

Ozar and Sokol have published a compilation of six value categories purportedly recognized by the dental profession in its approaches to treatment. The authors also describe how values are important in clinical decision making and propose a ranking of the values to help clarify the decision-making process when values conflict.[32] The values, in their hierarchical order, are as follows: *(1)* the patient's life and general health, *(2)* the patient's oral health, *(3)* the patient's autonomy, *(4)* the dentist's preferred practice values, *(5)* esthetic values, and *(6)* efficiency in the use of resources.

We include this account of the values of the profession because it is widely used by dental students and members of the profession to aid in resolving ethical issues in clinical practice. However, the very existence of these values as well as their ranking is controversial both within dentistry and outside it. In addition, this depiction of dentistry's values has some important differences compared with an earlier version coauthored by Ozar in 1988,[33] including the elimination of two of the original values and the addition of a new one. While changes in perspective are often helpful, for us it compounds the controversial aspects of this presentation. And for others who are newcomers to the field of dental ethics, it is important to present a balanced view of the role of values in ethical decision making. We wish that the Ozar-Sokol account could be as useful as it seems, but we believe that it primarily adds to the confusion. For now, however, it will be helpful to summarize their version of a possible list of values and to follow it with a critique that describes our concerns.

The Patient's Life and General Health

The sustaining of life and the promotion of overall health is the central concern of all practitioners and patients. Under normal conditions, dentists should not undertake treatment that will significantly jeopardize the life or health of patients. For example, a man with malignant hyperthermia who received serious facial trauma would have risked death had he been given general anesthesia for corrective surgery. That risk was deemed to outweigh the expected esthetic improvement that could result from the enhanced working conditions permitted under general anesthesia. In this case the oral surgeon therefore used local anesthesia. If one believed that the patient's life and general health always took precedence over other values, the only situation in which a dentist could take actions that risked the patient's general health would be if the dental treatment were for a condition that adversely affected general health even more, so that on balance, its correction could contribute to the improvement of general health.

The Patient's Oral Health

This value is invoked by dentists more frequently than any other and Ozar and Sokol believe it ranks next in line after the patient's life and health. Oral health, for the purposes of this discussion, includes appropriate and pain-free oral functioning. What is appropriate functioning will depend on such factors as age, stage of development, general health, and the patient's requirements for function. The concept of appropriate functioning, of course, requires subjective value judgments. The absence of pain is also an important aspect of the concept of oral health, even though the interpretation of pain is also subjective. Included as well are the basics of disease prevention and the maintenance of oral health. In the case of a patient with severe periodontal disease and poor past oral hygiene practices, it is valuable to stress the need for more strict home care standards before any treatment is started. In a patient who, for reasons of physical limitations, cannot possibly meet normal standards of cooperation, the dentist might conclude that it is unethical to begin any treatment whose success depends on patient cooperation. An example more directly related to oral function is one in which a patient requests fixed partial dentures involving teeth that are seriously compromised periodontally and are not expected to last more than a year or two. In such a case the dentist might consider it unethical to construct the restorations even though the patient might demand that it be done and be willing to pay.

The Patient's Autonomy

A third concept that is valued by patients and dentists alike is autonomy or freedom. In the context of health care, autonomy refers to the ability of patients to make their own health care decisions that reflect their own values and goals. When patients refuse further treatment on teeth and request that they be extracted, they are expressing autonomy. In a typical case, the tooth in question has received several other procedures and now requires root canal treatment and a crown. The dentist believes the tooth can be saved and disagrees with the patient's choice. In this situation, the tooth is already compromised, and although the dentist disagrees with the extraction, the request is reasonable and can be met. Many people find this ability to make autonomous (self-governing) choices valuable. Regardless of whether this capacity is valued, we shall see in Part II of this volume that many people hold to a moral principle that such autonomous choices must be respected.

On the other hand, Ozar and Sokol point out the complexity of respecting the autonomy of a patient.[32] If a patient, for example, were to request treatment that would appreciably compromise oral health, "and if the dentist acted on the patient's request out of respect for the patient's autonomy and did the procedure, the dentist would be acting unprofessionally."*

---

*Most aspects of our critique will appear later in the chapter. However, it is important to raise the question now about what Ozar and Sokol mean when they use the words *acting unprofessionally* in this instance. Under what circumstances is it unprofessional, for example, to compromise a patient's oral health by extracting multiple teeth that could readily be saved? Would the extractions always be unprofessional, or only when performed at the request of a patient? Even if most professionals would refuse to honor such a request, that still does not necessarily mean that extractions would be immoral. Would there be no morally valid reason for patients to request and the dentist to agree to the removal of multiple teeth that could be saved? In addition, if "unprofessional" means "is disapproved of by the profession," might not the profession be sometimes disapproving treatment that is morally justifiable? We believe that in assessing dentist-patient disagreements when patient autonomy is at stake, a more thoughtful approach should be taken.

The Dentist's Preferred Practice Values

During their formal education, dentists receive powerful messages regarding choices of treatment that often become incorporated in their values of preferred practice. Examples include the restoration rather than extraction of carious teeth (when possible), the use of crowns rather than amalgam restorations in compromised teeth, and the use of fixed restorations rather than partial dentures in situations where either is possible. In fact, some dentists place more value on their preferred practice values than on respecting patient autonomy. However, Ozar makes the point that the function of professions "is not to be measured by how attached a dentist might be to his or her patterns of practice, but rather by the benefits it secures to dentists and patients together."[32] If a dentist's preference for certain procedures is the basis for recommending them, there is no particular reason to assume that the patient would share those value preferences.

That said, there are inevitably some situations where a dentist's preferred practices contribute significantly to the patient's well-being. And conversely, in many situations where the patient chooses a treatment not favored by the dentist, the preferred practice values of the dentist ought to lose out.

Esthetic Values

Dentists recognize that facial and intraoral appearance are important to patients, and they routinely consider esthetic factors in their treatment recommendations. On the other hand, dentists are not likely to place their patients' concern for esthetics before considerations of pain-free oral functioning in the event of an incompatibility between the two. In addition, they understand that a patient's ideas of what is esthetically pleasing may differ from their own, and in most cases acknowledge that the patient's autonomy trumps their concept of esthetics. Even so, there are occasions where patients can make decisions about esthetic preferences that are terrible in everyone's eyes but their own. In dealing with such situations, which can ultimately have an adverse psychological effect on the patient, dentists must carefully consider how to approach such patients. They need to realize that, since value rankings are subjective, people will differ. They also need to realize that, while they should not impose their value judgments on patients, they normally retain the right to choose who they will accept as a patient. Except in special circumstances, they have a right to withdraw from practitioner-patient relations if what the patient is requesting is significantly contrary to their idea of the way dentistry should be practiced.

Efficiency in the Use of Resources

Finally, Ozar and Sokol consider "efficiency" to be a value. Efficiency is something that virtually all dentists perceive as essential for operation of a successful practice. Furthermore, as Ozar and Sokol put it, "There is nothing unprofessional in a dentist's working to control costs—in time, effort, or materials—provided the other central values are also given their due."[32] They think dentists should never be criticized for trying to improve efficiency. In addition, there are moral foundations for maintaining an efficient practice. With efficiency, one can do good and complicated things better, as well as faster. And with efficient use of resources, one can see more patients, which benefits the public at large. If efficiency can be accomplished without violating moral principles, it surely should be. But the interesting cases are those we will encounter in which, in order to maximize efficiency, some moral principle must be compromised. For example, it would often be more efficient to treat patients without taking the time to obtain an adequately informed consent, but consent is still an important moral requirement. Obtaining it may require sacrificing efficiency.

Critique and Commentary

Ozar and Sokol have provided the profession with a list of six values, hierarchically arranged, that are used as aids to clinical decision making. Their presentation, however, can be confusing and even misleading. It is not clear, for example, that all dentists follow the same ranking. It is not clear that they have to rank values similarly to practice good dentistry.

Do Dentists and Patients Rank Values Similarly?

One problem involves the perspective from which the values are viewed. Although we agree that it is important for professionals to understand the values that have influenced their concept of professionalism, they should also realize that some of these values may not be essential to promoting the welfare of patients. For example, preferred patterns of practice may not always serve the interests of patients.

The values of preferred patterns of practice are powerful influences on practice behavior that for some patients may be extremely beneficial, and for others inappropriate.

Moreover, even if it could be shown that dentists tend to rank values or the benefits of dentistry in a particular way, there is no reason to assume patients would use the same ranking. In fact, one should assume that dentists rank dental health differently than do laypeople—just as philosophers rank philosophizing more highly than others do. This does not make dentists or philosophers right in their value rankings. In fact, most probably—and naturally—dentists overvalue dental health in the way that philosophers overvalue philosophizing.

Is Efficiency a Value?

It is not even clear that all six items on the Ozar and Sokol list are really values. Values are "rational conceptions of the desirable." Efficiency reflects the idea that, with the available resources, it is better to produce more of the desirable than less. From that standpoint, how can it be classified as an independent value? Imagine, for example, a dentist being asked, "Would you rather promote general health or efficiency?" Efficiency is a way one can go about trying to achieve valuable ends. That is, one can pursue general health (or dental health or preferred dental practices, etc.) efficiently or inefficiently. If one values any of these things, presumably one would rather have more than less, so one would normally prefer pursuing them efficiently. However, trying to rank efficiency among the other five values appears not to have any coherent meaning.

Can Values Be Ranked?

In addition, some people reject the very notion that values can be ranked. They believe that a large amount of any one value will (and should) outweigh smaller amounts of other values. For example, a certain minute risk of life is taken whenever local anesthesia is used in the name of pain-free dentistry, yet most dentists believe that the risk is justified. Others may place patient autonomy above general health and oral health. Patients may elevate external (nondental) factors above all other values listed. Furthermore, as we shall see in chapter 3, according to some ethical systems, many of these values need to be subordinated to other ethical concerns that have nothing to do with these values at all.

Problems in Defining the Values

Besides any inherent difficulties associated with the process of ranking, some of the confusion may be attributed to the definitions of the values themselves. The most striking example is that of oral health. There are many ways to think about the meaning of the term. Is it the complete absence of oral disease, or does it mean that there is no disease requiring treatment at the present? Could oral health only exist in the complete absence of risk factors? Does a person who has a high caries rate but who has all new lesions promptly restored possess good oral health? Is a woman who is told by her dentist during a routine prophylaxis that there is a spot on a tooth that bears watching in good dental health? Suppose she is told there is a pinhole-sized cavity that needs attention, but the cavity isn't bothering her—does the absence of symptoms signify good oral health? Is a 70-year-old man who has had all of his mobile teeth extracted finally in good oral health, or does oral health require the restoration of function that could come with dentures? Which patient is in worse oral health: one with stained teeth that cause constant embarrassment or one with incipient periodontal disease that won't cause trouble for years? Should the definition of oral health be left to the insurance companies that decide what kind of treatment their policies will cover?

How Healthy Ought One to Be?

A closely related problem is how good an oral health a person ought to pursue. Arguably, "perfect" oral health—for example, no incipient caries, no early gingivitis, not even any risk factors—is not a realistic goal. Think how much brushing and flossing and how many visits to the dentist for monthly prophylaxes that would require. Yet once one abandons the ideal of perfect teeth, how far can one back away without drawing on value judgments and alternative cost considerations about which a dentist has no expertise?

The Mental Component of Oral Health

Another angle to the "oral health" dispute is whether the mental suffering that comes from cosmetic problems counts as a deficiency in oral health. Why should the mental suffering that comes from having functional difficulties resulting from a missing tooth count more than the mental suffering that comes from embarrassment from discolored teeth? Dentists certainly have an idealized concept of what counts as "good dentition," but identifying exactly what that is and whether patients should be pursuing that goal is more complicated than most dentists know.

One might think of these questions as being purely rhetorical. However, they make the point that the question of the meaning of oral health is complicated and that its answer is subjective. It is important to understand this complexity, because how we answer it affects how we practice dentistry. It can also affect the way we interact with patients who look at oral health differently than we do. It is much easier to deal with patients whose values are similar to one's own. Regretfully, they are not always the ones who need help the most.

References

1. Freidson E. The future of the professions. J Dent Educ 1987;51:140–144.
2. Bok D. Ethics, the university, and society. Harv Mag 1988;91:39–50.
3. Ethics committees double since '83 survey. Hospitals 1985;59:60–66.
4. Odom JG. Recognizing and resolving ethical dilemmas in dentistry. Med Law 1985;4:583–549.
5. Beauchamp TL, Walters L (eds). Contemporary Issues in Bioethics, ed 3. Belmont, CA: Wadsworth, 1982:655.
6. Levit KR, Lazenby HC, Cowan CA, Letsch SW. National health expenditures, 1990. Health Care Financ Rev 1991;13:29–54.
7. Levit K, Smith C, Cowan C, Lazenby H, Sensenig A, Catlin A. Trends in U.S. Health Care Spending, 2001. Available at: www.allhealth.org/recent/audio_03-17-03/TrendsHealthSpending.pdf/. Accessed 20 October 2003.
8. Stoline A, Weiner JR. The New Medical Market Place. Baltimore: John Hopkins Univ. Press, 1988:210.
9. Warner R, Segal H. Ethical Issues of Informed Consent In Dentistry. Chicago: Quintessence, 1980:115.
10. Jong A, Heine CS. The teaching of ethics in the dental hygiene curriculum. J Dent Educ 1982; 46:699–702.
11. Health Insurance Association of America. Source Book of Health Insurance Data. Washington, DC: Health Insurance Association of America, 2002.
12. Gallup G. The Gallup Poll, Public Opinion, 2001.
13. Christensen GJ. The credibility of dentists. J Am Dent Assoc 2001;132:1163–1165.
14. McCullough LB. Ethical issues in dentistry. In: Clark's Clinical Dentistry. Philadelphia: JB Lippincott, 1988:1–17.
15. Hasegawa TK, Lange B, Bower CF, Purtilo RB. Ethical or legal perceptions by dental practitioners. J Am Dent Assoc 1988;116:354–360.
16. Bebeau MJ, Speidel TM. Faculty and course development for a problem-oriented course in professional responsibility: Final report. Chicago: American Fund for Dental Health, 1983.
17. Holloway JA, McNeal DR, Lotzkar S. Ethical problems in dental practice. J Am Coll Dent 1985; 52:12–16.
18. Dummett CO. Ethical issues in dentistry. In: Reich W (ed). Encyclopedia of Bioethics. New York: Free Press, 1987:312–314.
19. Devine JA. If you don't care, who will? J Am Coll Dent 1984;51:8–11.

20. Cole LA. Dentistry and ethics: A call for attention. J Am Dent Assoc 1984;109:559–561.

21. American Dental Association Council on Ethics, Bylaws and Judicial Affairs. Principles of Ethics and Code of Professional Conduct, with official advisory opinions revised to January 2004. Chicago: American Dental Association, 2004.

22. American Dental Association, Office of Quality Assurance. Toward a broader understanding of ethics, self-regulation, and quality assurance. J Am Dent Assoc 1987;114:246–248.

23. Spaeth D. Dentist's role in peer review takes open mind. ADA News 1989;Nov 20:24, 26.

24. Sadowsky D. Moral dilemmas of the multiple prescription in dentistry. J Am Coll Dent 1979;46:245–248.

25. Hirsch A, Gert B. Ethics in dental practice. J Am Dent Assoc 1986;113:599–603.

26. Giangrego E. Child abuse: Recognition and reporting. Spec Care Dentist 1986;6:62–67.

27. Davis M. Dentistry and AIDS: An ethical opinion. J Am Dent Assoc 1989;19(suppl):9–11.

28. Bergamo FC. Ethics in the eighties. Spec Care Dentist 1985;5:204–205.

29. Wetle T. Ethical issues in geriatric dentistry. Gerodontology 1987;6:73–78.

30. Dunn WJ. Third-party coverage and ethical implications in dentistry. Compend Contin Educ Dent 1985;6:751–756.

31. Spaeth D. Dentists facing pressure. ADA News 1988;Sept 19:20–21.

32. Ozar DT, Sokol DJ. Dental Ethics at Chairside: Professional Principles and Practical Applications, ed 2. Washington, DC: Georgetown University Press, 2002:343.

33. Ozar DT, Schiedermayer DL, Siegler M. Value categories in clinical dental ethics. J Am Dent Assoc 1988;116:365–368.

chapter 2

The Structure of Professions and the Responsibilities of Professionals

In this chapter

Students who select the profession of dentistry give a variety of reasons for their choice.[1–3] Among them are the ability to earn a good income, the prospect of independent employment, and the opportunity to serve the public. However, when they first set foot in a dental school, most of them know little about professions in general or dentistry in particular. Furthermore, what they do know is almost certainly more closely related to dentistry's economic circumstances and working conditions than to any of its more esoteric aspects, such as the nature of the dentist-patient relationship.

It is not that money and how one earns it are not important or even crucial to choosing a career. However, these extrinsic considerations are but one aspect of the professional experience. It is at least as important to understand the scope of one's obligations to patients, to self, to the profession, and to society at large. In addition, it is vital to know how the various roles played by private practice, academia, professional organizations, codes of ethics, and licensing boards are all essential components of the dental profession.

In this chapter, we first discuss the historical development of professions in order to better understand their current structure and function. Next, we discuss the special obligations that professionals have to the people they serve. This is followed by a presentation of the characteristics of professions, as related to their historical development. Finally, in order to promote a more complete understanding of the relationships between professions and society, we consider some recent critcism of traditional views of professions.

A Brief History of Professions

The etymologic roots of the word *profession* have left their mark on all of its derivatives. Its original Latin meaning was "to profess," which signified one's willingness to make a public declaration of something that was important—and what usually was important was religion. For example, *Webster's Third New International Dictionary* first defined *profess* as the public act of taking religious vows. From that focused starting point, its meaning expanded to include open declarations of belief that are nonreligious. And for our purposes, "profession" also includes callings that require intensive preparation and high standards of achievement and that render a public service. Finally, however, its meaning has softened to include the less restrictive usage that many people give the term today: "a principal calling, vocation, or employment"[4]—in other words, almost anything that occupies most of one's time.

In the 16th century, the term *profession* was used for the first time to denote the special occupations of medicine, law, the divinity, and (sometimes) the military. These were the so-called learned professions. However, much of the population used the term to refer to everything from barbering to blacksmithing.[4] Thus, in at least one respect, not much has changed in the past four centuries. Nevertheless, over the years the restricted concept of profession has been the focus of a considerable body of literature that has attempted to define and characterize what professions are and how professionals ought to function.

From a developmental standpoint, it is clear that in the 16th century, professions were manned by members of the privileged class who had been educated in universities created many years before. In William F. May's words,[5] "'having a profession' provided a social location in life for the second, third, and fourth sons of aristocrats who, in a society committed to primogeniture, could not inherit portions of the estate that went exclusively to the eldest son, and yet who, as children of the aristocracy, should not have to work for a living and thus submit to the vulgarities of the marketplace. Thus the professions . . . provided the great families with an honorable social location for their surplus gentlemen." It follows, therefore, that the respect bestowed upon professions flowed only in part from the education they required and the value of their services. More important, their status stemmed from the privileged births of their members.

From that powerful beginning, the character of the "elite professions" changed but slowly over the generations that followed. With the onset of the Renaissance and the development of the middle class, increasing numbers of people—especially in England—entered occupations that more and more resembled the professions of the wellborn. Hence, the newcomers, too, wanted to be looked upon as members of a profession rather than as tradesmen.

To achieve that goal required a lot of work over a long period of time, guided by effective organization. Members of the would-be professions banded together to form associations, or guilds—certainly with no help from the state or anyone else—whose function it was to ensure survival. Over the course of generations, they performed whatever tasks were necessary to establish their credibility. For example, it was essential that adequate training and credentialing were both available and required for aspiring professionals, together with a license to practice. With these safeguards to the public in place or in development, the associations might then acquire enough power to negotiate with the state for favorable competitive positions in the marketplace. Their goal, in other words, was to restrict the practice of their particular occupation to members of their group. They also understood that they would not be taken seriously unless they demonstrated that they could provide dedicated service, administered with a sense of integrity.

This was the pattern for the development of professions in England. It also served as the prototype for what happened in the United States.* In these two countries, each hopeful occupation launched its own process for gaining credibility and sanctuary in the marketplace. And when an occupation became "successful" in establishing its legitimacy, it gradually became known and referred to as a profession.

In the United States, dentistry's attempts to be recognized as a profession moved ahead significantly in the 1830s,[6] thanks in part to the financial panic of 1837 and the unstable economic climate of speculation that preceded it. Businesses went

---

*The process was different in continental Europe, where the countries placed the stamp of authenticity on an occupation via its system of education. People were known as professionals if they attended state-supported institutions for their education.

bankrupt, banks collapsed, and unemployment escalated wildly.[7] Unlike in England, where people usually became dentists after lengthy apprenticeships and had done so since the 16th century,[8,9] in America there was no well-established system. Many American dentists were quite competent, often as a result of apprenticeship training. Nevertheless, because people could convert from the plough or the workshop to the dental chair in a few short months—often in a few weeks—dentistry loomed as a golden opportunity for unemployed people of all sorts to generate income quickly.[7] The collective competence level of the young profession soon plummeted, and concerns about the quality of care rose abruptly.

Although no national dental associations existed at that time, it was dentistry's good fortune that leaders emerged to organize their colleagues, all in the public interest against unscrupulous practitioners who advocated unorthodox treatment and who advertised aggressively and effectively.[6] In addition, influential practitioners turned their attention to three landmark ventures. One was to initiate a professional journal designed to "disseminate correct principles and expose error"[10]; it was called the *American Journal of Dental Science* and first appeared in 1839. Another effort was to establish schools specifically for the teaching of dentistry. In 1840, the world's first dental school, the Baltimore College of Dental Surgery, was created. The third effort was to create professional organizations, and again in 1840, the American Society of Dental Surgeons, the first national dental society, was formed. Leaders in the field also considered lobbying for legislation that would regulate licensure, but the prevailing political climate of individualism delayed those efforts for decades.[10] All these events are milestones in dentistry's movement toward recognition as a profession. All of the professions recognized today have experienced comparable landmarks, and for all of them, the process has been painstakingly slow.

Differentiation of a profession from other occupational groups is a complex social process. It requires society's acceptance of a special social status for the professional group. Assigning that status involves recognition of specialized knowledge not readily available to the general public and obtainable only through prolonged education. It also requires acknowledgment that the group has a special responsibility to promote the public interest and abide by a code of ethical conduct. Even after an occupation is widely regarded as a profession, the maturation process continues. In the United States, it was not until the late 1800s and early 1900s that the current economic prestige of the professions was established and their advantageous positions in the marketplace secure.[11] These were important milestones because they represented the overturning of a political tradition in the United States that resisted restrictions on entrepreneurs about how goods and services ought to be provided. For example, during the Jacksonian period of the 1830s and 1840s, Congress actually repealed legislation giving monopolistic advantages to medicine and law that had been enforced since the colonial days. The result was that an individual could practice any livelihood he or she wanted. For bonesetters, herbalists, and grocers/druggists, this was an open invitation to practice medicine. It took decades of political effort and appeal to the public interest before the earlier status quo was re-established.

In summary, from a developmental standpoint, a profession begins with the practice of a potentially distinctive body of expertise by a group of informally trained people. The expertise is viewed as having public value. The knowledge required of its practitioners expands with time, and during a long gestational interval, its members form organizations that promote their interests. In addition, they create systems for education, credentialing, and eventually licensure. The practitioners work to convince the public of their commitment and honor and of their ability to manage their problems and collegially maintain their discipline. The process is slow and untidy, but for the occupations that achieve their goal, the result is a rewarding career that serves important and highly valued roles in the public interest.

The process in general can be viewed as an unwritten pact with society, the basis of which is traditionally understood as follows: Professions are social institutions in that they provide services on behalf of the common good.[12] In return, they are granted a certain degree of power and autonomy with respect to their standards of practice, how their practitioners are trained and admitted to practice, and how the behavior of their members is monitored.[6,13] As long as society has confidence in the good will of the profession and believes it correctly serves the public interest, this arrangement is mutually advantageous.

There is one other point that should be made regarding the evolution of professions. Although reading about how occupations struggle to become professions helps us understand both their structure and their function, it can also be misleading. One gets the impression that after generations, maybe centuries, of hard work to become a profession, on some glorious day society formally grants the long-sought status. However, from the perspective of those who were in the midst of the struggles, nothing could be further from the truth. For example, in the 1830s, when the stage was being set for major advances in the professionalization of dentistry, those who practiced it already viewed themselves as members of a profession. They had no doubts at all. When dentists wrote or spoke about the challenges facing dentistry, the context of their concerns was their profession. Furthermore, when they took action to improve the quality of education or cope with irresponsible practitioners, they spoke of doing it to benefit their profession.[11]

The early 19th century dentists' conviction that they were indeed professionals acknowledges their recognition of the evolving definition of a profession. The next section provides direction for an increased understanding of the meaning of that term, while indicating that its definition is by no means agreed upon by all.

A More Complete Definition of a Profession

The definition of profession given previously covers some aspects of professionalism but ignores others, including self-regulation and collegial discipline. In fact, there is no consensus about what a profession actually is.[14]

Consider, for example, the differences between the definition offered by the American College of Dentists (ACD) and the definition that appeared in Paul Starr's book, *The Social Transformation of American Medicine*.[11] The ACD[15,16] defines a profession as: "[a]n occupation involving relatively long and specialized preparation on the level of higher education and governed by a special code of ethics." By contrast, Starr, a respected sociologist of the professions, defines it as: "[a]n occupation that regulates itself through systematic, required training and collegial discipline; that has a base in technical, specialized knowledge, and that has a service rather than profit orientation, enshrined in its code of ethics."

We find the Starr definition significantly more helpful. Although both definitions speak of the long and specialized education that is required, Starr's definition also includes the service orientation and self-regulatory aspects of professions.

Starr also points out that the behavior of professionals is regulated by "collegial discipline." Dentistry, for example, primarily functions through the self-restraint of individual practitioners. This is reinforced by the actions of associations* and the American Dental Association's (ADA's) Principles of Ethics and Code of Professional Conduct.[17] With respect to the latter, we disagree with the ACD definition. Rather than possessing the authority of governance, codes of ethics serve mainly as guides for conduct. There is little that dental associations can do to punish noncompliance; in many cases, codes of ethics provide no controlling influence other than suspension of membership in the organization—license to practice remains intact. In extreme cases, discipline is managed with the legal sanctions available to the state dental boards and with the malpractice system. This topic is discussed in the section on collegial discipline.

In addition, only the Starr definition cites the orientation to service rather than profit. Neither definition, however, deals with the relationship that professionals have with their clients or patients. This relationship, which is often said to be fiduciary in nature, is arguably the most distinctive aspect of being a professional and therefore is considered next.

Relationships with Patients: The Fiduciary Relation

Lawyers have different obligations to their clients than physicians have to their patients or veterinarians have to theirs. Likewise, the obligations of accountants, psychologists, engineers, or journalists differ because the goals of each profession differ, as do the services they perform.

---

*It seems that almost every organization has an association. In the Omaha, Nebraska, telephone directory, for example, there are 64 listings of "associations" representing everything from businesses and social services to the entertainment industry. And this does not include the American Dental Association, the American Medical Association, the American Bar Association, or the associations of other major national professions that do not have local offices. Associations are definitely not exclusive characteristics of professions. Yet arguably they deserve prominent mention because of the major role they played in the transformation of occupations into professions. Without them, there would have been no organized means to establish the credibility of fledgling professions and eventually to promote legislation to protect them in the marketplace.

However, they share a common characteristic—the fiduciary relationship. (With regard to principles of ethics, the fiduciary relationship is based upon the principle of fidelity, as discussed in chapter 7.)

A fiduciary relationship is based on trust and confidence that commitments between parties will be honored[18]; it exists whenever a doctor and a patient establish a professional connection. Because the patient should be an active participant in the relationship, these commitments are a two-way street. However, given the unequal knowledge and skills of the two parties, it is especially important that the health care provider be worthy of that trust.[19]

In the context of a fiduciary relationship, trust has two elements.[20] The first is competence. With dentistry in mind, patients expect dentists to be competent in executing their responsibility as oral health professionals.

The other element of trust transcends competence and moves to morality. The public trusts dentists to place their patients' interests higher than their own.

During their training, dentists are perpetually preoccupied with becoming trustworthy in the first sense. The achievement of competence is a long process and, for many, a painful one weighed down by periods of self-doubt. All dentists understand the responsibility of becoming clinically and technically competent. However, to fully understand the significance of putting the patient's interests above one's own requires some amplification.

First, it is important to note that trusting a professional is not the same as trusting a friend. Friends earn trust through years of demonstrating their worthiness. However, in the traditional understanding of the professions, a professional is someone who is to be given instant trust. In effect, patients trust that society is working properly. Whether or not they know it, patients trust that the profession's system of education, credentialing, and licensure has produced a competent practitioner. And even before that, patients also trust that the knowledge of the profession can help them.

Edmund Pellegrino, a physician-ethicist who has written extensively about the physician-patient relationship, explains it another way: "Trust in professional relationships is forced; it is trust generated by our need for help. When we need a doctor, lawyer, or minister, we have no choice but to trust someone, though we might prefer to trust none."[21]

This is important because of the vulnerability of those who need professional services, which derives from several sources. In all professional relationships, there is a baseline inequality of knowledge and skills. The dentist, for example, understands the problem and how to deal with it, while the patient may have trouble defining what the problem is or fully evaluating any treatment that might be provided. Vulnerability may be increased if the patient has a troublesome problem, such as pain, bleeding, or the consequences of trauma. Finally, perhaps especially in dentistry, fear and anxiety may lead to added vulnerability.

In considering patient vulnerability, keep in mind that a professional, etymologically speaking, "professes" to do good for another. The word *profess* has such a strong connotation of declaration and avowal that it essentially represents a promise to help. One promises to act not only with competence, but also with concern for the patient. Thus, because of the inequality of the doctor-patient relationship, and especially because of the vulnerability of patients, it is essential never to abuse that relationship.[22] In other words, patients trust that their vulnerability, in Pellegrino's words, "will not be exploited for power, profit, prestige, or pleasure."[21]

Having discussed the day-to-day commitments between professionals and their clients or patients, we now turn to the traditional ideals and orientation of professions and how they function. In doing so, we rely on Starr's three characteristics of a profession: specialized knowledge, service orientation, and self-regulation.

Characteristics of Professions

A Base in Technical, Specialized Knowledge

There is widespread agreement that one of the main characteristics of professions is the requirement of extensive, specialized university preparation.[4,20,23–25] Furthermore, the length and extent of the education adds to the dedication of professionals and increases the probability that they will practice it for the remainder of their working lives.[25]

For Eliot Freidson, a sociologist whose field is the professions, the "formal knowledge" generated by the educational process tends to separate professions from other occupations. He states that, "It has been shaped into systematic theories that explain facts and justify actions. It involves hypotheses, axioms, deductions, and models. . . . Members of professions are the 'agents of formal knowledge.'"[4]

The nature of the "formal knowledge" also means that it represents exclusive expertise that is understood only by members of the select group who have mastered and practice it.[26,27] As Freidson puts it, a profession "requires theoretical knowledge, skill, and judgment that ordinary people do not possess, may not wholly comprehend, and cannot readily evaluate."[26] Therefore, each profession provides a service that is essentially a monopoly in its area of expertise. Thus for competent service, the public, of necessity, must consult with members of professions—at least, that is the conventional view of the professions.[25]

The specialized nature of professional education has several relevant consequences according to the traditional understanding of the professions. One is that its complexity requires that professionals keep abreast of current developments through clinical and scientific journals and continuing education courses. Another is that few others besides professionals are in a position to teach it and to expand that knowledge through research. Similarly, in most disputes involving the validity of professional knowledge, who else but its membership can serve as arbiters?[24]

A Service Rather Than Profit Orientation, Enshrined in a Code of Ethics

Scholarly Viewpoint

In the traditional understanding of the professions there is substantial agreement that for an occupation to be considered a profession, the population at large must believe that its services have significant social value[26,27] and, as Freidson[26] puts it, are also "Good Work." To be so judged, one or both of the following two conditions must be met. One condition is that the services rendered must have intrinsic value that the public ranks very highly. For example, in medicine and law the preservation of health and life and the protection of self and property against the adverse actions of others both certainly qualify.[25]

The other condition is that the services are essential in the sense that they allow people to achieve their life goals. The services of medicine and law qualify from that standpoint. In contrast, Ozar uses the example of investment counseling, which is not universally thought of as a profession: "It is fully possible for people to achieve their goals in life without the particular benefits that investment counselors provide to their clients."[27]

Dentistry is thought to qualify as a profession because of the intrinsic value of its services and because the services allow people to pursue their life goals. Consider, for example, the important role that pain relief, caries prevention, the restoration of teeth, the reconstruction of occlusions, or the improvement of appearance has in this context.

In rendering these services, professions should be oriented to the service itself rather than to profit. This does not mean that profit is not desirable and even essential in dentistry or any other profession. Without it, one could not provide services, at least in the private practice model. However, the existence of professions is not based primarily upon profit. The daily activities of dentists, for example, are determined by the clinical conditions, anxieties, personal circumstances, and values of individual patients. Implicit in this idea is the expectation that the practice of one's profession is an end in itself–that there is intrinsic satisfaction and value to the professional in his or her performance of the work. There are said to be goods that are "intrinsic" or "internal" to the professions.[28] This, at least, is the traditional view of the professions.

How Professions View Themselves

According to sociologist John Kultgen, the important work of professionals concentrates on either of two areas. One is that of basic biological needs, from health and housing to interment of the departed. The other pertains to basic needs created by modern life, such as "education, transportation, sanity, order, legal counsel, energy, disposal of wastes, etc. The importance of the needs they meet distinguishes professional work from other highly skilled activities." How well the service is performed crucially affects the recipient's welfare. This is in contrast with the service of nonprofessionals, where incompetence can be quite upsetting but not central to the client's vital interests.[25] It is often believed that professionals are engaged in a special "calling" that bears obligations beyond those of ordinary employment. Because professions are of such critical value to society, they accept the responsibility of having a primary orientation to the welfare of the public at large.[26] For example, the ADA uses similar language in its Principles of Ethics and Code of Professional Conduct: "The dentist's primary obligation is service to the patient and the public-at-large."[17]

Codes of Ethics

Some, including many ethicists, see codes as representing professional standards that are obligatory from a moral point of view. However, ethicists realize that these standards are aspirational in nature and perhaps not acceptable to all members of a profession.

Others, including many professionals, view codes as representing a group consensus on how members should behave. That perspective may also be controversial; just because a profession agrees on a particular norm of conduct does not necessarily mean that it is satisfactory from a moral perspective. For example, the common practice of not criticizing or perhaps even discussing a previous dentist's faulty treatment may be appropriate conduct to professionals but an abrogation of veracity for the general public.

Because codes have generally been formulated without consultation with or representation of the public, the standards of professional behavior exist mainly from the standpoint of the professionals themselves.[19] And because professions and the public may not always agree on the standards of professional behavior, the issue cannot be easily resolved. For example, the preamble of the ADA document[17] says, "The *ADA Code* is, in effect, a written expression of the obligations arising from the implied contract between the dental profession and society." However, because there has been little representation from society in revisions of the Code, the result clearly presents the profession's view of how things are and ought to be.

The Functions of Codes

What are the intended functions of professional codes of ethics? One is to promote behaviors that are important in serving human goals. Primarily, this aspect guides practitioners in the management of challenging problems. The ADA Code,[17] for example, includes guidelines for the management of HIV-infected patients, along with opinions on confidentiality, patient abandonment, avoiding risky interpersonal relationships, and reporting abuse.

Another function of codes of ethics is to elevate professional standards of conduct. For example, the ADA's Principles of Ethics and Code of Professional Conduct[17] states that professionals have the duty to "treat the patient according to the patient's desires, within the bounds of accepted treatment," to "protect the patient from harm," to "promote the patient's welfare," and "to be fair in their dealing with patients, colleagues and society." These general principles are then amplified to a certain extent in the Code of Professional Conduct and the Advisory Opinions. Nevertheless, Beauchamp and Childress[29] point out that codes of ethics seldom "have anything to say about the implications of other principles and rules, such as veracity, respect for autonomy, and justice, which have been the subjects of intense contemporary discussion." In addition, the codes often do not appeal "to more general ethical standards or to a source of moral authority beyond the traditions and judgments of [professionals]. In some cases, the special rules in codes for professionals seem to conflict with and even override more general moral norms."

Codes also have social functions, such as maintaining the status of professions and strengthening their positions. These functions are oriented more toward the welfare of the profession than that of the public.[25]

To illustrate a code's social function, consider an example that has implications both for a profession and for its public. The ADA's Principle of Justice[17] states that: "the dental profession should actively seek allies throughout society on specific activities that will help improve access to care for all."* To its credit, the ADA has been involved in activities that do exactly what the code pronounces. It has worked with states and other organizations to promote access to care and improvements in the Medicaid system and has promoted access to care itself with its "Give A Kid A Smile" program. At the same time, however, there is increased public awareness that most dentists refuse to treat Medicaid patients. Despite the Code's call for the profession at large to "improve access to care for all," it is silent on the obligations of individual practitioners to this end.

What is the explanation for this dichotomy? A likely possibility is that the profession is primarily promoting its own interest rather than the public good. In doing so, its intentions may be to reassure the public that it is meeting its responsibilities. This is in spite of the fact that there is nothing in the ADA Principles and Code about the obligations of individual dentists to improve access to care. The absence of such a call from the profession to its members helps prevent individual practitioners from feeling pressured to participate in a payment system that they find onerous. Thus the "concealed intent" mentioned earlier may be interpreted as showing how the dental profession is trying to maintain and perhaps strengthen its status as a caring profession while at the same time not offending its membership.

All professions are concerned about fostering favorable public perception—a form of social ideology. Such doctrinaire concerns are expected and not inherently onerous, but when they appear in codes, they are often disguised (as in this example) under the aegis of a more lofty motivation. This is not to say that ideology should necessarily be equated with misleading statements; it can also represent genuine and accurate expressions of professionalism at its best.

The Notion of "Enshrining"

Finally, a comment should be made about the phrase, "enshrined in its code of ethics," which appears in Starr's definition. This should not be construed as meaning that the existence of such a code characterizes an occupation as a profession. On

---

*In 1992, when the first edition of this book was being prepared, the ADA Code had no specific statement about improved access to care for economically disadvantaged people. This apparently represents an important revision of the ADA's position on that issue, even if its call for action pertains only to the profession at large and not to individual dentists. Even so, the inconsistency is not surprising; changes in professions tend to be slow and incremental.

the contrary, many organizations that are not viewed as bona fide professions have codes of ethics, and, conversely, some recognized professions choose not to have them. Nor should one conclude that the enshrinement of an orientation to service in a profession's code of ethics offers any guarantee of enforceability. Nevertheless, the ubiquitous nature of codes and their reliance on voluntary compliance should not detract from the possibility that a well-conceived and well-executed code can help articulate the values and obligations of a profession.

Collegial Discipline and Self-regulation

Issues and Terms

The third characteristic of a profession is that it is self-regulating. This section deals with self-regulation in professions—its meaning and how it is expressed. One of the reasons Starr's definition was of interest to us was that it brings together the various aspects of self-regulation. That is, it acknowledges that the educational system is a significant part of self-regulation, as, by implication, are credentialing and licensing. Starr's definition then links it to collegial discipline, which, for some, is the more commonly considered component of professional self-regulation.

Self-regulation is widely recognized as a characteristic of professions.[20,25,26,30] To discuss self-regulation, we must also discuss autonomy, or the condition of self-governance of professions. Self-regulation is autonomy in action—the process by which professions express their autonomy. For example, in return for valuable services to society, defenders of the professions believe autonomy should be bestowed upon professions in the form of less governmental intervention than other groups might receive. Besides performing services, professions have also been expected to provide a certain degree of self-regulation, "not the least of which is the regulation of the behavior of the group's members."[13] As we will shortly see, the discipline of professionals is not the only form of self-regulation.

Autonomy can be viewed either collectively or individually. Collective autonomy pertains to the profession at large. It is often accompanied by legislative actions that ensure favorable competitive economic advantages for the profession. In effect, collective autonomy is society's recognition of the prestige, power, and credibility that the profession has earned over a long period of time.

Individual autonomy is enjoyed by the practitioners themselves. For most professionals, this is substantial because a profession's control over its membership is limited. As a result, most decisions and actions of professionals stem from their own moral viewpoints.[25]

Individual autonomy is particularly relevant to dentistry. A dated but interesting study of students' motivations to enter dentistry showed that autonomy and independence far outranked any other reasons for choosing it. Even prestige and income were far down the list. The authors concluded that "entering dental students would accept a career with less prestige, less money, and less opportunity to serve . . . because dentistry would afford them greater independence."[31]

Decades have passed since this study was published, and attitudes and values of dental students have surely undergone some alteration. However, the data coincide with current perceptions and therefore deserve consideration.

How Self-Regulation Occurs

Entering the profession In the section on the history of professions, we discussed why fledgling professions acted early in their development to regulate who became a member. Thus, this description of the process of self-regulation begins—in a recapitulation of history—with the educational system.

Consider the powerful influence that the profession has on the educational system. Most professional school faculty and administration are members of the profession, and dentistry is no exception. Most of the members of admission committees are dentists, and the profession controls the curriculum, how it is managed, and who graduates. Often there are tensions between members of the profession who are educators and those who are in practice, but in reality their shared tradition is much more profound than either group would sometimes like to admit. What is more, the educational program, besides offering the necessary clinical and basic science knowledge and technical competence, also inculcates the values and attitudes of the profession. In Kultgen's words, "The professional school is the primary socializing agency that initiates novices into the profession's subculture. . . . The development of professional conscience among new entrants into a profession is as important for the public welfare as technical competence."[25]

Entering practice When dentists graduate and become licensed, the process has the heavy stamp of the profession upon it. In dentistry, the receipt of a diploma means that one has graduated from an institution accredited by the ADA. The granting of a license by a state board of dentistry is almost exclusively controlled by prominent members of the profession, many of whom are appointed by state government at the recommendation of other members of the profession.

This illustrates the powerful role that the profession plays in these processes and the importance to the profession in maintaining its presence in them. Furthermore, this familiar system of licensure developed, in years past, only as the result of the profession's aggressive pursuits to obtain legal standing for its membership. Nowadays, when changes are proposed that affect the character of licensure, one can be sure that the professional association plays a prominent position in supporting or opposing the legislation. As Kultgen puts it, "In these ways the profession controls its controllers and insures that only those who conform to its standards are allowed to practice."[25]

Practice: The central phase This stage in the life of a professional is by far the longest, but it is influenced less by the profession with respect to attitudes and behavior than the earlier stages. Except for those who are active in professional associations, the profession's influence is mainly indirect, through its expectation of self-monitoring.

The profession maintains its presence in several other ways. One is simply that the attitudes and values of one's profession, indelibly imprinted during professional school, remain in place throughout life. These attitudes are reinforced by experiences with patients, which tend to foster a more mature understanding of the value and significance of what one does for others. Additionally, the profession exerts influence through its informal process of patient referral, wherein peer approval is expressed. There is also the process of continuing education, which is obligatory in most states and is substantially influenced by professional organizations. In a more subtle aspect of influence, members of a profession tend to spend time together socially as well as professionally.

Finally, the profession plays a role in disciplining its members. Peer-review committees are established by dental societies primarily to resolve disputes between patients and practitioners. Because in most states they function primarily as a mediating body, their enforcement of discipline must be considered marginal. However, the state boards of dentistry fulfill a disciplinary function that goes far beyond that of licensure. Based on complaints received from the profession and the public—usually the latter—the boards investigate and are sanctioned to levy punishments for the most egregious violations of their respective state dental practice acts. The only other recourse available to the public is the legal system—both legislation and malpractice—which remains independent of the profession.

Recent Criticism of the Professions

Thus far we have presented the classic understanding of the professions as occupational groups that rely on specialized knowledge, possess service orientation, and express self-regulation. Recently, this view has been called into question. Two different kinds of criticism of the notion of a professional have emerged. In order for both new and seasoned professionals to fully understand the relationships between their profession and society, it is as essential to know the criticisms as it is the more traditional and laudatory views.

Failure of Professionals to Live Up to Their Ideals

One group of critics views professions cynically, believing them to be devices for controlling the prestige and income of their members. These critics agree that professionals have specialized knowledge but believe that professionals take advantage of their special positions to exert monopolistic control over services people need, thereby controlling prices. The critics point to the professional control of advertising, for example, which until relatively recently was widely condemned by professional groups as unethical. They have claimed that such control, in fact, merely made it more difficult for laypeople to compare services and prices and thus made dentistry more profitable.

Another failure in living up to the ideals of one's profession is the presence in every professional group of people who take advantage of their position to pursue their own interests. Such behavior is unethical and often illegal. Criticisms of the ability of professions to identify and discipline the small minority of professionals who abuse their status are covered later in the section on self-regulation.

Criticisms of the Ideals

We think the more interesting criticism of the professions is more subtle and more provocative. It first accepts the claims about professions that virtually all professionals try to be reasonably good servants of the public interest who do what is right for their patients or clients. The criticism, however, is about the very concept of a profession and whether the traditional view can be sustained.

The traditional view rests on the distinction between a profession and a mere occupation. A profession, as we described, deals with specialized knowledge, is committed to the public welfare, and engages in self-regulation through the educational and disciplinary processes. An occupation is a way of earning a living—working as a laborer, an employee, or an entrepreneur.

Critics now say that the distinction between a profession and an occupation is more complicated. Some laborers, for example, require specialized knowledge and often advanced university degrees. Businesspeople are expected to have some degree of commitment to the public welfare through leadership in civic affairs and contributions to worthwhile community projects (and not merely because of the good publicity). They are also expected to conform to minimal standards of good conduct, which are sometimes expressed in a code of ethics. They do wrong, for example, if they engage in false and misleading advertising. They cannot justifiably lie about their product, even if sometimes they are not expected to go out of their way to point out its shortcomings. (It is noteworthy that traditional professional ethics has accepted one kind of lying—the "white lie" a clinician tells to a patient or client for the purpose of relieving anxiety.)

Clinical professionals also are confronting the limits of their public altruism—not merely in generating income, but also in acknowledging that the professional's duty to family, friends, or self may justifiably limit the duty to serve the client or the public. Most important, the critics of the professions want a more realistic assessment of self-regulation.

Specialized Knowledge
The most obvious problem with the "specialized knowledge" characteristic is the realization that fields such as dentistry are so complex that even the most dedicated professional is frequently pushed to and beyond the limits of his or her knowledge.

There is a second problem as well. Professionals were presumed not only to have specialized knowledge of a field, such as oral and maxillofacial surgery, but also to know what would best serve the client's interest.

Recent criticism of the professions challenges this presumption. While the need for technical, factual knowledge is inescapable, critics claim that it is impossible to know what serves someone's interest just by mastering the technical facts. They claim that deciding what is best always requires a value judgment that cannot be derived from the facts themselves.

This applies as much in deciding what is best for the dentition of the patient as in any other field. If one type of restoration is predictably going to last longer but has a less esthetic appearance, it is an open question which is the "best dentistry." Everyone wants durable restorations, but everyone also has some degree of concern about appearance. Deciding what is "best" requires going beyond knowledge of the facts to consider the goals of the patient, his or her economic means, and so forth.

The problem becomes even more complex when one factors in the interests of patients beyond their dentitions. The cost of the highest quality restoration may place it beyond the reach of some patients, who may have to choose between the best quality dentistry and food for their children. What is best for the patient's teeth may not be what is best for the patient or the patient's family. Even the most knowledgeable dentist may still end up not knowing what is best for the patient.

Part of the problem is that the relationship between client and practitioner has become increasingly anonymous. When consulter and consultant get together, the reasons for the relationship usually do not involve the consultant's knowing anything about the interests of the client. In other words, the relationship is largely accidental. Furthermore, and perhaps more important, the overall welfare of a client is quite complex, with many influences, ranging from health, psychological, and legal to educational and religious, all of which impossibly complicate the professional's understanding of the client's values or needs. No one would expect a professional to have insights into the client's complex personal makeup.[32]

Consider the case of a dentist who routinely takes an annual set of bitewing radiographs as part of a regularly scheduled preventive visit. The dentist, no doubt, believes that they benefit the patient and involve little risk. The patient, however, may evaluate the benefits and risks quite differently. The patient may have greater fear of x-ray exposure, for example. Or the patient may have other potential uses for the $35 the dentist will charge. Without knowing the patient's attitudes about x-ray exposure and the alternative use of the money, the dentist really is not in a good position to know that those radiographs are what is best for the patient. At most, the dentist may know what would maximize the patient's "dental welfare," but he or she cannot know what is in the interest of the patient's overall well-being.

Orientation to the Public Interest

Another criticism of the traditional view of the professions focuses on the claim that professions are oriented to the public interest rather than self-interest. The initial problem is that the healing professions have never really accepted a commitment to the "public interest." They have focused on the welfare of the individual patient—sometimes to the exclusion of the welfare of the community. The emergence of public health dentistry, for example, has only partially reoriented the profession's focus from the individual patient to the community.

Furthermore, even if we take this commitment to the welfare of the patient to be the real service orientation of the professions, problems remain. Although scholars accept service as a component of professions, there are differing views about how well professions meet that obligation. Until the latter part of the 20th century, sociologists tended to look at professions "as honored servants of public need." More recently, policy-makers have viewed professions as "over-narrow and insular in their vision of what is good for the public." With the passage of time, the evaluations have become increasingly unfavorable. Rather than concentrating on their accomplishments, critics have pointed out their preoccupation with acquiring political influence and improving their relationship with the "political and economic elites."[33]

These presumed preoccupations, critics say, are expressed as important conflicting interests, including "wealth, prestige, power, and autonomy."[32] Professions ensure that their interests are met by providing expert services to those who can afford to pay for them. If they were to expand their services to humanity at large, their ability to fulfill their own interests would diminish. However, at present, society's hierarchical nature is such that as long as upper income groups receive services, minimal benefits for the lower ranks will be sufficient to "quiet social unrest." This approach is deeply ingrained in the fabric of professions and is part of their historical tradition. And although it is in conflict with the concept of caring for the needs of society, the critics' position is that it is nonetheless inevitable.[33]

Finally, the service orientation raises the question of whether a profession has a basis for actually knowing how and in what way the public can be served. In chapter 10 we consider cases in which a dentist or a dental group has more than one way of serving the public. One approach may produce the greatest overall expected benefit, while another might serve a particularly needy but relatively small group. When it comes to choosing the proper moral strategy for serving the public interest, the profession and the public may not always have the same inclinations. It is not enough just to be oriented to public service; the professional must also have a basis for deciding who should be served and on what basis. This brings us to the problems with the third characteristic of professions: self-regulation.

Collegial Discipline and Self-regulation

The system of self-regulation operates in dentistry and other professions through a combination of self-restraint and collegial discipline. Everyone recognizes that the system is largely unenforceable. However, most members of a profession adhere to its aspirational qualities enough so that it continues to function as a cohesive unit. If there were to become a widespread division between the practices of its membership and its stated goals and standards, the profession would be at risk of unraveling.[11,25]

Thus, in the interests of maintaining the functional integrity of a given profession, one would hope that its members would value their colleagues' respect and work to justify it. The opinion of critics, however, is that collegial relationships may represent little more than professional socialization and the exchange of clinical knowledge. In other words, critics say that collegial self-regulation has little value in terms of protecting the public. If it really worked, the public would view professions as more trustworthy.[20]

To correct the problem, members of professions would have to be much more prepared to identify ethical transgressions of their colleagues, including incompetence.[25] Almost all professional codes agree with this position. The ADA Code, for example, states that dentists have an obligation "to report to the appropriate review-ing agency . . . instances of gross or continual faulty treatment by other dentists."[17]

The problem is that reporting a colleague is a daunting task. No one wants to "squeal" on another professional, and no one wants to pay the price of being viewed as a turncoat to one's profession—especially if one lives in a small commu-nity. There is also the widespread feeling of "There, but for the grace of God, go I."[26] One hears stories about being sued by the errant colleague and about the time involved in testifying before the state board or other organizations.

Underlying these issues, all of which are distinctly unpleasant anyway, are addi-tional cautions from the ADA Code. Most of its Advisory Opinion consists of admo-nitions to dentists to make sure that criticism is justifiable. Little is presented on one's commitments and how to fulfill them. Furthermore, the last sentence of the Adviso-ry Opinion warns, gratuitously we think, that dentists who make unjustified criti-cisms run the risk of being the object of a "disciplinary proceeding."[17]

The preceding remarks are not intended to single out dentistry as a bad example of the way that a profession handles self-regulation. No profession wants to see its membership criticized, especially when the complaint comes from one of its own. At the same time, professions are not structured to provide officially sanctioned disci-pline, except in particularly serious instances. Thus, if there is to be control, it can only work privately and informally from one colleague to another in an environment of mutual respect. Such encounters are difficult, but their potential influence is sig-nificant. As difficult as the problem is, if professions fail in their trustworthiness to deal with it adequately, they fail also to shield the public from harm. Critics point out that the system under which professions now operate provides little opportunity for redress in case of failure. In such circumstances where self-regulation is inadequate, the system needs additional external controls of an as yet unspecified nature.

Thus far we have expressed concern that the process of collegial discipline and self-regulation may not always work as well as it might because members of the profession may experience psychological and social pressures to avoid what these processes would require. There is also a deeper concern: Although acting "profession-ally" seems as a general concept to be a noble and uncontroversial idea, exactly how professionals should act is a matter of some disagreement both inside and outside the profession.

The Variable Goals Within Professions Another issue for critics is that because of the complexity of professions, no single set of goals prevails consistently through-out a profession. This means that the opinion or recommendation of a given pro-fessional may not be credible. When professionals concentrate on one aspect of their profession and become highly skilled in it, they come to value that approach above others. Their conviction in its effectiveness is so powerful that they become strongly committed to it—some would say overcommitted. For example, the goal for some dentists is the prevention of disease, while for others it is the restoration of compro-mised dentitions. Most practitioners have goals that focus on care for individual patients, while some work to benefit communities. This is not to imply that all dentists do not acknowledge the contributions to the welfare of patients made by all branches of dentistry. It is only that one cannot resist valuing one's area of expertise more than other valid approaches.

Conflict Between a Profession's and Society's Goals   At its best, professional self-regulation would presumably make dentists conform to the standards seen by the profession as the ideals of the practice of dentistry. However, what if society's views about the way dentistry should be practiced do not match those of the profession?

One example of this is advertising. We have seen that the professions traditionally tended to treat advertising as unethical, in part because it seemed beneath the dignity of professionals to behave like mere businesspeople. We have learned, however, that some sectors of the public, particularly the Federal Trade Commission, have a very different view. They defend advertising as promotion of free speech and claim that the public is better off if appropriate forms of advertising occur than if they are prohibited.

This is just one example of behaviors about which professionals and laypeople have disagreed. Dentists, like other healing professionals, seem to favor serving the public by following a course that does as much overall good as possible while some sectors of the lay population might prefer a policy that gives special attention to the worst-off patients. In the past, dentists have also tended to disagree with the broader society about whether incompetent, dishonest, or impaired dentists should be exposed publicly or managed within the professional nexus.

All of these are examples of cases where the profession and the broader public disagree about what constitutes ideal dentistry. Collegial discipline and self-regulation at their best promote the profession's vision of dentistry. But from the point of view of a public that does not always agree on the details of that vision, collegial discipline and self-regulation are counterproductive. Hence, there has been a recent movement to involve the lay public more in matters of licensure and discipline, not because dentists cannot be trusted to put forth their best efforts, but rather because their best efforts may promote dental practices that do not quite fit with the public goals.

The process wherein members of a profession both set the standards for professional behavior and exert disciplinary influence on its membership is an example of *collegiality*. In its best sense, collegiality is one of the ideals of professionalism that greatly enhances the life of a professional. However, it can also restrict the options of the patient, or perhaps future patients, to remedy their problem appropriately, either by clinical treatment or through legal action. When protective collegiality results in patients who are not fully informed of their conditions, it violates the profession's implicit fiduciary relationship with society.[26]

With the mention of the fiduciary relationship with society, we conclude the discussion of the criticism surrounding the traditionally recognized characteristics of professions. The next section presents questions critics have raised about the fiduciary relationship, primarily from the standpoint of the client or patient and the individual professional.

Concerns About the Fiduciary Relationship

The fiduciary relationship as paternalism

Some people take issue with the concept of making decisions that are in the patient's best interest. One concern is that although the idea of fiduciary relationship sounds good, it usually emerges as paternalism. That is, when clinicians recommend treatment that is in their patient's best interests, all too often the recommendations are exclusively from the perspective of the health care providers, and the views of the patients about their own interests tend to get lost.[23,34]

Is the trust of patients justified?

This has led some critics of traditional notions of trust to observe that it no longer makes sense to trust professionals—not because professionals are self-serving, but because they lack some of the crucial information needed to warrant trust. There are two different senses in which people should not be trusted. Some cannot be trusted because they have a track record of cheating or failing to fulfill responsibilities. This is not what we are suggesting. The second sense in which people cannot be trusted is in their lack of perspective needed to act in a client's best interest. If knowing what is best requires knowledge of the patient's beliefs, values, and priorities, and if contemporary practice circumstances do not normally permit the dentist to have that information, then the dentist should not be trusted with making unilateral decisions about what interventions promote the patient's well-being, even if the dentist is a fully responsible professional devoted to his or her patient's welfare.

Response to the Concerns

In our view it is important to listen to critics of the fiduciary relationship, just as it is to hear the criticisms of other characteristics of professions and professionalism. Professions, like other social institutions, are not perfect. The important thing for members of professions to consider is how to more effectively meet their obligations to patients and clients. With that in mind, here are some responses to the criticisms.

Even though it may be impossible to know the interests of the patient, there is another interpretation of acting in the patient's interest that may be considered. It essentially acknowledges the impossibility of knowing the patient's interest and says, in effect, don't worry about it. Instead, what one should do is first be fully aware of biases and self-interests that tend to influence one's clinical decisions. Only when that is done can one make sure that those influences do not interfere with meeting obligations to patients.[35] The other point to remember, of course, is that decisions about treatment are not the dentist's to make. That prerogative belongs to the patient, the implication being the need for mutuality in the expression of recommendations, concerns, and viewpoints.

As to the previously expressed concern about the tendency toward overcommitment to one's own area of expertise, there is the counterargument that professionals should *not* be value-neutral. Health professionals, for example, ought to be advocates for the clinical welfare of their patients even though they realize that there are many interpretations of what that welfare is and whether in the end it should prevail in the patient's choices. It is an appropriate and central function for them to promote the medical aspect of the patient's well-being. Even so, as suggested earlier, the role they play should be collaborative and based on respect for the patient's personal autonomy. This includes respecting the views and decisions of the patient even when they disagree with the patient or believe that he or she has made personally harmful choices.

It is undeniable that the professions have provided great benefits for people. Their supporters accept the ideals that they profess, are satisfied by their accomplishments, and see them as working for the good of society. Their detractors, however, believe that they have failed to fulfill their promise and that their lofty ideals are really a smokescreen that conceals their efforts to maintain the status quo.[25]

Our view is that while members of professions do not always live up to their stated ideals as fully as they claim, many professionals have genuine desires to serve that, when expressed, should not be considered hypocritical. And even if noble ideals that are publicly proclaimed do not completely represent the views and conduct of the profession, they still serve as worthy aspirations to all concerned.

References

1. Bartlett LH, Ervin SA, Guo IY. A view of the profession: From dental student to practitioner—a 10-year perspective. Tex Dent J 1997;114:19–22.
2. Cohen R, Coburn D. Motivations for studying dentistry among first-year dental students. Med Educ 1977;11:139–150.
3. Hallissey J, Hannigan A, Ray N. Reasons for choosing dentistry as a career—a survey of dental students attending a dental school in Ireland during 1998–99. Eur J Dent Educ 2000;4:77–81.
4. Freidson E. Professional Powers: A Study of the Institutionalization of Formal Knowledge. Chicago: University of Chicago, 1986:242.
5. May WF. Money and the professions: Medicine and law. William Mitchell Law Rev 1999;25: 75–102.
6. Bebeau MJ, Kahn JP. Ethical issues in community dental health. In: Gluck GM, Morganstein WM (eds). Jong's Community Dental Health, ed 5. St Louis: Mosby, 2003:425–445.
7. Asbell MB. The professionalization of dentistry—Part 1. Compendium 1993;14:992,994,996.
8. Bishop MG, Gibbons D, Gelbier S. Apprenticeship in the nineteenth century, and the development of professional ethics in dentistry. Part 1. The practical reality. Br Dent J 2002;193:261–266.
9. Bishop MG, Gibbons D, Gelbier S. Ethics; 'in consideration of the love he bears.' Apprenticeship in the nineteenth century, and the development of professional ethics in dentistry. Part 2. Hippocrates' long shadow. Br Dent J 2002;193:321–325.
10. McCluggage RW. A History of the American Dental Association: A Century of Health Service. Chicago: American Dental Association, 1959:526.
11. Starr P. The Social Transformation of American Medicine: The Rise of a Sovereign Profession and the Making of a Vast Industry. New York: Basic Books, 1982:514.

12. Gorovitz S. Professions, professors, and competing obligations. In: Pellegrino ED, Veatch RM, Langan JP (eds). Ethics, Trust, and the Professions. Washington, DC: Georgetown University, 1991:93–112.

13. Buchanan A. The physician's knowledge and the patient's best interest. In: Pellegrino ED, Veatch RM, Langan JP (eds). Ethics, Trust, and the Professions. Washington, DC: Georgetown University, 1991:177–192.

14. Freidson E. The theory of professions: State of the art. In: Dingwall R, Lewis P (eds). The Sociology of the Professions. New York: St Martin's, 1983:19–37.

15. American College of Dentists. Ethics Handbook for Dentists: An Introduction to Ethics, Professionalism, and Ethical Decision Making. Gaithersburg, MD: American College of Dentists, 2000:20.

16. Gurley JE. The Evolution of Professional Ethics in Dentistry. St Louis: American College of Dentists, 1961:113.

17. American Dental Association Council on Bylaws and Judicial Affairs. Principles of Ethics and Code of Professional Conduct with official advisory opinions revised to January 2004. Chicago: American Dental Association, 2004.

18. Rule JT, Veatch RM. Ethical Questions in Dentistry. Chicago: Quintessence, 1993:282.

19. Veatch RM. A Theory of Medical Ethics. New York: Basic Books, 1981:387.

20. Barber B. The Logic and Limits of Trust. New Brunswick, NJ: Rutgers University,1983:190.

21. Pellegrino ED. Trust and distrust in professional ethics. In: Pellegrino ED, Veatch RM, Langan JP (eds). Ethics, Trust, and the Professions. Washington, DC: Georgetown University, 1991:69–89.

22. Zaner R. The phenomenon of trust and the patient-physician relationship. In: Pellegrino ED, Veatch RM, Langan JP (eds). Ethics, Trust, and the Professions. Washington, DC: Georgetown University, 1991:45–67.

23. Barber B. Some problems in the sociology of professions. Daedalus 1963;92:671.

24. Goode W. "Professions" and "non-professions." In: Vollmer HM, Mills DL (eds). Professionalization. Englewood Cliffs, NJ: Prentice Hall, 1966:33–43.

25. Kultgen J. Ethics and Professionalism. Philadelphia: University of Pennsylvania, 1988:394.

26. Freidson E. Nourishing professionalism. In: Pellegrino ED, Veatch RM, Langan JP (eds). Ethics, Trust, and the Professions. Washington, DC: Georgetown University, 1991:193–220.

27. Ozar DT. Virtues, values, and norms in dentistry. In: Weinstein BD (ed). Dental Ethics. Philadelphia: Lea & Febiger, 1993:3–19.

28. Pellegrino ED. The internal morality of clinical medicine: A paradigm for the ethics of the helping and healing professions. J Med Philos 2001;26:559–579.

29. Beauchamp TL, Childress JF. Principles of Biomedical Ethics, ed 5. New York: Oxford Univ. Press, 2001:7.

30. Millerson G. The Qualifying Professions. London: Routledge and Kegan Paul, 1964.

31. Kohn N. Motivation for a professional career. In: Vollmer HM, Mills DL (eds). Professionalization. Englewood Cliffs, NJ: Prentice Hall, 1966:81–87.

32. Veatch RM. Is trust of professionals a coherent concept? In: Pellegrino ED, Veatch RM, Langan JP (eds). Ethics, Trust, and the Professions. Washington, DC: Georgetown University, 1991: 159–173.

33. Larson MS. The Rise of Professionalism. Berkeley, CA: University of California, 1977:309.

34. Childress JF. Who Should Decide? Paternalism in Health Care. New York: Oxford Univ. Press, 1982:250.

35. Brock DW. Facts and values in the physician-patient's relationship. In: Pellegrino ED, Veatch RM, Langan JP (eds). Ethics, Trust, and the Professions. Washington, DC: Georgetown University, 1991:113–138.

chapter 3

Basic Ethical Theory

In this chapter

- The Meaning of Morality
- Possible Grounding of Ethics

The Meaning of Morality

The cases in this book deal with ethics. So before looking directly at the problems they pose, we need to have some basic understanding of the meaning of morality and ethics. It will also be helpful to know how moral claims are justified and what some of the major positions are in ethics. This chapter and the next will outline some answers to these questions. In chapter 5 we will explore ways to solve ethical problems as posed in clinical cases.

The Meaning of Ethics and Morals

Distinguishing the Factual from the Evaluative

Many questions faced in dentistry can be viewed as questions of fact. A dentist may want to know whether an amalgam or a composite resin restoration is likely to last longer or whether a pulp is infected. These are questions that we can assume, at least for now, can be answered by good dental science.

There are other kinds of factual questions relevant to dentistry as well. Dental patients may want to know the cost of different kinds of restorations, whether a procedure will be painful, or whether a crown will be cosmetically noticeable. Dentists may want to know whether the law permits a waiver of liability when a patient asks for a procedure the dentist cannot endorse. These are not exactly questions of dental science, but nonetheless they are what we can consider matters of fact.

One can know all of the relevant scientific facts about dentistry and still not know how to proceed with clinical dentistry. It is impossible to know whether a dental procedure is good or bad, right or wrong, without turning to the realm of evaluation. It is only with the combination of knowledge of the relevant facts and some framework of evaluation that one can know what is clinically appropriate. In short, to know what to do, the decision-maker has to know what a desirable outcome is.

Recognizing that an evaluation is taking place is not as easy as it may seem. Deciding that one approach is better than another will in itself require an evaluation. Deciding that a treatment has side effects does so as well. By saying that a treatment has a side effect, we are acknowledging it is undesirable. Even the claim that a dental procedure is "indicated" is a claim with some evaluative component; it is a claim that, all things considered, the procedure offers a better mix of risks and benefits than does any alternative. Evaluations are ubiquitous in dentistry as in all clinical professions.

Identifying Evaluations

One way to recognize an evaluation is to look for evaluative terms: "good" or "bad," "right" or "wrong," "desired" or "undesired." Sometimes the evaluations are slightly disguised, as when a treatment is "recommended" or "ordered." In addition, the phrases "risk," "harm," "side effect," "treatment of choice," and "medically indicated" all signal an evaluative judgment. Sometimes evaluations take the form of declarative sentences that are really value judgments in disguise, for example, "You don't want to chew on that side for an hour" or "the dentist is dedicated to the welfare of the patient." These statements imply the value judgments that it would be bad to chew too soon or that a "good" dentist is dedicated to the welfare of the patient. One of the keys to dental ethics is learning to recognize the evaluative judgments that occur in all clinical decisions.

Moral and Nonmoral Evaluations

Of course, not all evaluations are moral or ethical; they might simply be matters of personal taste or preference. One person may find a gold crown attractive; another may find it garish. Although both have made evaluations, we do not consider either to have made a *moral* evaluation. Some evaluations are merely matters of societal preference. Others are esthetic evaluations. Still others may be cultural or religious without being moral or ethical.

A moral or ethical evaluation must meet certain characteristics. First, it must be an evaluation of a person's actions or character. Even among evaluations of actions or character, not all evaluations are moral. A dancer may be graceful, a dentist may show great manual dexterity. Any value judgment made about an inanimate object—a painting or a partial restoration—will not be a moral judgment (although one may certainly make a moral judgment about the person who did the painting or made the restoration).

The distinction between moral and nonmoral evaluations is not always a sharp one, but most people tend to think of an evaluation as moral or ethical when it meets most, if not all, of the following five characteristics.

Ultimacy Perhaps the most critical characteristic of moral or ethical evaluations is that the standard by which the judgment is made is deemed ultimate, ie, there seems to be no higher standard by which one might judge. The judgment has what the philosopher John Rawls calls "finality."[1,2] If we say that lying to a patient to cover up a bungled restoration is immoral, we mean that it is wrong by the highest, most definitive standard that we can imagine. That standard might be "the eyes of God" or some secular equivalent based in reason or on the moral law of nature. By contrast, if when asked why you believe a behavior is right you claim that your favorite textbook said so, or that your friend or community said so, we would be justified in asking why you consider these to be the ultimate standard of reference. When we say something is morally good or bad, right or wrong, we are saying it is so by the most ultimate standard of reference we can imagine.

Universality Moral or ethical evaluations are often also said to be universal.[1] By this we mean that if other people are considering exactly the same action or character trait in exactly the same situation, they ought to come to the same evaluative conclusion. If we say that Dr Jones's lying to cover up a mechanical exposure in a particular patient is morally wrong, we mean that everyone should consider this lie by Dr Jones to be immoral. Used in this way, the term *universality* does not imply rigidity or legalism. It is not the view that all lying, no matter what the circumstances, is always wrong. It is conceivable that Dr Jones might be thought to be right in lying in some extreme circumstance—to save his life or the life of someone else. The claim made here is that when we say an evaluation is a moral evaluation, we believe that anyone considering an act (like a particular lie) ought to come to the same evaluation that we do.

In this sense moral evaluations are different from matters of personal taste or even societal judgment. We do not consider it a contradiction if one person likes gold and another does not. These preferences we treat as a matter of taste about which people may disagree without contradicting one another. If, however, we say that someone was morally wrong to extract a sound tooth on a particular occasion, we imply that anyone considering that act on that occasion ought to come to the same conclusion.

From this standpoint, moral judgments are like scientific judgments. Any two people considering exactly the same event at the same time ought to agree on their account of it. Of course, this does not mean that people actually do always agree on moral judgments any more than they agree on scientific judgments. It is only that, for matters believed to be universal, there cannot be contradictory accounts that are true simultaneously. If two people give contradictory accounts of the same event at the same time, at most only one can be right.

Altruism or neutralism   Another characteristic of moral evaluations is that they are neutral or "general." Judgments cannot be tailored to the advantage of the person making the judgment. The dentist should not recommend a fixed partial denture only because the amount of profit is greater than that for a partial denture. A rule that permitted dentists to recommend a course solely because it was the most profitable would not satisfy the criterion of neutrality unless one were willing to accept a rule saying that all trusted advisors could recommend action based solely on personal profit. Principles and rules of morality cannot be crafted to promote the advantage of the person stating them.

Publicity   Another criterion that tends to make evaluations moral is that one must be willing to publicly state the evaluation and the basis on which it is made. This rules out judgments that rely on secretiveness to produce the desired effect. For example, a pediatric dentist contemplates telling a young child that drilling probably will not hurt when he knows that it almost certainly will. He considers that a white lie in this case will avoid anxiety for the child and is therefore justified. However, if it were publicly known to patients that this dentist followed a policy of lying to make patients feel better, his goal would be defeated. According to the criterion of publicity, a policy such as this is a moral policy only if it can be made known publicly.

Ordering   Finally, any set of principles, rules, or character assessments should provide a basis for ranking conflicting claims. Ethical problems often arise in professional practice when one is caught between two competing obligations. For example, the dentist wants to do as much good as possible by restoring a certain tooth, whereas the patient, appealing to autonomy, wants to have it extracted. A systematic ethical account should be able to tell which claim has moral priority and why.

These five criteria—ultimacy, universality, altruism or neutralism, publicity, and ordering—constitute criteria of an ethical system and provide a way to distinguish moral from nonmoral judgments. If an evaluative claim that is made about human conduct or character meets these five criteria, it will be a moral or ethical claim.

Distinguishing the Moral and the Ethical

So far we have distinguished factual claims from evaluative judgments and distinguished those judgments that are not moral or ethical from those that are. We should also clearly understand the two terms that are used to apply to judgments that meet the criteria we have just outlined. We have variously called these evaluative judgments *moral* or *ethical*. But what is the difference?

Some people, considering that the term *moral* has the same root as *mores* or customs, use *moral* to apply to social customs or habits. In English, however, mores are distinguished from morals. Mores, in fact, are not considered to be in the realm of the moral. Customs or societal practices, after all, can be well established without necessarily being moral. Mores refer to the well-established practices of a society; they are not necessarily grounded in some ultimate source of judgment beyond which there can be no appeal. For example, a particular culture may consider a woman who wears a short skirt to be immoral, even though we, as outside observers, recognize that this judgment merely reflects current social consensus.

Another attempt to define moral equates the moral with deeply held, even religious, convictions. While moral positions may be deeply held and may be grounded in religious traditions, they need not be either deeply held or religiously grounded. Moreover, ethical positions also may be deeply held and religiously grounded. Thus, whether the conviction is deeply held or religious does not seem to be a basis for separating the terms *moral* and *ethical*.

There is another sense in which people have tried to distinguish the moral and the ethical. Our unreflective, ad hoc judgments can be called *moral judgments*, while more systematic, reasoned accounts of these judgments are sometimes referred to as an *ethic*. If this distinction correctly distinguishes the two terms, then morality refers to specific judgments while ethics refers to the disciplined, systematic, reasoned theory that might support the specific moral judgments. In this sense, all people make moral judgments, but only some can provide an ethical account that supports the moral judgments. Ethics is the systematic reflection on morals.

In this book we use the term *moral* to refer to specific judgments and the term *ethical* to refer to systematic reflection. There is no hard-and-fast separation between the two, but when referring to an ad hoc judgment by a dentist, patient, or society, we will call it a moral judgment. When we are examining a more systematic theory of moral rightness or wrongness, as in the code of ethics of the American Dental Association, a religious group, or a philosophical school, we shall speak of ethics.

Possible Grounding of Ethics

If moral judgments and the ethical systems that stand behind them have their grounding in an ultimate standard beyond which there is no appeal, just what might that ultimate grounding be? Much of the history of ethical theory has been devoted to answering that question. Several foundations of ethics have been proposed.

Cultural Relativism

When people first begin to reflect on their moral judgments, it is not uncommon for them to suspect that what we call ethics is really nothing more than the judgments of our culture. For something to be considered moral, according to a position often called *cultural relativism*, it must simply meet with the approval of one's culture.

Undoubtedly, the judgments of different cultures differ widely over matters believed to be moral. We are talking not only about skirt length and sexual practices but also about basic beliefs regarding the rightness of lying, killing, breaking promises, and injuring others. One possible explanation is that when people live in different cultures, they express the judgments of their cultures.

Upon examination, this position of cultural relativism poses serious problems. First we must distinguish between *descriptive relativism* and *normative relativism.* Descriptive relativism is a factual claim that people in different cultures have differing views about matters believed to be moral. Almost no one who has witnessed more than one culture denies that such differences do, in fact, exist.

Normative relativism is a claim regarding the ultimate source of moral norms: that there is no single universal foundation of moral judgments. Cultural normative relativism is the view that moral judgments are grounded only in each culture's collective opinion. If, however, representatives of two different cultures disagree about what appears to be a moral matter, then we cannot automatically conclude that ethics is just a matter of cultural opinion. More work needs to be done to reach the conclusion that the reason they differ is that the ultimate standard of moral judgments is nothing more than the views of the various cultures.

First, we need to be sure that the people from the two cultures in disagreement are really considering the same events. Consider the important problem of inflicting pain on laboratory animals for purposes of research such as developing new dental techniques. If we are considering small mammals, not all cultures have the same factual beliefs about what is happening to the animals. If one culture believes that extracting teeth in unanesthetized animals hurts the animals and another believes that it does not, then it is shortsighted to assume that, if they have different moral judgments about the use of animals, they disagree ultimately over matters of ethical principle. They could both believe that it is wrong to hurt animals but that it is acceptable to extract teeth painlessly for justified research. We cannot attribute differences between cultures to real differences in moral positions until we know that the differences relate to moral judgments and not simply to beliefs about the facts.

Second, even if we are convinced that the moral positions of two cultures are really different, that difference surely does not establish the truth of the claim that moral judgments are grounded only in culture. Even if it can be shown that one culture believes that it is moral to hurt animals for human betterment and another believes that it is not, it does not show that the ground of their positions is nothing more than their cultural views. There could be some other basis—the will of a god or some other universal rationality beyond their culture—to which both are appealing. They might simply disagree on what the will of God is or what reason requires. In fact, when two cultures disagree about something that each thinks is worth fighting about, they both must believe that there is, in principle, a single cross-cultural basis for resolving the dispute. Otherwise, why fight?

It is possible that some issues that a culture perceives to be ethical really are not. A culture could misclassify the nature of the judgments it makes. Some people in our culture consider homosexuality immoral while others consider it a variation, but hardly immoral.

If some issues are falsely perceived by certain cultures to be matters of morality, then that does not indicate that all matters believed to be moral are really only cultural.

Personal Relativism

One problem with cultural relativism is that it seems possible to say without contradiction that an action conforms to the standards of one's culture but is still morally wrong. For example, someone living in the antebellum southern slave culture could have said, "My culture believes slavery to be morally right, but it is really wrong." If that can be said without contradiction, then culture cannot be the standard of morality. Moreover, even if one accepted cultural relativism, it would be extremely difficult to determine the relevant culture. Each individual is identified with a religious culture, a national culture, an ethnic culture, a familial culture, and an educational culture. In fact, we are all composites of many cultural and subcultural groups. We might not be able to identify one single culture for making ethical judgments even if we wanted to do so.

An alternative is to appeal to the judgments of the individual as the standard for making ethical judgments. According to *personal relativism,* a behavior or character is considered good or right when it conforms to one's personal standard of goodness or rightness. The individual, not the culture, is the standard of reference according to this view.

This position is somewhat harder to assess than cultural relativism. We can at least identify what the standard is. But do we really want to say that hurting animals is morally wrong for a person when and only when it violates that person's personally held standard of morality? Do we really want to claim that morality is nothing more than conformance to personal standards of right and wrong? That would make it logically impossible for anyone to be morally wrong in his or her judgment. Of course we could consider that the actions of others were wrong, but we would have to hold that they are wrong to each of us only because they violate our individual standards.

That of course is not inconsistent with their being morally right for the one engaged in the questioned behavior (because they are in conformance with his or her standards). Personal relativism reduces morality to conformance with one's own code or standards. Each person becomes his or her own ultimate standard of judgment.

It might be true that there is no ultimate standard for any ethical judgments, that we are really fooling ourselves by searching for something more universal. But personal relativism is a difficult position to maintain. It means, for example, that there is no contradiction between my holding that it is right for me to lie, cheat, and steal while at the same time someone else holds that under the same circumstances it is wrong for me to lie, cheat, and steal. For most of us, morality is a matter of right and wrong that is not grounded in either cultural or personal standards. The appeal is beyond these levels and that is why morality is different from matters of taste or preference and why matters of morality are worth arguing. That is what makes professional ethics something more than cultural conformity or personal style. What could be the grounding of ethics if it is to be more fundamental, more ultimate, than are personal and cultural standards?

Professional Codes

If cultural and personal standards of morality do not provide a sufficient basis for professional ethics in dentistry, what other options are available? Historically, professions have generated their own codes of ethics and have been responsible for adjudication of ethical disputes among their members. Could we say that, at least for professional ethics, the profession provides the ultimate standard of judgment in ethics?

As early as the time of Hippocrates in ancient Greece, groups of physicians wrote their own codes of ethics. Hippocratic physicians, in particular, drafted their own code, which, as the professions gained their independence during the Middle Ages, became the foundation for an independent ethical code for the health professions.

The Hippocratic Oath consists of two separate parts, an oath of loyalty to the profession and a code of conduct.[3] It contains some esoteric elements that make little sense today—pledging by the Greek gods and goddesses and even a prohibition on surgery, for example. But it also contains what, according to some, remains to this day the essence of the ethics of a health professional. The health professional pledges to work always for the patient according to his or her ability and judgment. It includes a vague, perhaps controversial, pledge of confidentiality and equally vague opposition to giving deadly drugs and "pessaries" to produce abortion.

Let us examine whether the Hippocratic Oath, or some updated version of it, could provide the ethical foundation for the health professions or whether the American Dental Association's code could serve as a summation of the profession's views of the standard for ethical behavior of dentists. The issue is whether the professional understanding of the dentist's ethical obligations can be the ultimate foundation that we have been seeking. Some believe that by its very nature a profession creates its own ethical standards. That is a controversial, implausible position, however. One version of this view is that the profession is the single, universal source of an ethic for dentists. That raises problems, however, especially for dentists who are members of religious groups who claim that God is the source of all morality or for those who subscribe to secular ethical systems outside the profession.

Another version holds that the profession is only one possible source of an ethic for dentists. Other groups may also formulate their own understanding of what the norms for dentists should be. For example, while professional dental associations reached one position on the ethics of advertising, some lay groups have reached different positions. This brings us back to cultural relativism and raises new problems. What members of the dental profession believe to be the ethical duty of dentists could differ from that which other groups believe is the duty of dentists. There seems to be no reason why those outside the profession should yield to those inside in establishing what the norms are. Moreover, dentists are also members of groups outside the profession. They belong to churches that have ethical positions; they may subscribe to one or another major ethical theory (utilitarianism, for instance). Some of those groups may have positions on professional conduct that differ from that of the professional association, which could mean that the dentist would support two contradictory ethical positions simultaneously.

Another possibility is that the grounding of the norms expressed by dentists in their code is actually more universal, but that members of the profession have the unique ability to know what the norms are. This raises the question of whether the process of becoming a dentist (or any other professional) uniquely qualifies one to know the ethical norms as they apply to one's profession. Agreement within the profession about what the norms are is just one among many possible ways in which the ethical norms for a profession can be determined.

With increasing frequency, disputes are arising over what the proper ethical duties for the dentist are in dealing with those outside the profession. For instance, there is disagreement on what should be done when the dentist believes that the patient would benefit from a violation of confidentiality or a less-than-expected disclosure of information. Sometimes there is disagreement about what a dentist should do when the interests of society conflict with those of the patient. Especially when we realize that it is not always obvious exactly who speaks for the profession, the idea that the profession should always be the final standard for settling such disputes is becoming increasingly controversial.

Universal Standards

If cultural groups (including professional groups) as well as personal opinions are not adequate standards for grounding moral judgments, what else could provide that ultimate foundation? For members of religious groups, especially monotheistic religious groups, the answer is clear: An action or character is ethical when it conforms to the moral standards of the god of the religious group. Members of such groups believe that if their god approves of an action, or if the action conforms to the moral laws created by their god, then, by definition, the action is morally right. Of course, not everyone will agree with the believer's understanding, though for that person the ultimate foundation has been found. The foundation is universal in the sense that the believer holds that everyone ought to accept his or her standard as ultimate.

Secular thinkers also may accept some universal standard, perhaps locating it in reason. Kant,[4] for example, thought that ethics was ultimately grounded in reason, while the empiricists believed it was grounded in nature knowable through experience.[5] Others have held moral norms to be universal and knowable through intuition rather than reason or experience.[6] All of these views share the notion that when someone makes a moral judgment, he or she is making a claim that has its grounding in some universal source that, in principle, everyone should share. Of course, not everyone will necessarily agree with such a moral judgment, but when a disagreement about a specific ethical judgment occurs, there is a contradiction—at least one view must be wrong.

Other ethical theories have attempted to reject this understanding of the grounding of morality without reducing ethics to pure relativism. Some have held that moral statements are really not objective statements relating to any universal standard at all, but are merely expressions of emotion,[7] efforts to evoke agreement,[8] or prescriptions for the behavior of others.[9] In the end we must recognize that there is probably no single theory about what the ultimate foundation of moral judgments is. If there were, we probably would no longer have moral disagreements.

As we proceed to analyze the cases in this text, however, we need to understand that we are examining how a behavior, policy, or character trait would be assessed by some standard viewed as ultimate. The fact that we cannot always agree on these judgments is not evidence that there is no such ultimate standard. In the end each of us will have to judge the issues raised in these cases for ourselves, but that is not the same as saying that personal opinion is necessarily the ultimate standard by which we judge.

The problem in ethics is, in many ways, similar to that in science. For most issues the correct answer is quite clear to all—or at least to those who have spent some time reflecting on the issue. In some difficult cases even those who have struggled long and hard cannot agree on precisely what the proper account is. Each person individually has to decide on his or her own, but that should not be taken to imply in ethics any more than in science that there is no account that is more appropriate or more correct than any other. It could well be that some claims made in the name of ethics are really only matters of taste (about which we believe that people can disagree without contradicting one another), but that does not imply that all ethical claims are ultimately only matters of opinion.

Alternative Theories of Normative Ethics

Having explored the nature and meaning of ethics and the ways in which moral claims could be identified and justified, we need to say a word about some of the major systematic positions about what makes actions, policies, rules, or character traits right and wrong, good or bad—what is called *normative ethics*. We must put aside the preliminary issues of meaning and justification and which reference point we use in making such claims.

Normative ethical theories are now addressed specifically in studies of health care ethics,[10–16] but the basic issues will be similar in any kind of normative ethical theory. There are three general kinds of judgments in normative ethics: judgments about which kinds of actions or rules are right (*action theory*), which nonmoral things are good or bad (*value theory* or *axiology*), and which traits of character are desirable (*virtue theory*).

Action Theory

The most obvious normative ethical questions raised by the cases in this volume have to do with whether the behavior of dentists or others is morally acceptable. Sometimes these judgments are made about specific instances of behavior; sometimes they are made about more general rules that govern behavior. In either case, they are part of a theory of right action, or what we call action theory.

A theory of right action articulates general principles that tend to make actions right or wrong according to the ultimate moral standard of reference. These principles necessarily are general because they have to be limited to a manageable number that are understandable to the ordinary person. They are principles such as beneficence (doing good), nonmaleficence (avoiding harm), veracity (truth telling), fidelity (including keeping promises), respect for autonomy, avoidance of killing, and justice. Much of the work of ethics is in converting these general principles to judgments about specific situations.

A general theory of right action may include the view that these general principles should be applied to specific actions through the use of rules. Rules of thumb, for instance, help translate principles into specific judgments, but some ethical theories insist that rules be taken more seriously than that. In these theories, rules define practices such that the practices themselves are judged by the principles, rather than on a case-by-case basis. These views are called *rule-based theories*. Conversely, theories that propose applying the principles more directly to individual actions (perhaps using rules only as guidelines or as rules of thumb) are called *act-based* or *situational theories*. The concepts of rule-based and act-based theories are discussed further in the next two sections.

Utilitarianism and consequentialistic theories One major group of theories that is particularly dominant in the ethics of health professionals, including dentists, holds that what really matters is the *consequences* of actions. The dominant principles for such theories are beneficence and nonmaleficence, where doing good and avoiding harm are considered the only morally relevant features of actions.

Of course, there can be great differences about *(1)* what counts as a good or a harm, *(2)* whether these are objectively determined or merely based on the preferences of those being affected, and *(3)* the priority between doing good and avoiding harm.

Much of Catholic moral theology is *consequentialistic* in that it judges actions to be right or wrong, in part based on whether the actions conform to the *telos,* or natural end of the human person. Secular consequentialistic theories may look at more mundane, this-worldly consequences. *Utilitarianism* is perhaps the most well-known example. According to utilitarians, the definitive principle of ethics is that an action is right if it does as much or more good than any alternative action. This notion is sometimes expressed as doing "the greatest good for the greatest number."[17,18] In the classical utilitarian theories, this is calculated simply by considering the net amount of good (good minus harm) for each person and then summing over all persons affected.

Health care ethics, including dental ethics, places great emphasis on consequences. For example, in the case we use in chapter 5 as our prototype for case analysis, a dentist was asked to see a patient who had been in an automobile accident that caused dental injuries. Because of the patient's threatening demeanor, the dentist wondered about his obligations to treat him, despite evidence of legitimate need. The dominant ethical notion, as we have seen, is that the health professional is to benefit the patient and protect the patient from harm according to the clinician's judgment. While this is essentially a consequentialistic approach, there is a catch: The only benefits and harms that count are those to the patient.

The justification for this limit is not easy to grasp. Some might argue that we have a rule-based utilitarianism operating. Over the centuries we may have discovered that if each clinician does what he or she believes is best for the patient, then, in aggregate, the greatest overall good will result. That would be a rule-based utilitarian ethic in which the rule that clinicians should ignore the consequences for everyone other than the patient is defended on the belief that in the end more good will be done than if any other approach were used.

While that might work in some cases, it seems unlikely that ignoring the interests of everyone but the patient will normally produce the greatest aggregate social benefit. Another possibility is that defenders of the ethics of clinicians do not exactly subscribe to a purely consequentialistic ethic. They may believe that the correct principle for clinical health care is that only the consequences for the patient count morally. From this perspective, it might be deemed immoral to trade off the patient's welfare against the welfare of others.

Exactly why such a trade-off would be immoral would be a puzzle to a pure consequentialist such as a utilitarian (unless it just worked out to be the best way to maximize the total amount of good done). To many clinicians, however, limiting their attention to their individual patients seems to make moral sense. They may believe that it is inherent in the nature of the practice of the health professions to focus only on the patient or that a promise has been made by the professional to society to limit attention in this way. If so, they are not completely consequentialists. They are "consequentialists with a catch"; they also abide by some principle that discriminates among consequences to tell them which consequences are morally relevant.

Deontological theories Many ethical theories include principles that tend to make actions right yet do not focus solely on maximizing good consequences and minimizing bad consequences. For example, some theories hold that respecting autonomy is a right-making principle of action even when doing so does not produce the best possible consequences. Other principles that do not focus on maximizing net consequences include the principles of veracity or honesty, the principle of fidelity (including keeping promises), the principle that it is wrong to kill, and the principle of justice (goods should be distributed in a fair or equitable manner).

Whenever the right action, rule, or practice is determined at least in part by principles other than those that focus on maximizing net good consequences, the theory is termed *deontological*. The term comes from the Greek for "duty." Such theories, which can differ widely among themselves, share the notion that what is right is not determined solely by what produces the most net good in aggregate.

As with consequentialistic theories, the principles can be applied directly to individual actions on a case-by-case basis (act-deontology) or can be mediated through a set of rules (rule-deontology). Thus it is important to note that consequentialistic ethics is not necessarily more case-oriented or situational. It is perfectly possible that one can be a rule-utilitarian or an act-deontologist.

Prima facie duties and duty proper It is possible then for there to be more than one ethical principle in a normative theory of what makes actions or practices right. Whenever there is more than one principle, we need to distinguish between our *prima facie duty* and our *duty proper*. A prima facie duty is a duty taking into account only one moral principle. One's duty proper is one's duty after taking into account all relevant principles and applying some theory of how to reconcile conflict among principles. Thus it might be a dentist's prima facie duty never to hurt a patient even though inflicting pain may be understandable and necessary after taking into account the duty of beneficence for the patient and the duty to respect the autonomy of the patient. One's duty proper takes into account all moral principles, whereas one's prima facie duty considers only one moral dimension at a time.

Value Theory or What Counts as a Good

All consequentialistic theories and many deontological theories are concerned about producing good outcomes and avoiding bad outcomes. Any ethical theory of right action that includes any consideration of consequences•–either one that focuses on maximizing net good or one that is concerned with distributing goods justly—must have a further element. There must be an account of what counts as a good or a harm. Some theories focus on subjective preferences; others make some attempt to determine benefits and harms objectively.

One critical element in these theories is how dental and medical goods relate to other kinds of goods, including economic, social, psychological, familial, legal, and spiritual. This poses an interesting problem for dentists. Dentists might plausibly be thought to be experts on one particular kind of health care good: "oral well-being." Even this claim is controversial. It is not clear, for example, whether a dentist has any expertise in deciding what counts as a dental good. If a patient presents a problem that can be fixed effectively and economically but with some remaining cosmetic problem, or if it can be fixed in a more costly but esthetically pleasing way, it is not clear that there is any "correct" dental choice about which a dentist can exert expertise. Likewise, the choice between a short-term and a long-term solution is obviously not one that a dentist can make with expertise. Even the notion of "oral well-being" may be one about which reasonable people disagree and about which dentists may not have any real claim to expertise.

When we realize that rational people do not want to maximize their "oral well-being" in isolation from other kinds of well-being, the problem becomes even more complicated. Certainly no one profession can claim to know what will maximize the general well-being of a patient, let alone the overall well-being of the society at large. Nevertheless, for utilitarian theorists and other theorists who include principles of beneficence and nonmaleficence, an answer to these questions must be found.

Virtue Theory

A third kind of normative ethical judgment must be distinguished from principles and values. Sometimes in health care ethics we are at least as interested in the character of the actor as in the behavior itself. Virtues are persistent dispositions or traits of character that are judged in different ethical theories as good or bad. In recent clinical biomedical ethics, virtue theory is undergoing something of a renaissance.[19–22] Virtue theory is distinguished from action theory because it focuses on the ethics of the character of the actor rather than the morality of the behavior. Many virtues of actors correlate with principles of right action. For example, beneficence has as its correlate the virtue of benevolence. An action is beneficent if it produces good consequences; an actor is benevolent if he or she wills to do good (even if that is not the end result). It is possible to be benevolent (to will the good) without actually being beneficent (doing the good). In such cases we may have to decide which is more important, doing the good for a bad motive or doing harm even though it is done with a good motive. Whatever our judgment on these matters, it will be important to realize that the two kinds of judgments, while both counting as moral judgments, are substantively different.

In this text we focus primarily on the ethics of actions and therefore must clarify the principles that indicate what makes actions or practices right, keeping in mind that we can also assess the virtues of the actors involved. It is to a characterization of the principles of right action that we now turn.

References

1. Rawls J. A Theory of Justice. Cambridge, MA: Harvard University, 1971.
2. Beauchamp TL, Childress JE. Principles of Biomedical Ethics, ed 5. New York: Oxford University, 2001.
3. Edelstein L. The Hippocratic Oath: Text, translation and interpretation. In: Temkin O, Temkin CL (eds). Ancient Medicine: Selected Papers of Ludwig Edelstein. Baltimore: John Hopkins University, 1967:6.
4. Kant I. Groundwork of the Metaphysic of Morals. Paton HJ (trans). New York: Harper and Row, 1964.
5. Hume D. An Inquiry Concerning the Principles of Morals. New York: Library of Liberal Arts, 1957.
6. Moore GE. Principia Ethica. Cambridge, England: Cambridge University, 1903.
7. Ayer AJ. Language, Truth and Logic. London, England: Victor Gollancz, 1948.
8. Stevenson CL. Ethics and Language. New Haven, CT: Yale University, 1944.
9. Hare RM. The Language of Morals. Oxford, England: Clarendon, 1952.
10. Beauchamp TL, Walters L (eds). Contemporary Issues in Bioethics, ed 6. Belmont, CA: Wadsworth, 2003.
11. Pellegrino ED, Thomasma DC. The Philosophical Basis of Medical Practice. New York: Oxford University, 1991.
12. Jonsen AR, Siegler M, Winslade WJ. Clinical Ethics: A Practical Approach to Ethical Decisions in Clinical Medicine. New York: Macmillan, 1982.
13. Engelhardt HT. The Foundations of Bioethics, ed 2. New York: Oxford University, 1996.
14. Emanuel EJ. The Ends of Human Life: Medical Ethics in a Liberal Polity. Cambridge, MA: Harvard University, 1991.
15. Brody B. Life and Death Decision Making. New York: Oxford University, 1988.
16. Veatch RM. A Theory of Medical Ethics. New York: Basic Books, 1981.
17. Bentham J. An introduction to the principles of morals and legislation. In: Melden AI (ed). Ethical Theories: A Book of Readings. Englewood Cliffs, NJ: Prentice Hall, 1967:367–390.
18. Mill JS. Utilitarianism. In: Melden AI (ed). Ethical Theories: A Book of Readings. Englewood Cliffs, NJ: Prentice Hall, 1967:391–434.
19. Hauerwas S, Pinches C. Christians Among the Virtues: Theological Conversations With Ancient and Modern Ethics. Notre Dame, IN: University of Notre Dame, 1997.
20. MacIntyre A. After Virtue. Notre Dame, IN: University of Notre Dame, 1981.
21. MacIntyre AC. Dependent Rational Animals: Why Human Beings Need the Virtues. Chicago: Open Court, 1999.
22. Hursthouse R. On Virtue Ethics. New York: Oxford University, 1999.

Ethical Principles

In this chapter

Ethical dilemmas often arise when the issues depend more on moral evaluations than on clinical skills or scientific judgment. For example, a practitioner may wonder if it is morally acceptable to refuse to see an objectionable patient, to avoid seeing someone else's patient in an emergency, or to not tell a new patient about some harmful dentistry done by a previous dentist. In each instance the opposing alternatives represent positions in debates that depend on ethical principles.[1]

Over the last two decades, principles such as autonomy, nonmaleficence, beneficence, and justice have been accepted as basic principles.[2–4] Briefly stated, these principles require that all actions (including those by health care providers) demonstrate:

1. Regard for self-determination (respect for autonomy)
2. The avoidance of doing harm (nonmaleficence)
3. The promotion of well-being (beneficence)
4. Fairness in the distribution of goods and harms (justice)

Other principles are sometimes included with those listed, including veracity, fidelity, avoidance of killing, and perhaps privacy and confidentiality.[1] Some of these may be combined, or one may be treated as derivative from another. Autonomy, veracity, and fidelity are, for example, sometimes combined into the principle of respect for persons. Confidentiality may be derived from the general principle of fidelity.

It is the purpose of this chapter to introduce these principles, emphasizing autonomy, nonmaleficence, beneficence, and justice. In case discussions in later chapters, these principles will be amplified and applied to dental situations so that the roles of the other principles will become clear.

Autonomy

The moral principle of autonomy provides the underpinning for broad concepts such as the right to privacy, freedom of choice, and the acceptance of responsibility for one's actions.[2–4] It is the moral principle that supports one's freedom to think, judge, and act independently without undue influence.[5] Although the notion of autonomy grew out of the Western idea of political self-rule, in medical ethics it gives rise to a duty to permit individuals to make informed decisions about factors affecting their health. Issues of autonomy, especially as they pertain to questions of informed consent, are at the heart of many ethical dilemmas that occur in dentistry.

An autonomous person is one who acts intentionally and whose actions reflect a thoughtful and individualized choice based on adequate information. Such a person functions without undue external or internal influences that could affect the outcomes of decisions. It seems highly unlikely that even the most autonomous person will meet those standards all the time. Sometimes decisions are made without access to the necessary information, occasionally even without awareness that the information is needed, and sometimes internal factors such as pain may distort one's ability to make informed decisions.

For these reasons it is preferable to speak of autonomous acts rather than autonomous people. Just as a so-called autonomous person may make choices that are not autonomous, a nonautonomous or partially autonomous person may make autonomous choices in certain circumstances.[6] A mentally disturbed, institutionalized person may make informed decisions about the choice of friends and other aspects of daily life but probably is totally incapable of weighing the risks and benefits of sterilization. An 8-year-old child is only partly autonomous but is perfectly capable of understanding that the application of dental sealants would probably prevent the harms associated with occlusal caries later.

Considering the generally unequal relationship between health care provider and patient, the patient cannot make autonomous choices unless the health care provider respects the patient's right to be adequately informed and then acts accordingly. This makes clear that there are two different aspects to the issue of autonomy: autonomy itself and the respect for autonomy. Autonomy refers to the self-direction of the individual. Respect for autonomy refers to the recognition that others have rights to hold and act on personal values and beliefs. Respect for autonomy is part of the Kantian view that each person has intrinsic worth and possesses certain rights that others are obliged to respect. It is an extremely important principle in health care.[7,8] In dentistry, a patient who values the preservation of her teeth may be deprived of that opportunity if her dentist assumes she will want an abscessed tooth removed because he believes she cannot afford root canal treatment.

The principle of autonomy sometimes conflicts with other principles. A patient's preference may be for the extraction of her last 10 maxillary teeth and the construction of a denture. If the patient is adequately informed about the importance of retaining the natural dentition, the decision is autonomous even if the patient's choice is not the one that the dentist believes most promotes her well-being. The dentist may see clearly that periodontal therapy and partial dentures will maximize functional benefits. In this situation the dentist has to decide whether to do what the patient wishes or what the dentist believes will benefit her the most.

The management of such conflicts is a source of controversy. Some view autonomy as the highest-ranking principle, one that must remain inviolate. That is a position only an extreme libertarian would maintain, however. Many people recognize that autonomy must be limited, at least in some cases in which autonomous action will do harm to others. However, even if autonomy is subordinated to patient benefit, the dentist would have to be able to determine what will really serve this patient's interests (rather than merely what would serve the dentist's interest in a similar situation). That may be very hard for the dentist to do.

More controversial is the case in which acting autonomously will upset others or offend their moral standards. One such case is the earlier scenario where the patient's preference for dentures and the extraction of 10 salvageable teeth conflicts with the standards of the dentist who sees that better function can be obtained with more conservative approaches. (The dentist, however, may not be able to take the patient's agenda adequately into account. The patient, for example, may want to get the dental problem resolved in what seems to her a more final way. She may want to end the anticipation of further problems with her remaining teeth. It is very difficult for a dentist to be able to take into account all the concerns of the patient.)

The resolution of these conflicts depends on an understanding of the priority of the principles. Some people hold that autonomy has equal priority with beneficence, nonmaleficence, justice, and the other principles.[9] According to this view one can make a moral choice only after assessing the implications of all the relevant principles. Others give autonomy an absolute priority over beneficence when only the welfare of the autonomous actor is at stake while sometimes compromising autonomy when the rights or welfare of others is affected.[4] Conflicts over autonomy can be quite dramatic, as with an adult Jehovah's Witness patient refusing blood transfusions despite the possibly mortal consequences. The patient's decision may be substantially autonomous based on the belief of the need to execute a divine command. On the other hand, if the patient were a child who was not yet autonomous, there would be no direct conflict between autonomy and doing good. If there were any conflict at all, it would be between the welfare of the child and the autonomy of the parents. In such cases the autonomy of the parents is generally not taken to be decisive; the transfusion might be ordered by a court. This action would protect the child until he or she could express autonomous choice. Many people believe that autonomy can be overridden only to protect the interests of those who are not substantially autonomous or to protect the legitimate interests of others.[10]

Nonmaleficence

The principle of nonmaleficence holds that an action is wrong insofar as it inflicts harm on others. This principle is commonly thought to be a cornerstone of the Hippocratic Oath, appearing as an admonition to "above all, do no harm." However, the Hippocratic Oath itself, though stating that the physician should benefit the sick and protect them from harm, does not give supremacy to nonmaleficence.[11]

The exact meaning of "harm" and the relative position of nonmaleficence in relation to other principles are the subjects of some controversy. Harm, for example, has referred to matters ranging from emotional distress, property damage, and the loss of liberty to pain, disability, and death. The exact meaning often depends on the context of one's interest.

The principle of nonmaleficence encompasses several rules of conduct such as those elaborated by Gert.[12] They include not causing pain, disabling, stealing, committing adultery, or depriving others of pleasure. In many cases lying and the deprivation of freedom of action and opportunity may be perceived as harms as well. In other cases they might still be thought to be wrong because they violate the principle of autonomy or veracity even if they do not harm.

Almost all of these rules are relevant to the practice of dentistry, some more clearly than others. Issues of nonmaleficence abound in dentistry, as in all professions. A general dentist with limited surgical skills considers performing a biopsy herself rather than referring the patient to an oral surgeon. An oral surgeon wonders about referring a patient with a small (probable) squamous cell carcinoma of the skin to a plastic surgeon or doing the biopsy himself. A dentist is instructed by a patient to remove all remaining teeth and construct dentures, but the dentist sees better possibilities. All these examples involve issues of concern for harming the patient in one way or another.

Discussions of nonmaleficence become linked with issues of beneficence, which is the principle of enhancing welfare.[2–4] Some philosophers separate the two principles, considering them to be sufficiently different to warrant separate treatment. Others consider the two principles to be inextricably bound together under the heading of beneficence. In the interest of maintaining clear discussion, they are considered separately in this book.

Beneficence

Beneficence is the principle that actions are moral insofar as they produce benefits or enhance welfare.[2] Together with nonmaleficence, it is one of the two principles concerned with making the consequences of actions as good as possible. They can be called the "consequence-maximizing" principles. Some people view these as simply two sides of the same principle; they view harms as nothing more than the negative of benefits. They may combine the two by subtracting the amount of expected harm from an action from the expected benefits or by setting up a hierarchy. Other people keep the two consequence-oriented principles separate.

William Frankena[13] is an example of a philosopher who views nonmaleficence as a subdivision of beneficence. He believes that the rules of beneficence require that one:

1. Ought not to inflict evil or harm
2. Ought to prevent evil or harm
3. Ought to remove evil
4. Ought to do or promote good

This presentation of beneficence leads off with what other philosophers would call nonmaleficence: the avoidance of inflicting harm. In any case, it is clear that the rules are part of a continuum relating to the welfare of others. Some philosophers argue that the rules are listed in a hierarchy: the higher the place on the list, the more stringent the obligation.

In medical and dental contexts, harm refers to the pain, suffering, and disability of injury and disease. If one followed the priority of Frankena's list in treating dental caries, the greatest obligation would be to avoid inflicting harm. For example, there could be no justification for doing a restoration when a tooth is caries free. It would leave the person worse off.

Using Frankena's ranking, the next most important obligation would be to prevent harm, such as by preventing new caries lesions. This suggests the moral priority of an effective preventive program in the office. Under this hierarchy, prevention ranks higher than the elimination of harm, the third of Frankena's considerations. Therapeutic interventions such as the removal of harmful caries lesions and the placement of restorations fall here.

Last comes the promotion of good. An example would be the use of cosmetic bondings that improve upon a basically normal and acceptable situation in a patient who desires cosmetic interventions.

The debate over these obligations involving harms and benefits is far from over. An absolute priority of avoiding harm would lead to an absurdity. No dentist could ever cause pain in his or her patient even to do great good. That would mean the use of no handpiece and no local anesthetic—even though they would prevent much greater harm.

Because of these doubts, there is good reason to reject a hierarchy of obligations related to beneficence. Even those who are advocates of a hierarchy of obligation concede that in many strict interpretations, nonmaleficence cannot supersede beneficence in any absolute way. The discomfort of local anesthesia injection is necessary to avoid the much larger pain of extraction, and the harm of the removal of alveolar bone is necessary to gain access to an impacted third molar and get the benefit of the removal of a dentigerous cyst.

Beneficence is interwoven with nonmaleficence in a continuum that extends from doing no harm to the prevention and removal of harm and the doing of good.

Despite the relation between the concepts of not doing harm and doing good, there is an important difference in the nature of the action required. In most instances nonmaleficence requires only restraint from harmful acts. An example is the restraint from recommending esthetic bonding when it is obvious that the patient does not believe there is an esthetic problem.[14] Beneficence, on the other hand, requires positive action that places certain demands on the time or other resources of the individual.

The nature of the beneficence-based obligation that people have to one another in general society is controversial. Some philosophers argue that although we are strictly required to avoid doing harm, we have no special requirement to promote the interests of others. Others believe that if we are in a situation where our acts can provide good for others, then, assuming certain conditions are met, it is our obligation to act beneficently.

A pure utilitarian theory includes only the principles of beneficence and nonmaleficence. One of the criticisms against utilitarianism is that it seems to elevate doing all of the good that one can possibly do to a strict moral duty when we normally would consider there to be some limit on what is morally required of us. Pursuing every possible increment of good is normally thought to be beyond the call of strict moral duty.

By contrast, most ethical theories consider beneficence an obligation that is prima facie. It may be overridden by other, more compelling considerations. In fact, some approaches to the problem of conflict among ethical principles so radically subordinate beneficence that it would never be justified to violate someone's autonomy simply to do him or her good or to violate the principle of veracity simply because of the good it would do.

This view of beneficence describes the circumstances in which all of the helping professions find themselves. In medicine and dentistry, beneficence has traditionally been considered the cornerstone on which the profession functions.[15] Its central role is generally affirmed by professional codes of ethics from the Hippocratic Oath to the American Dental Association's Principles of Ethics and Code of Professional Conduct. This can lead to the overriding of an autonomous person's decisions in order to make that person better off.

Paternalism

The overriding of the substantially autonomous patient's wishes for the purposes of benefiting the patient is called *paternalism*. This practice follows the pattern of how parents treat children. Paternalistic acts are done in the name of beneficence and are well intentioned. Sometimes the health care provider may not even be aware that this behavior can create an ethical conflict because it violates the principle of autonomy. An example is seen with a patient who has a congenitally missing second premolar that, in this case, could be treated either with a fixed partial denture or by orthodontic space closure. The patient asks if the space could be closed orthodontically without compromising the occlusion and function. The dentist, however, is so convinced that managing these problems with fixed partial denture techniques is better for the patient that he dismisses the orthodontic option and persuades the patient to go with the three-unit fixed partial denture.

Balancing Benefits Against Harms

Whether one views beneficence and nonmaleficence as two separate principles or as two aspects of the same principle, a dentist will often be in the position of engaging in actions that include benefiting and causing harm. This situation occurs when, in the process of providing benefit, it is necessary to inflict harms to a greater or lesser degree. This frequently occurs with silent understanding of both the patient and the dentist, as with the injection of local anesthetic to avoid the larger pain of cavity preparation. This requires a method of balancing benefits against harms. Sometimes the balancing process is more difficult, as when mandibular resection is being considered in the presence of a malignant ameloblastoma.

The balancing process requires that the patient's values and viewpoints be taken into consideration because they influence the nature and amount of the good produced. Problems sometimes arise from variations in patient values or conflicts with the values of dentists. One patient may define "good" as having all teeth caries free forever. Another may view "good" as having all carious teeth promptly restored. Those two different interpretations of "good" require quite different approaches on the part of the dentist. The first patient requires as good a preventive program as the dentist can offer. The second patient apparently values primary prevention less and is more concerned about the early diagnosis and treatment of new caries lesions. This type of situation will be discussed in later chapters, including the issue of whether the dentist has the right or responsibility to try to change patients' values through education.

Several different strategies for combining benefits and harms have been proposed. The most common is to mentally assign quantities to the amount of good and the amount of harm and then subtract the amount of harm from the amount of good to arrive at a net good. This approach is sometimes called "arithmetic combining" because it involves adding and subtracting.

Using another strategy called "geometric combining," the decision-maker estimates the amount of benefit and harm, calculates the benefit/harm ratio, and chooses the course that has the best ratio.

An alternative to the arithmetic and geometric forms of combining benefits and harms would be to give an absolute priority to nonmaleficence. Sometimes the moral slogan *primum non nocere*, which is usually translated as "first of all, do no harm," is understood to be a moral injunction to first make sure no harm is done to the patient before attempting to do good. Taken to its extreme, this would, as we have seen, prohibit any dental interventions that cause any harm, even if the harm is necessary to do great good for the patient.

Problems in Relating Benefits and Harms

At least three different types of ethical problems in health care are related to beneficence and nonmaleficence.[3] The first (and the most frequent in dentistry) includes conflicts experienced by professionals as they consider balancing good against harm for the same patient. This is seen in questions about prescribing drugs to patients suspected of being drug abusers, in the management of possible child abuse, and in deciding whether painful, risky oral surgery procedures are worthwhile.

Another problem includes conflicts between patients and professionals over what constitutes a good treatment result. An example is a request from a patient for a cosmetic mandibular osteotomy when the oral surgeon visualizes the benefits as being minimal.

The third problem arises when the involvement of a third party possibly changes the nature of the professional's beneficence. The third party may be the one responsible for a person with Alzheimer disease, an insurance carrier, or both.

Justice

The principle of justice has to do with three closely related ideas: *(1)* treating people fairly, *(2)* giving people what they deserve, and *(3)* giving people that to which they are entitled. These ideas are not only different, they may lead to conflict. Consider the problems if you were responsible for the just allocation of dental care in our society and had to do so knowing that the resources were inadequate. The implications of those three ideas would have to be deliberated.

One way of treating people fairly would be to give everyone an equal chance for access to the dental health care system, as with flipping a coin. Although this approach might be considered fair in the sense that everyone's chance would be equal, it could be criticized as unfair because it fails to consider other characteristics of people, such as their needs, interests in dental health, and willingness and ability to pay for dental services.

If you decided to allocate dental care on the basis of what people deserved, you would have to figure out which characteristics of people qualify them to more dental care and which ones qualify them to less. Do people deserve more dental care because they need more, because they want it, because they are employed (or unemployed), because they can afford it, or because of other characteristics?

Issues of fairness and giving people what they are due are primary concerns of justice. The issue of entitlement is also frequently brought up. On the broadest scale is the debate about whether everyone is entitled to a minimum level of health care, including dental services. In our dilemma over the allocation of scarce dental resources, it might be possible to serve everyone only if services were restricted to the elimination of pain and infection and the minimal restoration of function (provided that one could successfully define *minimum*).

Alternatively, one could take the view that dental health care is not an absolute entitlement, but that some groups of people deserve entitled access to the system based on inadequate opportunity to otherwise receive the care. In that instance decisions would have to be made about the more entitled groups. Should they include the poorer people with the greatest dental problems? The handicapped? Decisions would then have to be made about how to handle the larger group now receiving dental services, those who want the services and who are also able to afford them.

This discussion shows the major role that justice has in discussions of public policy. The principles of beneficence, nonmaleficence, and respect for autonomy also play a role in these discussions. How these principles relate to the principle of justice will depend on one's strategy for resolving conflict among principles. One approach would be to balance these competing claims. Another would be to attempt to order the principles in some fashion. As mentioned earlier, one approach is to balance autonomy and justice but to rank these jointly over beneficence and nonmaleficence.[4]

Similarly, justice, though particularly relevant in public policy discussions, also plays an important role in decisions that must be made in the dental practitioner's office. Is a patient who is not in your practice entitled to emergency care (especially in the middle of the night)? Should compromise treatment be instituted when full fees cannot be afforded? Should you accept a request to provide limited free services to a nursing home just when your practice is getting busy? How should you treat an adolescent with a disfiguring amelogenesis imperfecta who is on medical assistance that does not cover esthetic treatment? How should a dentist respond to the simultaneous needs of several patients, especially when the worse-off patients cannot be helped as much as the better-off ones?

Justice is also at issue in dental offices in more subtle ways. Consider the dentist who enjoys the challenges and the rewards of fixed partial denture therapy. He reaches a point in his practice where he is able to maximize his patient contact with those patients requiring multiple-unit fixed partial dentures. The periodontal needs of his patients are almost exclusively left to the care provided by his hygienist. This allocation of his personal resources presupposes a concept of personal justice that allows the setting aside of his obligations to the periodontal needs of his patients and the devotion of most of his time to extensive fixed partial denture work.

Distributive Justice

The term *distributive justice* is used in managing the issues of societal distribution of benefits and burdens. It pertains to a just allocation of many different aspects of life that include voting rights, salaries, taxes, minorities' rights, women's rights, health care, military service, garbage collection, and education. Distributive justice tries to link interests, ambitions, and capabilities with moral views about how society should distribute its benefits and obligations. Discussions of justice related to voting rights and garbage collection in the United States are largely resolved. However, with issues like health care where scarce resources are major factors, debates about distributive justice are very pertinent.

It is important to realize that although distributive justice helps define choices and make proposals for the distribution of benefits and risks, it does not necessarily fully answer questions about which groups should get the benefits and which should assume the burdens.

The Formal Principle of Justice

A basic idea underlying the principle of justice is the *formal principle of justice,* which is said to have originated with Aristotle. It states that "equals must be treated equally, and unequals must be treated unequally."[16] As a good starting place for discussion, there is common agreement about this principle, largely because the principle is so vague. It gives no guidance whatsoever about who is equal and who is unequal. It also does not tell us on what basis unequals should be treated unequally.

Consider the formal principle of justice in relation to the question of who gets dental care under funds provided by an organization such as the Veterans' Health Administration. Not all veterans are equal from the standpoint of characteristics relative to dental care. Some are young, and some are old. Some are healthy, and some are sick and hospitalized. Some have toothaches, and some do not. Under the formal principle of justice we should agree on such points as: *(1)* all similarly situated sick and hospitalized veterans (equals) should be treated the same and *(2)* veterans with missing teeth and veterans with intact dentitions (unequals) should be treated differently because their needs are different. However, the formal theory of justice does not provide any framework for thinking about which of those characteristics deserves the most consideration in the allocation of resources.

Moving beyond this formal principle of justice requires additional work. If justice is like respect for autonomy, beneficence, and the other principles, presumably it conveys a special prima facie, morally right-making consideration that will feed into final judgment about one's duty proper. Exactly how it fits in will depend on how one balances or ranks the principles that we are considering as well as how one interprets the principle itself.

At this point it is important to determine what might be the specific element of the decision that we call justice. Keeping in mind that considerations of autonomy and of doing good are already accounted for by other principles, we might begin by examining a standard list of possible substantive elements that would make a distribution just.

Rescher[17] presents the following alternatives, which are pertinent for distributive justice:

1. To each person an equal share
2. To each person according to need
3. To each person according to effort
4. To each person according to contribution
5. To each person according to merit
6. To each person according to free-market exchange

Some of these, however, are already taken into account under the rubrics of autonomy and beneficence. Presumably, the reason why Rescher suggests "contribution" as a criterion has to do with beneficence. Such a distribution would maximize the good done by rewarding those who contribute most. Likewise, rewarding merit (as distinct from effort) also seems based on consideration of maximizing the good. The reason we might consider free-market exchange seems to have something to do with respecting autonomy. Effort, need, and the notion of equal share, however, do not seem to be linked either to beneficence or to autonomy. They come much closer to what we mean by justice in the sense that there is some moral consideration other than respect for autonomy or production of aggregate good that is morally relevant to the distribution of goods.

However, these all may be elements of a single concept of justice. The distribution of dental care in equal shares or according to need both seem closely linked to our concept of justice. In fact, these may simply be two ways of saying the same thing. Surely, one central element in a principle of justice (elements not already captured by the principles of beneficence and autonomy) is the distribution of resources based on need.

That leaves consideration of effort. We incorporate effort into our concept of justice, and we seem to believe that those who voluntarily try harder deserve more than those who do not. These facts could lead some to advocate that with respect to dental care, the distribution of resources should be based on need provided that, in the case of substantially autonomous persons, those who have made no effort to retain dental health somehow have less of a claim. Put in more general terms, a prima facie principle of justice in health care requires that all people have a right to opportunities for equal dental health.

Figuring out what is an opportunity for dental health will be extremely controversial. Limits placed on the basis of failure to maintain dental health presumably would be unreasonable for persons who are not competent (such as children), for those whose dental problems are genetically determined, or for those who are now substantially autonomous but developed dental problems or dental habits before they became autonomous adults.

Three Theories of Distribution

It is often difficult to find a unifying theme that underlies policies of distribution in many institutions. We can get some sense of how justice relates to autonomy and beneficence when we consider different social positions on how resources should be distributed for the distribution to be ethical. To answer that question we need to consider the proper relation among the utility-maximizing principles (beneficence and nonmaleficence), autonomy, and justice. Three alternative answers to the question of what counts as an ethically right distribution dominate the contemporary discussion. The *utilitarian* has as its goal the maximizing of the aggregate net good for the society; the *libertarian*, the objective of respecting freedom; the *egalitarian*, the objective of giving people equal opportunities to have needs met.

Health care policies in the Western world reflect some elements of all three theories of distribution. We want the best health care possible for all based on need, but at the same time we sense we are spending too much money on it and advocate cost-containment policies. We endorse the principle of equal access to health care but continue to support a competitive free-market atmosphere.

Utilitarian Distribution

The *utilitarian* theory of distribution, basing allocation on utility, incorporates the principles of beneficence and nonmaleficence. Some proponents of utility believe that distribution based on need will emerge as the pre-eminent obligation because meeting great needs often produces greater good per unit of resources. Critics say this theory ignores personal needs and the concerns of minorities. Key phrases used by utilitarians are "magnitude of risks," "amount of public benefit," and "risks of failure."[5]

Libertarian Distribution

Libertarians believe that economic benefits, including health care, should be allocated on the basis of respecting autonomy. They believe that right distribution is attained when health care is determined by free-market exchange.

Under the libertarian standard, need is not a factor. This does not mean that libertarians would not take steps to provide health care for those who need it. However, their actions would be on the basis of freely given charity rather than on the principle of justice.

At present, and in the recent past, the libertarian theory of distribution has partially determined the health care policy of the United States. US policy is not exclusively libertarian, however, as can be seen by the existence of federal, state, and local programs designed to provide health care services to needy groups of people.

Egalitarian Distribution

The *egalitarian* theory of distribution holds that an independent principle of justice is morally determinative. This theory is based on the observation that many features of our lives are determined largely by accidents of birth and circumstances. One can grow up wealthy or poor, with a cleft palate or with perfect features, with a tendency for chronic disease or with a good constitution. To the extent that any of these are true they are undeserved—either good or bad. If such features of people's lives are undeserved, then those committed to an egalitarian principle of justice hold that society should take steps to make people more equal.[18]

Extreme egalitarians call for the distribution of all goods and services so as to produce opportunities for equality. However, most egalitarians are more moderate and put limits on the nature and extent of benefits under discussion. Debate inspired by moderate egalitarian views has led to proposals for a two-tiered health care system. The first tier is the provision of adequate, but not complete, health services to everyone. Equal access is a primary feature with allocation of services made on the basis of need. The second tier is the purchasing of additional services (more expensive and perhaps optional) by those who can afford them and want them.[19] The first tier would be based primarily on the principle of justice; the second tier would be based primarily on autonomy.

Other Ethical Principles

These four principles—autonomy, nonmaleficence, beneficence, and justice—together have received predominant attention in contemporary health care ethics. Other principles, however, are included in many medical ethical theories and may prove decisive in some of the cases we consider in this book.

Veracity

One characteristic of actions, rules, and practices that tends to make them judged right is that they involve telling the truth and not lying. The Hippocratic tradition judges truth-telling to patients based on considerations of utility—whether the truth would help or hurt the patient—but since 1980 the American Medical Association has been committed to dealing honestly with patients without regard to whether honesty also produces benefit and avoids harm.[20]

Some people believe that the core underlying ethical principle that supports veracity is really the Kantian principle of respect for persons. According to this principle, people are to be treated as ends and not as means. They deserve respect that is incompatible with dealing with them dishonestly. That same respect for persons also may underlie the moral principle of autonomy, as well as the next two principles we shall consider: fidelity and avoidance of killing. As a practical matter it probably makes no difference whether we speak of one overarching principle of respect for persons that has four separate elements (autonomy, veracity, fidelity, and avoidance of killing) or whether we speak of four separate principles, each of which is prima facie morally relevant.

Fidelity

Another aspect sometimes subsumed under the rubric of respect for persons is fidelity. This is the belief that it is morally right to keep promises and other commitments, both implied and explicit. Fidelity may be the source of duties of health professionals to their patients (even when abandoning them would do more good on balance). Fidelity is believed by some to be the foundation of the duty of confidentiality. According to them, health professionals make a promise to patients to keep certain information confidential. Breaking confidence is really breaking faith. Of course, much will hinge on exactly what is promised, a question we shall take up in the cases in chapter 7.

Avoidance of Killing

A crucial principle for biomedical ethics has historically been that it is wrong to kill. Sometimes this is put in terms of the sacredness of life; other times a sharp distinction has been drawn between active killing and forgoing treatment, with only active killing being proscribed by the principle of avoidance of killing. According to this view, it is not intrinsically wrong to forgo treatment (although for most patients, forgoing may violate the principle of beneficence). Some ethical theories base the prohibition on killing on the principle of nonmaleficence. They claim that what is wrong with killing people is that it sets back their interests. The important implication is that, in special medical cases where people would actually prefer to be killed, it would be morally acceptable to kill them. By contrast, if killing is independently morally wrong, then even mercy killing is deemed unethical. Even though killing is a major concern in medical ethics, it is not normally an issue in the practice of dentistry. We therefore will not devote further attention to this principle.

Gratitude

Other principles sometimes surface in ethical theories that also include lists of principles. Philosopher W. D. Ross[21] held that gratitude was such a principle. It was a way of showing respect for people who previously helped you. You have a duty, he believed, to repay such help even over and above any good that will come to you or the other party.

Reparation

Finally, Ross also held that if one is responsible for injury to another, there is a duty of reparation to make amends.[21] Again, he held this true regardless of the calculation of the good or harm that making reparation would do.

This list of principles—the consequence-maximizing principles of beneficence and nonmaleficence plus the principles that identify right-making characteristics of actions other than producing good consequences—constitute the basis for systematic reflection on ethical choices that a dentist must make. In the chapters in the second and third parts of this book we look at the implications of these principles for dentists who are confronted with difficult moral dilemmas. Before doing so, however, we need to develop a format for systematic review of case problems.

References

1. Childress JF. The normative principles of medical ethics. In: Veatch RM (ed). Medical Ethics, ed 2. Boston: Jones & Harcourt, 1997:27–48.
2. National Commission for the Protection of Human Subjects of Biomedical and Behavioral Research. The Belmont Report: Ethical Principles and Guidelines for the Protection of Human Subjects of Research. Washington, DC: US Government Printing Office, 1978.
3. Beauchamp TL, Childress JE. Principles of Biomedical Ethics, ed 5. New York: Oxford University, 2001.
4. Veatch RM. A Theory of Medical Ethics. New York: Basic Books, 1981.
5. Gillon R. Philosophical Medical Ethics. New York: John Wiley & Sons, 1986.
6. Faden R, Beauchamp TL, King NNP. A History and Theory of Informed Consent. New York: Oxford University, 1986.
7. Childress JF. Paternalism in Health Care. New York: Oxford University, 1982.
8. Engelhardt HT. The Foundations of Bioethics, ed 2. New York: Oxford University, 1996.

9. Brody B. Life and Death Decision Making. New York: Oxford University, 1988.

10. Dworkin G. Moral autonomy. In: Engelhardt HT, Callahan D (eds). Morals, Science, and Sociality. Hastings-on-Hudson, NY: Hastings Center, 1978:156–171.

11. Edelstein L. The Hippocratic Oath: Text, translation and interpretation. In: Temkin O, Temkin CL (eds). Ancient Medicine: Selected Papers of Ludwig Edelstein. Baltimore: Johns Hopkins University, 1967:6.

12. Gert B. Morality: A New Justification of the Moral Rules. New York: Oxford University, 1988.

13. Frankena WK. Ethics, ed 2. Englewood Cliffs, NJ: Prentice Hall, 1963.

14. Gilbert JA. Ethics and aesthetics. J Am Dent Assoc 1988;117:490.

15. Pellegrino ED, Thomasma DC. For the Patient's Good. New York: Oxford University, 1988.

16. Aristotle. Nicomachean Ethics, Book III. Ostwald M (trans). Indianapolis: Bobbs-Merrill, 1962: 118–120.

17. Rescher N. Distributive Justice. Indianapolis: Bobbs-Merrill, 1966.

18. Rawls J. A Theory of Justice. Cambridge, MA: Harvard University, 1971.

19. Fried C. Equality and rights in medical care. Hastings Cent Rep 1976;6:29–34.

20. American Medical Association. Code of Medical Ethics. Chicago: American Medical Association, 2001.

21. Ross WD. The Right and the Good. Oxford, England: Oxford University, 1939.

chapter 5

Format for Resolving Ethical Questions

In this chapter

- Protocol for Ethical Decision Making
- Analysis of the Case of the Suspicious Dentist
- Our View

Case

- The Case of the Suspicious Dentist

Case 2: The Case of the Suspicious Dentist

Dr Alex David has a general practice in a midwestern city. Most of his patients are middle-class business and professional people. Late one afternoon, Mr William Worthy entered Dr David's waiting room, unannounced, as a referral from the chiropractor next door. He said that he had been in an automobile accident the day before that resulted in back and dental injuries. He wanted a dental examination for his insurance company and then, presumably, he would follow up with treatment.

Superimposed on this entirely straightforward story were the disturbing appearance and behavior of Mr Worthy and the two thuglike men who accompanied him. Dr David thought all three of them looked like trouble. Mr Worthy in particular was irritable, agitated, and threatening, and he wanted medication, specifically Valium. While Dr David was interviewing Mr Worthy, his friends left the waiting room and entered the treatment area. They wandered through the hall, entering several operatories. Their unauthorized entry and their suspicious demeanor alarmed the office staff and Dr David. After two or three requests, Mr Worthy's friends re-entered the waiting room.

At his first opportunity, Dr David called the chiropractor, who confirmed the basic story. The chiropractor said that he, too, had been concerned when the trio had entered his office. He therefore had called the hospital where Mr Worthy was treated following the accident, but everything checked out.

When Dr David found time to examine Mr Worthy, the patient's anxiety and tense oral musculature made the examination difficult. Mr Worthy jumped at every touch. He said he had a lot of pain in his teeth but could not be specific as to location. He again stated his need for Valium to help him relax, and Dr David reluctantly saw his point.

The examination itself was inconclusive. Several cusps were fractured. Electric pulp testing and thermal tests were ambiguous, and it was hard to interpret percussion. Other pathoses (caries and periodontal disease) existed that were not related to the trauma. Radiographs did not help either. Altogether, the picture was confusing. Dr David thought the pain could be from the fractured cusps, but the amount of pain did not coincide with the clinical picture. On the other hand, he knew that the full consequences of trauma are often not seen until much later.

Dr David decided to prescribe a small amount of Valium to cover the next 5 days, and he agreed to see Mr Worthy again at that time. Dr David was concerned about drug dependency, but Mr Worthy denied regular use of Valium or any other drug. Dr David's hope was that the pain response was primarily due to anxiety and would be substantially modified by the Valium and by time. His plan for the next visit was to seal the exposed dentin on the fractured cusps to confirm the source of the pain. If that did not help, referral to an endodontist was the next step. Long-range management of the fractures would involve restorative procedures and root planing to start to control the periodontal disease.

The plan was acceptable to Mr Worthy, and he agreed to return in 5 days. Two days later, Mr Worthy called Dr David to say he was in real pain and demanded more Valium. Dr David considered what to do. He really did not have time in his schedule to see Mr Worthy that day, but he also did not want to prescribe more Valium. What he really wanted was to not accept Mr Worthy into his practice because of his suspicious and fear-provoking demeanor. However, large parts of the story seemed legitimate. Dr David admitted that if Mr Worthy had shown up in a three-piece suit and alone, instead of in dirty chinos and a leather jacket and with his disreputable friends, he would have a much different outlook on this case.

DISCUSSION:

In addition to the judgments about the benefits and harms of various examination and treatment options, there are at least two aspects of this case in which the decisions do not depend entirely on clinical or scientific facts. First, there is a conflict between genuine concern for personal safety on the one hand and an obligation to help the patient on the other. There is also a question as to the advisability of giving Valium to someone who might be dependent on the drug. These are problems that have ethical implications and require ethical reasoning for their resolution.

In approaching the analysis of ethical issues, we suggest that better ethical decisions will occur if an established method of analysis is used. An orderly approach to decision making will allow us to take into consideration variations and conflicting views that may exist among personal values, conscience, religious convictions, professional codes of ethics, legal constraints, and the viewpoints of patients. A five-step approach to ethical decision making in dentistry is presented in the following section.

Protocol for Ethical Decision Making

In considering any dilemma, first make sure that the resolution of the issues actually depends on ethical considerations. Sometimes what appears to be an ethical dispute really hinges on disagreements or misunderstandings of the facts of the case. Determine that there is clarity and agreement on all of the relevant facts. Once that is accomplished, follow these four steps.[1,2]

Step 1: Determine the Alternatives

List the possible alternatives. Keep in mind the possible consequences to the patient, yourself, and others. This will be dealt with further in step 4. Include all aspects of the circumstances in your considerations, including dental, medical, social, and psychological. At this stage include all options that are possibilities, even those that seem immoral, as long as they could be plausible to the patient or to some health professional. There will always be some options that are beyond reason for everyone considering the alternatives. Eliminating these from consideration already involves a moral judgment. To keep such judgments to a minimum, at this point include all options that any relevant decision-maker considers plausible.

Step 2: Determine the Ethical Considerations

Consider the ethical implications of each alternative. Identify the ethical principles involved and determine the role of beneficence, nonmaleficence, respect for autonomy, justice, and other principles. Once you have determined the role of beneficence and nonmaleficence, estimate which produces the greatest balance of good over harm.

Step 3: Determine the Considered Judgments of Others

After you have begun to apply the principles to the alternatives, as a guide to your deliberations and a check against your own judgment, consider what your professional group believes to be ethical in this situation. Its view may or may not be morally correct, but this at least tells you what your colleagues have concluded in similar situations. You may also wish to consider the statements of codes of dental ethics from other countries or the codes of other health professions on similar topics as well as the views of other organizations—religious, civic, political, or social—that might have ethical views relevant to the question at hand.

If as part of becoming a professional or a member of these other groups you have made certain morally binding commitments, keep in mind that those commitments must be evaluated in the context of the principle of fidelity and in its implication that it is right-making to keep such commitments. Thus the promises that you have made in the process of assuming certain roles may be relevant to deciding what ethically ought to be done.

Step 4: Rank the Alternatives

Sometimes the process of working through the last two steps will establish that one of your alternatives satisfies the ethical requirements of the case better than all of the others. Often, however, your analysis will show that various principles, rules, or values (and the courses of action that follow from them) are in conflict. In these situations additional analysis is sometimes required. One approach is to determine your general position regarding conflict among principles and to apply it to the specific case. For example, some people attempt to rank certain principles as having priority over others. Other people simply consider all principles equally weighty and attempt to make an intuitive judgment about how to resolve conflict. Still others prefer to reason by analogy from cases for which moral judgments are clear. On the basis of such analysis, select the course of action that best resolves the conflicts.

Analysis of the Case of the Suspicious Dentist

Before we proceed with the ethical analysis of the case, we should first make sure that we are clear on the relevant facts of the case. Sometimes merely clarifying the facts will reveal that an apparent ethical conflict was really a dispute over the facts. In other cases, such as this one, real ethical disagreement about what ought to be done probably remains even if we agree on the factual matters.

This case was a problem for Dr David because he felt threatened by Mr Worthy and his friends. He felt they were "casing" the premises, and he had an understandable concern about what any one of them might do. Thus, there seems to be a real basis for Dr David's concern. He was also irritated by the patient's request for drugs. Over the last several years, requests for drugs by addicts have become a familiar problem, and this situation could be exemplary. On the other hand, there was no doubt that Mr Worthy had clinical problems related to his automobile accident.

One of the clinical problems was whether Mr Worthy's pain was clearly from irreversible pulpal pathosis. If so, then Dr David could solve his problems by referring Mr Worthy to an endodontist. Another problem was whether Mr Worthy's pain was severe enough to mandate his being seen right away. If so, then Dr David had to act accordingly.

In Mr Worthy's case, the answers to these questions are not readily apparent. However, in other situations a careful look at the facts of the case may provide answers based on factual rather than ethical considerations. For example, two dentists may agree that it would be wrong to prescribe aspirin with codeine for dental pain following an extraction for a former addict but perfectly reasonable to do so for a patient who has never been addicted. A dispute about the correctness of a prescription for aspirin with codeine may really be nothing more than a dispute over whether the patient was a former addict.

Determining the Alternatives

Once we are sure that we agree on the relevant facts of the case, our next step is to identify the alternatives. Dr David thought about the clinical ambiguities and considered several alternatives:

1. Refuse all further treatment and suggest that the patient find another general dentist
2. Refer the patient to an endodontist without further clinical contact. Give him some names and possibly help him to make an appointment
3. Prescribe Valium by phone and have the patient keep the original appointment
4. Refuse to prescribe Valium and rearrange the schedule to see the patient today

Identifying the Ethical Considerations

Beneficence and Nonmaleficence

In considering these choices in terms of the ethical considerations, several points can be made. First, some of the options do not directly benefit the patient. That is, they tend to violate the obligation of beneficence insofar as it requires benefit to the patient. The refusal of treatment in option 1 is an obvious example. Although the patient may follow the dentist's advice and seek care elsewhere, he does so at more inconvenience to himself than is necessary. He might also delay contacting another dentist, which could be detrimental to him in the long run.

On the other hand, when option 1 is assessed in the light of the full implications of the principle of beneficence (taking into account benefits to parties other than the patient), the dentist should consider whether he can do more good for others by not accepting the patient. If, for example, he was caring for another emergency case at the time, he might conclude that beneficence required not taking this patient, at least at the moment. He might even consider beneficence to those who are not his patients. He might, for instance, be concerned about using his time for some other good purpose. Or he might be concerned about protecting his staff from harm.

Autonomy and Other Ethical Principles

Another major principle to consider is the principle of autonomy. While autonomy is often relevant in recognizing the right of the patient not to enter a professional-patient relationship, it also can imply the right of the dentist to be autonomous. This would have to be assessed in light of any promises made as well as the claims of justice that the patient might have. Any other principles including fidelity and justice as well as truth-telling (veracity) that may have bearing on the case need to be considered.

Referring the patient to an endodontist (option 2) can certainly be expected to benefit the patient, because of the special skills possessed by endodontists in the diagnosis of dental pain. This is especially true if the dentist expedites matters by offering him aid in identifying a practitioner and helping him to make contact. On the other hand, if Dr David's original plan is sound, a referral may not prove to be necessary. Also, a referral will be more costly to the patient (or to the insurance company). If the referral to the endodontist at this time would be expected to further benefit the patient dentally, it would be more ethically acceptable. As it stands, Dr David's motives, should he refer now, are more along the lines of dumping the patient. The ethics of any such plan would have to take into account the implications of other principles, including veracity. It would, for example, be dishonest to deceive the endodontist about the nature of the patient being referred.

Option 3, to prescribe Valium by phone and have the patient keep the original appointment, is controversial on two counts. First, it assumes there is some good reason why the patient cannot be seen on the day of the call, when, in fact, the only reason may be the dentist's desire to avoid the patient. Second, if the dentist decides to prescribe Valium at this time, he deems the risks to be worth it. This belief cannot be based on clinical or scientific knowledge but rather is founded in a pre-established group of attitudes about drug addiction, its progress, and its treatment.

Decisions founded on such attitudes deserve ethical commentary. To not prescribe Valium could be said to be exercising nonmaleficence on the belief that, if Mr Worthy is an addict, additional Valium will add to his burden. On the other hand, prescribing Valium would have to be justified either by beneficence (on the belief that additional Valium will not be harmful even if Mr Worthy is an addict) or by autonomy (on the belief that Mr Worthy should have the right to be self-determining in the use of Valium). To select one course of action over the other is to endorse one set of beliefs and to reject the other.

All of these comments have been made with the interests of the patient in mind. A final ethical commentary from that standpoint pertains to option 4. This alternative, which combines the refusal of Valium with rearrangement of the schedule to see the patient the same day, might seem to maximize the potential benefits while minimizing the potential harms. On the other hand, the principle of fidelity implies that promises made to other patients in the form of appointments have at least a prima facie claim. Moreover, rearranging the schedule will have to come at the expense of harms to others—at least inconvenience, perhaps greater or more prolonged suffering, and possibly poorer-quality dentistry to other patients.

Considering the Views of Others

When the judgments of other groups are applied to this case, there seems to be no conflict between what the patient wants and the professional values regarding standards of care. Conflicts of that sort sometimes arise when a patient wants a tooth removed and the dentist, knowing the tooth can be saved, feels strongly about the value of maintaining the intact dentition; no such conflict exists here.

However a conflict may exist between the American Dental Association's (ADA's) Principles of Ethics and Code of Professional Conduct and any alternative that involves getting rid of the patient. Section 4.B of the Code states that: "[d]entists shall be obliged to make reasonable arrangements for the emergency care of their patients of record."[3] Essentially the same statement is made pertaining to patients not of record. Therefore, this section makes clear the ethical obligation to reasonably treat Mr Worthy. The definition of "reasonable" is left to one's own judgment.

Ranking the Alternatives

The ranking of the alternatives has been simplified by the previous discussion, at least insofar as the patient's interests are concerned. By refusing to prescribe Valium and arranging to see the patient today (option 4), the benefits are greatest and the potential harms are least, both for short-term and long-term considerations. Although referring the patient to an endodontist seems reasonable, it might be unnecessary, add to the expense, and lessen the probability of the patient having all of his dental needs addressed.

Option 3, besides having the risks of prescribing Valium, also has the disadvantage of delaying the patient's treatment for several days, which potentially could be harmful. Therefore, it could possibly be eliminated from consideration, depending on one's views about the risks of doing harm should the patient already be addicted.

Option 1, the refusal of all further treatment, is eliminated on the basis of conflict with beneficence to the patient. On the other hand, Dr David might believe that the refusal of treatment would eliminate, or at least lessen, the risks to his person and property by the presence of this troublesome patient. Dr David had major concerns about Mr Worthy's potential for trouble, and he could feel that his obligations to himself, his family, his staff, and his other patients outweigh his obligations to this patient. Dr David has to make the decision, considering all principles on a prima facie basis, as to which of the obligations is more compelling.

Our View

We conclude that option 4 is the most plausible even though it could put the dentist at some risk. Evidence of a substantial risk, however, is not so compelling that option 1's refusal of further treatment is warranted. The facts of Mr Worthy's accident were authenticated both by the chiropractor and the local hospital. In addition, the patient's behavior, even his request for Valium, were judged by Dr David, however reluctantly, to be at least plausible under the circumstances.

Parenthetically, we should say that we don't like option 1 for another reason: We think that telling the patient to find another dentist on his own does not qualify as making "reasonable arrangements," which is required by the ADA Code whether or not Mr Worthy qualified as a patient of record. We make the argument that because Dr David had already seen the patient and developed a plan for treating the emergency problem, Mr Worthy was already a patient of record. In this instance it doesn't matter; "reasonable arrangements" are required for emergencies, patient of record or not. It would be reasonable to provide the patient with the name and number of a hospital dental service, and perhaps even more helpful to provide a direct referral to another general dentist—as unlikely as that is in this situation. But offering no help at all does not qualify as reasonable.

Option 2 would be justified only if there were a sound clinical basis for referral to an endodontist: Patient benefit would require the referral. Otherwise, such a referral would violate the requirements not only of patient benefit but of veracity as well. In this case, however, Dr David had already decided for himself that referral to an endodontist was premature at that point.

But suppose that Dr. David genuinely believes that treating Mr Worthy further would seriously jeopardize his staff or even other patients? If that is his fear, then he has no choice but to refuse further treatment, unless he wants to arrange for additional security during further visits, which seems unlikely. After all, he has no obligation to treat a patient who might well put him, his staff, and his patients at risk of harm. If he makes that choice, however, it seems essential to us that he take an active role in helping Mr Worthy make an appointment with a suitable practitioner or hospital service—preferably the latter, since to which esteemed colleague will he refer this risky patient? Furthermore, if Mr Worthy happens to be an addict the hospital service would theoretically place him in an institution that could help him deal with that problem. In fact, we believe that if Dr David were to help connect Mr Worthy with a good hospital dental service, it would be quite an ethically acceptable option, even if the assumptions of risk to staff and others were less. However, we still prefer option 4 because we think that the relationship between private dentist and patient offers a better opportunity for continuity than does the hospital situation, where the prospects for follow-up care may be more difficult.

One final point pertains to the question of whether Dr David has the right to refuse to treat Mr Worthy if the latter was not his patient. That clearly would have been the situation if Dr David had not yet seen the patient. In addition, others might argue that one brief visit does not mean that Mr Worthy was Dr David's patient of record. If such was the case, then clearly, from the ADA Code's perspective, Dr David "may exercise reasonable discretion" in selecting patients for his practice. However, if he chooses to not accept Mr Worthy, he still has an obligation for beneficence and thus to at least make "reasonable arrangements" for Mr Worthy's care. This puts us back to Dr. David's actively helping his patient make an appointment at a hospital dental service. Anything less is unreasonable. Furthermore, if Dr. David knows that Mr Worthy will receive competent care, it eliminates the necessity to even consider the highly questionable act of prescribing Valium to someone who is a potential addict and not even a patient of record.

Conclusion

This case presents an example of an approach to making decisions about ethical problems. The analysis is given in its fullest form for purposes of illustration; obviously, not all cases require such lengthy analysis. In addition, a case presentation represents a static moment in time; some of the issues raised here might be solved easily by gathering further information. For example, a clearer picture of Mr Worthy might show him to be less or more of a problem, and his questionable status as a drug addict might be resolved. Also, Dr David had no information about Mr Worthy's previous dentist, if any, at the time of his dilemma. That piece of information might have been helpful in making a decision.

The case is unusual in that it contains a risk of personal harm for the dentist. Therefore, the major conflict was between that risk for the dentist and the principle of beneficence for the patient. This case was provided as an example of the need to make decisions when there are conflicting principles and concerns. Secondary issues also existed. One issue was the question of nonmaleficence for the possibly drug-addicted patient. Another was Dr David's possible obligations to his other patients. A third was dealing honestly with the endodontist to whom the patient was referred.

References

1. Ozar DT. Model for ethical decision making. Informal distribution through PEDNET, 1989.
2. McCullough L. Ethical issues in dentistry. In: Hardin JF (ed). Clark's Clinical Dentistry. Philadelphia: JB Lippincott, 1988:1–17.
3. American Dental Association, Council on Ethics, Bylaws and Judicial Affairs. Principles of Ethics and Code of Professional Conduct, with official advisory opinions revised to January 2004. Chicago: American Dental Association, 2004.

Part II
General Principles
in Dental Ethics

Doing Good and Avoiding Harm

In this chapter

Cases

Ethical problems in dentistry, like ethical problems in general, can sometimes be approached by looking at which general principles are at stake. Two of the most obvious are that actions tend to be right insofar as they produce good results and wrong insofar as they produce bad or harmful ones. Sometimes these two notions are referred to by their more technical names—the principles of beneficence and nonmaleficence, or the principles of doing good and not doing bad.

In some people's ethics these are the only principles that count, while in others' there are additional features that lead to calling an action morally right or wrong. In later chapters in Part II of this volume we look at some of these other principles, including the principles of autonomy, truth-telling, fidelity, and justice. These latter principles hold that independent of whether one's actions result in good or bad, they can be judged wrong morally if they involve lack of respect for the autonomy of others, telling of lies, breaking of promises, or unfair allocations of benefits and harms.

Even if one focuses only on questions of doing good and avoiding harm, however, matters of moral controversy can arise. The cases in this chapter were chosen because they pose questions about what is the morally right thing for a dentist to do based solely on judgments about doing good and avoiding harm.

Traditional ethics has held that the dentist should do what will benefit the patient and protect the patient from harm. This idea can be traced all the way back to the Hippocratic Oath, in which the health professional pledges to apply measures "for the benefit of the sick according to my ability and judgment. I will keep them from harm and injustice."[1]

In a similar vein, the American Dental Association's (ADA's) Principles of Ethics and Code of Professional Conduct holds that "professionals have a duty to act for the benefit of others. Under this principle, the dentist's primary obligation is service to the patient and the public-at-large. The most important aspect of this obligation is the competent and timely delivery of dental care within the bounds of clinical circumstances presented by the patient, with due consideration being given to the needs, desires, and values of the patient."[2] Included in virtually any professional ethic is the idea that doing good counts morally in favor of an intervention and doing harm counts against it.

This might seem so obvious that it is nothing more than a moral platitude. Still, there is room for dispute over how the doing of good and harm relates to morality in dental practices. First, it is controversial how benefits relate to harms. For instance, is it always acceptable to do harm to a patient provided it is accompanied by a greater amount of benefit? Second, there are controversies in deciding just what counts as a benefit in dentistry. The patient's view may be quite different from that of the dentist. Third, even if we know what counts as a dental good or harm, we may have ethical problems in relating these dental consequences to other (nondental) benefits and harms. A patient may purposely reject an offered dental benefit in order to invest time or money in something else he or she desires. Fourth, controversies sometimes arise over the moral duty of a dentist regarding benefits and harms for nonpatients, either former patients or those who have never been patients. Finally, there are many instances in which the interests of patients conflict with others who are not patients. This includes the interests of the dentist as well as the interests of the society in general. In this chapter we look at moral problems involved in relating benefits and harms, in the principles of beneficence and non-maleficence.

The Relation of Benefits and Harms

One classical problem in health professional ethics is how benefits relate to harms. While the Hippocratic tradition simply asks the health professional to do good for the patient and protect the patient from harm, other moral codes in health care give a special priority to avoiding harms. The slogan *primum non nocere* (first of all, do no harm) is one of the most widely used in health care ethics.[3,4] It is often interpreted to mean that avoiding harm has a special moral priority over doing good. The dentist, according to this view, should only strive to do good for the patient when he or she has first of all made sure no harm would come to the patient.

On the other hand, many individuals, drawing on the original form of the Hippocratic tradition, treat benefits and harms as being on a par. They see them as being equally weighty, so that the harms can simply be subtracted from the benefits when deciding which action does the most net good. They would consider the possible good from each course (taking into account both the amount and probability of good) and subtract the possible harm. A closely related way of reasoning about benefits and harms is to calculate the ratio of benefits to harms. This is often done formally in what is called a benefit-cost or benefit-harm analysis, but it is done intuitively by dentists constantly during the course of dental practice.

One major problem with this reasoning is that benefits and harms are often notoriously hard to quantify. We surely are not concerned only about monetary costs. We need to take into account pain and suffering, as well as the satisfaction of a well-functioning dentition, esthetic pleasure resulting from attractive teeth, and so forth. Surely, estimates of benefit and harm are only approximations, but such estimates are made constantly in all decisions in life, including complex decisions in health care.

The first problem we encounter is what we should do with these estimates of benefit and harms after we have made them. Do we simply subtract the harms from the benefits for each possible course of action, do we calculate the ratios, or do we strive first of all to make sure that as dentists we do not harm our patients while trying to help them?

Case 3: The Patient Scares the Dentist

Dr Joanne Heller, a pediatric dentist, had been treating Sylvia Maldin for several months, and the treatment was now finished. Sylvia was a 12-year-old girl with extensive dental caries who had been referred by a general practitioner because she had physically refused all treatment. Dr Heller had been able to work with her effectively, partly through conventional communication skills, which led to an increase in Sylvia's trust, and partly with some pharmacological help.

Dr Heller had been using combinations of Demerol and Atarax. Her strategy, over time, was to gradually reduce the dosage in a weaning process. She considered her experience with Sylvia to be a good one. She liked Sylvia, and she knew that she had helped Sylvia to overcome some significant problems in coping with dental care, which hopefully would carry her through a lifetime.

As Sylvia was getting ready to leave after her last visit, she thanked Dr Heller for what she had done, especially for showing her how helpful drugs could be in overcoming difficult situations. Sylvia thought, for example, that drugs could help reduce her anxiety in confronting new situations, meeting new people, or coping with the stress of taking examinations. She asked if Dr Heller could prescribe some more drugs for her that she could use in those situations.

Dr Heller tried to impress upon Sylvia that she could not legally or ethically do what Sylvia asked and that to do so could harm her. Sylvia expressed her disappointment and said that she regretted having trusted Dr Heller as a friend. But in the end, Sylvia said, it probably did not matter; she thought she could get what she needed in the schoolyard.

Dr Heller was shocked and appalled by Sylvia's comments. It had never entered her mind that she was in any way harming her patient. Now her certainty that Sylvia had benefited from the treatment wavered.

DISCUSSION:

When Dr Heller is deciding between possible treatment plans, she will list, at least mentally, the potential benefits and harms of alternative courses of action and the probabilities of their occurrence. A drawback to this method is that one must be sure to identify all of the possible benefits and harms. In this case Dr Heller did not anticipate the subtle but important risk that she could be teaching her patient to be a drug abuser.

The first question the case raises is whether Dr Heller was at fault for failing to anticipate this risk. Should she have been on the alert based on the fact that she knew Sylvia was an unusually difficult patient (so difficult that the general practitioner referred her to a specialist)? Of course, if she should not be expected to take into account the risk, it is hard to hold her at fault. What is the extent of the dentist's obligation to anticipate such risks?

At this point it is fair to say that most pediatric dentists would be reluctant to use sedation in the way that Dr Heller did. Sedation over multiple appointments is usually reserved for children in the 2- to 5-year-old bracket. Older children such as Sylvia, who are difficult to manage clinically, often represent more complex emotional problems that would best be handled under general anesthesia or intravenous or other forms of deep sedation, in which the goal is to complete all necessary treatment in as few visits as possible. Nevertheless, there are risks from general anesthesia and other forms of deep sedation. Depending on the evaluation of the alternative risks and benefits, Sylvia, her parents, and Dr Heller may be within reason in choosing the option that they did as long as the risk of future abuse was so remote that it was appropriately ignored.

Assuming that she did anticipate the risk and could attach some probability to it, another kind of ethical question arises. Should Dr Heller simply calculate the potential benefits and the potential harms and choose the course of action that is expected to produce the greatest possible net benefit, or is there some other way that she should reason them through?

In some interpretations of health care ethics, the practitioner takes as his or her motto, "First of all, do no harm." Avoiding harm done by one's own hand is morally considered the first priority. Even if as much or more good were done, according to this view, it would be wrong to do the harm. For example, in medicine it seems obviously wrong to kill one person even if in doing so we could obtain several organs for transplant that would save a number of lives. We do not simply calculate the number of lives saved and subtract the one life taken to conclude that the killing would be justified. Some people have argued that the reason it seems obviously wrong to kill one person to save many is that actively doing harm is morally worse than, or more significant than, doing good.

In this case, if Dr Heller should have anticipated the possibility that she would be encouraging her young patient to become a drug abuser, should that be seen as something the clinician should avoid at all costs, or should she try to calculate the amount of harm and compare that harm to the potential benefits of using the drugs?

In calculating the expected benefits and harms, we would normally estimate their seriousness and multiply by the probability (at least as a mental estimate). For Dr Heller one such calculation might be that the important benefit of Sylvia's long-term willingness to accept regular dental care could have a 70% chance for success. On the other hand, one might estimate that the extremely serious harm of encouraging drug abuse might be as much as 5%. Although the estimates are subjective, the process can be very helpful in focusing on the implications of harm.

If we give special priority to avoiding harm to patients, what should we make of the fact that virtually all dental interventions risk at least modest, short-term harm? Even modern dentistry hurts sometimes. Would an absolute priority for not harming the patient make even a needle stick immoral? After all, that needle is, for many patients, the most severe mental and physical pain that they experience in the dentist's chair. Surely, we do not want to give such high priority to avoiding active harm of the patient that the dentist is totally immobilized.

There is one other concern that needs to be addressed. What, if any, are Dr Heller's obligations to Sylvia and her parents once she recovers from the shock of Sylvia's departing comments? Is she required to take steps that might help circumvent Sylvia's inclination to use drugs? Should Sylvia's parents be called in for a conference, or should Dr Heller respect Sylvia's confidentiality? If Dr Heller does decide to call them in, should she tell Sylvia beforehand of her intentions? How should she describe what has happened, and what should she recommend the parents consider doing? How should she portray her own role in precipitating what happened? These questions also arise in chapter 7 when confidentiality is the topic.

Case 4: A Choice Between High-Risk Surgery and Continued Disfigurement

Mr Carl Bengstom, age 38, was referred to Dr Jose Gutierrez, an oral and maxillofacial surgeon at a large research-oriented hospital on the West Coast. Mr Bengstom suffered from polydermal myositis, a connective tissue disorder with severe systemic effects. Therapy for polydermal myositis is largely palliative and, for Mr Bengstom, had included prednisone for many years. More recently he also took methotrexate on a monthly basis. Of importance in this case was delayed healing, especially in his lower extremities. He had a tendency to get ulcers in this area, and they took an exceedingly long time to heal.

Mr Bengstom's life was very difficult, and he was miserable most of the time. One of his main problems was his appearance. His face was severely distorted because of the overgrowth of his maxilla. The distorted growth involved significant asymmetry and a very long maxilla from a vertical perspective, which resulted in an extremely large overbite. In addition, there was essentially no masticatory function; the only contact between his maxillary and mandibular teeth was a single point on one cusp of the maxillary and mandibular second molars.

Adding to Mr Bengstom's problems was the extensive destructive resorption of the condylar heads of the mandible as seen radiographically. There was only 1 mm of bone between the middle cranial fossa and what remained of the condyles. This finding increased the risk of any surgery in the condylar area. There were two broad choices for Mr Bengstom: have nothing done or undergo extensive maxillofacial reconstruction.

Dr Gutierrez thought about what he should tell Mr Bengstom about his options for treatment. Certainly one possibility was not to do any surgery at all. The risks of failure of the surgery were high, especially because of Mr Bengstom's healing difficulties. Furthermore, if postoperative infection were to occur, it could be life-threatening. The possibilities of relapse also had to be considered in view of the nature of the disease. Another problem was whether to insert prosthetic replacements for the diseased condyles. Two surgeons he consulted favored this approach. However, Dr Gutierrez decided that if he undertook the case he would not use prosthetic condyles because he thought it would be unwise to employ a foreign object in a patient with healing problems.

Despite these substantial risks, if surgery were done, there was also the possibility of a major improvement in appearance and function. Dr Gutierrez's approach would be to do a Le Fort I horizontal maxillary osteotomy, in which the maxilla is disconnected from the rest of the skull and separated into three pieces: an anterior wedge-shaped section and right and left posterior portions. He would then reduce the vertical length of the maxilla and correct its asymmetry and reattach the shortened maxilla to the skull in its new position. If all went well the mandible would be able to rotate forward and re-establish occlusion.

Knowing that Mr Bengstom could be overwhelmed with the prospects of facing such intrusive surgery, Dr Gutierrez thought about how to present the possibilities to his patient.

DISCUSSION:

This case reveals the complex interplay of technical objective and personal subjective factors. The task of the decision makers is to determine the benefits and harms of doing the surgery and those of avoiding it. Moreover, because there are alternative ways of doing the surgery, the benefits and harms need to be assessed for each. Deciding potential benefits and harms extends well beyond the scientific data. One of the most critical factors in this case may be the mindset of the patient. How well can he tolerate the mental agony of his present condition? How well can he handle the mental challenge of risky surgery? Likewise, in choosing among the variations in the surgical techniques, different subjective risks and benefits may be assessed differently depending on the character traits and values of the assessor.

This is a case in which resolution heavily depends upon the values of a significantly vulnerable patient. Clearly, such a person is severely compromised in his ability to objectively assess the alternatives presented to him. An important issue, therefore, is the extent to which the professional should help the patient participate meaningfully in the assessment of benefits and risks.

In such circumstances, the professional needs to be especially sensitive to how the possibilities for treatment are portrayed. Arguably, the doctor can never truly be in the position to fully understand the patient's values and to know what is in the patient's best interests.

Nevertheless, the doctor can look for ways to help the patient to at least lessen the harms associated with making a bad decision. The patient can be asked if there is a person or people who could participate in the discussion of treatment possibilities, perhaps a spouse, a parent, a sibling, a trusted friend, or a member of the clergy. Important information can be put in writing for future consideration. A second opinion can be suggested.

Even if the dentist and patient can determine the benefits and risks of the alternatives, the problem is not resolved. The dentist or patient (or both) may believe that there is a special duty not to harm. This could incline either of them to resist taking the chance of causing severe harm to the patient, possibly leading to a situation in which the dentist might insist on avoiding a risk of harm even if the patient thought the risks were worth it. Dr Gutierrez could plausibly believe that there is a serious risk of harm, but that, in his assessment, the benefits will be great as well. He could opt for the course that will maximize the net benefit, or he could give special weight to not harming the patient. Giving special priority to avoiding harm has very conservative implications. It would logically lead to never taking any risks. Most people prefer the moral stance of giving benefits and harms equal weight—mentally subtracting the harms from the benefits and choosing the course that produces the most net good. However, that still requires a subjective judgment about how much good will arise from the alternatives. Deciding whether to give special weight to avoiding harms is a matter of which ethical theory one uses. That is normally not part of a dentist's expertise.

In this case, it sounds like the surgeon's view is that for maximum impact on appearance and function, there is only one way to go. But in stating that, Dr Gutierrez ought to acknowledge that he is not considering other factors, such as risk of failure, risk of disease progression, and psychological effect on the patient.

What Counts as a Dental Good

However the conflict about how to relate benefits to harms is resolved, somehow the dentist and patient must determine what counts as a benefit or a harm. In dentistry the most relevant benefits and harms will be what we can call dental goods and dental harms, respectively. These are the benefits and harms that the codes of dental ethics normally have in mind when they commit the dentist to doing good for the patient.

Deciding what counts as a good or bad dental situation is more controversial than it may appear. Presumably an intact, functioning dentition counts as a good dental situation; caries lesions, missing teeth, pain, and vertical bone loss count as bad. But often the sorting of good and bad is much more complex. Is a well-functioning partial denture as good as natural teeth that are severely compromised? If not, how much worse is it? Is a time-consuming, expensive inlay better or worse than a four-surface amalgam restoration—and just how much better or worse? Does a well-functioning but discolored tooth count as bad in the calculation of overall dental good? If so, how bad? How does it compare with a crazed, chipped enamel surface that causes no problem now but probably is destined to in the future? How does one compare short-term and long-term benefits and harms?

During education in dental school, through the years of practice, and with the assistance of clinical research, certain patterns of answers begin to emerge that sometimes appear as a professional consensus. Often, however, patients may not share these judgments. This can lead to disagreements between patients and professionals about what is the best course of action to resolve a dental problem. It can even lead to disputes about whether a problem exists.

At this point, three closely related problems need to be distinguished. In some cases, a patient may concede that she agrees with the dentist's judgment of what would be the best thing dentally. The patient may still disagree about the recommended course of action. She may, for example, acknowledge that a three-unit fixed partial denture is best but consider it too expensive. She may want to sacrifice what is best dentally for some other nondental good that is competing for her scarce resources to maximize her overall good. Cases like these will be discussed later in this chapter.

Another group of cases involves problems in which the patient and dentist agree about what counts not only as the dental good for the patient, but also as the overall good. Still, a patient might insist that he should have the moral right to act autonomously, to choose to sacrifice his own welfare. A parent who rejects a recommendation for a needed full-mouth reconstruction in order to save resources to use for his children might fit this situation, as might a patient who chooses to take a modest risk for a research project. This group of cases, in which autonomy and patient welfare are in conflict, will be the subject of chapter 8.

Still another group of cases involves conflict over the concept of the dental good itself. The cases presented here all involve disputes over what is best dentally for the patient. The disputes may arise between dentist and patient or between professional colleagues. The problem in these cases is to determine the extent to which there is an objective basis for deciding the best thing to do dentally and whether knowledge of dentistry alone can resolve the conflicts. These problems are illustrated in the following cases.

Case 5: Agree to Disagree

At the age of 35, Mrs Margaret Tilden resumed treatment in Dr Joanne Stump's office. She had been Dr Stump's patient 10 years previously and then had changed dentists. For a while she had been without care altogether. In the recent past her priority had been rearing her children. Dr Stump remembered her as someone who was quite fearful of dentistry.

Mrs Tilden's oral condition was not good. She had several deep periodontal pockets and at some point a gingivectomy had been performed. Caries was extensive. Although no teeth needed extraction, restorative treatment would require endodontic treatment on four teeth and crowns on six teeth. Extensive periodontal care was also required. Even with this much attention, she might well lose her teeth later in life unless she significantly changed her home care practices and maintained regular dental care. Dr Stump thought Mrs Tilden would benefit from this care even if she ultimately required dentures.

Mrs Tilden wanted all of her teeth removed now. Root canal treatment was out of the question because of fear and also because of the expense. Dr Stump was definitely opposed to that plan, especially for someone Mrs Tilden's age. From the standpoint of alveolar bone retention, the longer the dentures could be postponed, the better off Mrs Tilden would be.

Dr Stump considered whether to perform the treatment as requested. She also wondered how far she should go to convince Mrs Tilden to accept her choice.

Case 6: Interrupted Treatment

Mrs Alice Andrews, age 55, entered Dr Theodore Fuller's practice wanting to save her remaining teeth. Dr Fuller was a periodontist-prosthodontist with extensive experience in the use of implants. Mrs Andrews's main problem was in the maxillary arch, where she had only six remaining teeth, all in the posterior segments. All of her teeth had about 50% bone loss and required considerable periodontal therapy. When that was complete, Dr Fuller planned to place two implants in the anterior segment and finish with complete maxillary reconstruction.

Shortly after the periodontal treatment was started, Mrs Andrews developed a brain tumor and underwent surgery for its removal. Although it was malignant, it was thought to have been completely excised. However, she was left with a facial nerve deficit and the left side of her face was immobile.

Mrs Andrews returned to Dr Fuller while she was still convalescing and wanted the treatment completed. Dr Fuller was skeptical. Access to the oral cavity was extremely limited because of the paralysis, which made the technical aspects of the surgery and subsequent prosthodontics very difficult to perform. Her teeth were more mobile than before and were even depressible, a finding that made the prognosis more questionable. In addition, she seemed depressed and in a weakened condition. This concerned Dr Fuller more than anything else, because he was not sure she could withstand the procedure. As an alternative he could extract her teeth and fabricate conventional dentures. Although this approach would be considerably less stressful for Mrs Andrews, considering her facial paralysis, the outlook for success was poor. Furthermore, Mrs Andrews was determined to proceed with implants. Dr Fuller recognized that some intervention was necessary, but he did not like either alternative.

Case 7: Surgeon's Dilemma

A 65-year-old man with a history of cardiac problems was referred to an oral surgeon by a dentist in a rural community about an hour away. The dentist's request was for the removal of one badly decayed molar. However, the patient asked that the surgeon also remove the adjacent tooth. The tooth in question had a large caries lesion, but it could have been easily restored. Other teeth were also noted to be in bad repair. When the surgeon said he thought he should call the referring dentist about removing the adjacent tooth, the patient said the surgeon could if he wanted to, but it wouldn't change anything as far as he, the patient, was concerned.

The patient's cardiac problem was limited to angina. There was no history of rheumatic heart disease or subacute bacterial endocarditis. The patient requested antibiotics, stating that all previous dentists had given him antibiotics. The surgeon knew that antibiotics were not indicated in this case. He explained the reasons why they should not be given, but the patient was adamant in his request. With conflicts both in the selection of teeth for extraction and the administration of antibiotics, the surgeon considered how to respond.

DISCUSSION:

All three of the cases in this section present situations in which the patient disagrees with the dentist's recommended treatment plan. It would appear that the dentist, as the trained professional, ought to be able to determine what is best for the patient and that the patient is hardly in a position to disagree. However, patients do disagree, and for varying reasons. In these cases the patients seem to be concerned about their dental health but disagree with the dentist about what constitutes the best dentistry.

Keep in mind, too, that dentists often disagree with each other. The professional consensus about treatment choices previously mentioned is a generalization that admits to many exceptions that further complicate the determination of what counts as a dental good. For example, in managing the problem of a missing posterior tooth, the restorative dentist, the oral and maxillofacial surgeon, and the orthodontist—each genuinely committed to the welfare of the patient—may each value and be convinced of the merits of the approach that they have mastered. Considering the range of viewpoints so enthusiastically championed among the clinical experts, it is not surprising that the values and interest of the patients are sometimes overlooked.

In the case of Mrs Tilden, the woman who wanted all of her teeth removed, the patient's values are clearly different from the dentist's. Mrs Tilden is now in a position to want dental care, but she obviously does not like taking care of her teeth. She may anticipate correctly that her teeth will have to be extracted in favor of dentures sooner or later and prefer to get it over with. She also expresses what appears to be more than the usual fear of root canal therapy.

The question here is whether it is better dentistry in some objective sense to attempt the maxillary restorations even if it involves more time, pain, and psychic trauma. Is this simply a matter of taste and preferences, or is there some sense in which a dentist can say it is better dentistry to try the restorations first? Some might believe that providing the restorations does more good, but if Mrs Tilden says she is better off with the extractions, it is not clear how a dentist could establish that she is wrong.

And from Dr Stump's standpoint, given her conviction that saving Mrs Tilden's dentition at this time would clearly be in Mrs Tilden's dental interest, how should she handle the impasse that now exists between her and her patient? How should she go about explaining her position? In the event that Mrs Tilden disagrees with her, what responsibilities does Dr Stump have to her patient?

The same problem in reverse arises in the case of Mrs Alice Andrews, the woman with what may be a terminal brain tumor. She is firm in her conviction to go ahead with extensive implant therapy, but the dentist resists. Mrs Andrews's motivations are unclear. Dr Fuller, however, is concerned both about the prospects for clinical success with the implants and Mrs Andrews's ability to physically and psychologically withstand the procedure. To make matters worse, he also thinks that conventional prosthodontics will not work well either.

There appear to be two very different ways to think about resolving this case. First, from one standpoint, there seems to be no way to determine the objectively best dental course. If Mrs Andrews says she is better off enduring the burdens of the extensive dentistry and understands the risks, proving she is wrong seems impossible. What is the best for her is simply a matter of taste and personal preference, no matter how strong the convictions of either party are.

In addition, the question of what is objectively the best dentistry raises an issue about the basic nature of dentistry: Is it an art or a science? If one views dentistry (and medicine) as a science, then such questions as implants versus dentures could be determined through clinical trials or other empirical research. And even if such evidence is not now available, the fact that it is amenable to such an approach clearly suggests dentistry is a science.

On the other hand, if dentistry is an art, then patients are not the automatic, predetermined recipients of technical reasoning. To consider it an art is to never forget that patients are not diagnoses or treatment plans—nor for students are they requirements for graduation. If dentistry is practiced as an art, one draws heavily from science, but one's actions are tempered by the patients and their circumstances. Recent thought on these matters supports the idea that one can never conclude what is best for the patient strictly from scientific studies. Even after science establishes what the outcomes are likely to be, a value judgment still must be imposed on the outcomes. Science can never tell us which outcome is better; at best it can tell us what the outcomes are going to be.

The other perspective on Mrs Andrews's case suggests that from the standpoint of beneficence, Dr Fuller's work is not yet done. As a starting point, he needs to decide what *he* thinks ought to be done and why. Then his role is to help Mrs Andrews as best he can with the choice she has to make. Meeting this goal requires an atmosphere of mutuality and dialogue. Mrs Andrews needs to feel encouraged to talk about why she wants to have implants so badly. And Dr Fuller certainly needs to express his views about the risks and benefits of each approach and what his choice would be. He also needs to tell her where he is coming from. Are his feelings based on extensive experience and success with implants? Has his training automatically oriented him toward implants? Does he especially pride himself on removable prosthodontics? Is he particularly oriented toward providing the best possible functioning occlusion?

Our view is that the first perspective without the second is incomplete. While it is essential to understand the frailty of scientifically based clinical decision making, it is also necessary to build on that understanding to promote an atmosphere of mutual respect and forthright exchange of information so that the best possible decision can be made. With that in mind, what are the issues that Dr Fuller needs to discuss with Mrs Andrews? How should he go about handling the discussion?

The man with the cardiac problem who wanted a restorable carious tooth removed and wanted antibiotics poses a similar problem. Here it is important to probe far enough to understand exactly the nature of the dispute. For example, why does the man want an antibiotic? Has he simply confused this dental situation with a previous problem in which an antibiotic would plausibly offer significant benefit? If so, perhaps patient education is needed. On the other hand, he may hold correctly that with an extraction there is always some risk of infection. He may desire to guard against even a small risk. What would be the basis of the dentist's objection to the antibiotic? It is incorrect to say that it will offer no conceivable benefit. Thus, a dentist may believe, based on his values, that the patient would be better off without the antibiotic, but he has no scientific basis for proving it. On the other hand, he may be worried about the societal effects of overuse of antibiotics (the eventual development of resistant strains). However, then he is trading the welfare of his patient for the long-term benefits for the society. Likewise, there is no scientifically correct answer to the question of the extraction. On what basis can a dentist say that it is better dentistry to restore the carious tooth rather than to remove both teeth at the same time, thus minimizing the trauma for the patient?

Compare the assessment of the dental good in these three cases and those in the previous section. There seems to be no objective basis for deciding what promotes the patient's dental well-being. Is the best dentistry the dentistry that maintains a functioning dentition no matter what the cost to the patient, the pain and psychic trauma, and the inconvenience? Or are there other standards that we might use in deciding what is the best dentistry?

Dental Good Versus Total Good

The cases that we have just examined make clear how difficult it is to determine what is good for the patient even if we focus exclusively on the dental good. An argument can be made that even in the sphere of dentistry, determining the good is inherently a subjective process about which no amount of dental knowledge can ever definitively determine what is the good for the patient. Thus, dentists disagree not only among themselves, but also with their patients about what is dentally best for the patient.

From the patient's point of view, however, there are many things on the agenda besides dentistry. Sometimes the dental good gets subordinated to other benefits that have nothing to do with dentistry or any other kind of health care. The following cases involve disputes between the dental good and other benefits. In analyzing these cases, watch for what the dentist and the patient consider to be the benefits at stake. On what basis should such disputes be resolved? Is it reasonable to strive for what is best dentally even if it means accepting what is less-than-best in other areas of life?

Case 8: Partial Refusal of Treatment

Mrs Donna Perdaris was a very well-to-do patient of Dr Lynn Decker. Mrs Perdaris's husband, a prominent trial lawyer, was also a patient. Mrs Perdaris needed extensive care that included fixed partial dentures on both maxillary and mandibular arches and the extraction of the four maxillary incisors because of extensive bone loss. Crown preparations were completed for all teeth in the maxillary arch and a full acrylic resin provisional splint was inserted. The provisional splints were to be in place for a few months, during which time conservative periodontal treatment was to be completed. Periodontal surgery would follow.

While Mrs Perdaris was wearing the provisional restorations, her husband had a serious accident and a prolonged hospitalization. When he was discharged, Mr and Mrs Perdaris went to one of their out-of-state homes while he recovered. Mrs Perdaris's splint fractured three times while she was away. Each time she flew home to Dr Decker for repair.

Mrs Perdaris asked Dr Decker if she could make her something that would not break. Perhaps she could make the provisional restorations out of the same durable and esthetic materials as she ordinarily would use for the final restorations. Mrs Perdaris would, of course, be willing to pay for these extra services. Her main concern was that when traveling abroad on some planned extended visits she would not need to be concerned with breakage or her appearance. She promised to complete all needed treatment after her life got back in order.

Dr Decker wondered what to do with this unusual suggestion. She had never done such a thing before, and it was contrary to the usual best principles of care. She also had increasing doubts about the sincerity of Mrs Perdaris's stated intention to complete periodontal care at a later time. If she did not follow through, the long-range prognosis would certainly be poor. On the other hand, Dr Decker was also convinced that Mrs Perdaris genuinely feared the periodontal surgery. Perhaps over the course of several visits, Mrs Perdaris's fears could be reduced to the point where she would be willing to go through with the surgery. In addition, Mrs Perdaris needed the restorative treatment and seemed to trust Dr Decker.

DISCUSSION:

This case presents an interesting mix of judgments about dental and other benefits. If pressed, could Mrs Perdaris make a case that the course she was pursuing served her dental interests? She would have to rely on an argument that dental interests are served, in part, by following a course that relieves anxiety. If Mrs Perdaris simply said that all she really wanted was splints without the periodontal surgery, would Dr Decker be acting unethically by providing the portion of the treatment Mrs Perdaris is willing to accept?

The case becomes more complicated if Mrs Perdaris admits up front that the course she is pursuing is really not ideal dentistry. How should Dr Decker respond if Mrs Perdaris says straightforwardly, "I have more important things in life than dentistry. Right now it is important for me to be with my husband, and we simply enjoy traveling very much." It is possible that what is in the patient's overall interest conflicts with what is in her dental interests. If so, is there any reason why a dentist should feel ethically bound to refuse to provide what patient and dentist agree is less-than-ideal dentistry?

In considering this question, it is helpful to see what views have been expressed in general medical situations regarding the refusal to comply with a patient's wishes. One such situation occurs when the physician is confronted with a request that he or she objects to on moral grounds. Examples include amniocentesis as an approach to the parental choice of sex and a request to use an untested drug for cancer treatment. In such cases the physician's role would only be to refuse to participate in such treatment, not to criticize the patients or to keep them from receiving such treatment from others. Thus, providing what is requested is not part of physicians' generally recognized obligations; the patient's autonomy should not supercede.[5] In dentistry, an example might be a refusal to do multiple extractions for a young person in the absence of any pathology. How comparable is Mrs Perdaris's situation with this criterion?

Another situation is one in which physicians should not refuse treatment if by doing so the condition would become worse. Because the case under discussion here involves treatment in progress, does the issue of avoiding harm come into play? If Dr Decker were to refuse Mrs Perdaris's request, would it be considered abandonment? Is the preferred position one in which there is no option but for dentist and patient to have discussions designed to chart a course of action that is clinically acceptable and that Mrs Perdaris can comply with—especially since she has recently been through difficult times with her husband's illness?

Case 9: Mrs Miller Wants Dentures

A 60-year-old woman, Mrs Leona Miller, was a new patient for Dr Andrew Press. His examination showed that although her mandibular arch was not in bad shape, only 12 teeth remained in the maxillary arch, and six were in such bad shape that they needed to be extracted. Also, Mrs Miller's oral hygiene was not good. She had a partial denture in hand, but she had not worn it for a few years because of the deteriorating condition of her mouth. The other six teeth clearly could be saved, but it would require a fair amount of restorative and periodontal therapy. This was Dr Press's recommendation.

Mrs Miller, on the other hand, wanted all of her remaining maxillary teeth removed. Her previous partial denture had never really been satisfactory, and she had friends telling her how good their dentures were.

Dr Press hated to make dentures for this patient. He knew only too well their limitations and problems. Mrs Miller was adamant and refused Dr Press's solution. He debated whether to do as she wanted.

DISCUSSION:

This appears to be another case in which the dentist must determine whether the dispute with the patient is about the understanding of the facts or about values. It may be that Mrs Miller has an unrealistic optimism about dentures and an unnecessary pessimism about the partial denture based on a very limited experience. On the other hand, she may have more complicated value differences with her dentist. She may, for example, really be concerned about the costs of the restoration. If so, she has to compare the value of the partial denture to the value of all the other things she could do with the money. That surely takes her well beyond the values of dentistry.

Assuming that Dr Press and Mrs Miller discuss the real likelihood of outcomes and reach an understanding about the facts and Mrs Miller still prefers the dentures, what reason is there for Dr Press not to cooperate? Assuming it is rational for Mrs Miller to trade off goods in one area of life for goods in another, wouldn't it be rational for her to choose less than the best dentistry in order to have some resources to do other things she values highly in other spheres of life?

Suppose that Dr Press decided not to make dentures for Mrs Miller— essentially declining to accept her as a patient. As he gives her this information, does he have any responsibilities to her beyond saying that he will not treat her and why?

Case 10: Crown Versus Clothes

Mrs Kathleen O'Brien was a 32-year-old mother of three who had recently entered the practice of Dr Virginia Fogel. Several years earlier Mrs O'Brien had fractured the mesiobuccal cusp of her maxillary right permanent first molar. Her dentist had placed a three-surface amalgam restoration in the tooth, and it had been trouble-free since then. Dr Fogel examined Mrs O'Brien's mouth and told her that although the restoration in that tooth looked good, it would probably be better to place a crown. Sooner or later the restoration was likely to break down anyway, and taking care of it now could avoid more extensive problems later on.

Mrs O'Brien did not exactly dispute Dr Fogel, but she wanted to avoid paying $750 for the crown. She needed to have money available to buy food and clothes for her children and her budget was tight. She asked a friend who was a dentist to take a look at her tooth. His opinion was essentially the same as Dr Fogel's: The restoration might last for years, or it might fracture tomorrow. Mrs O'Brien would be better off getting the crown done now.

The dentists' opinion worried Mrs O'Brien, but she decided to keep her restoration.

DISCUSSION:

It appears that Mrs O'Brien does not dispute the dentists' opinion that getting the crown would be better dentistry. However, she is not sure that maximizing her dental health will also maximize her overall well-being. Are there times when it is rational for patients to choose less than the best dentistry? If so, how should the dentist respond when patients make such choices?

The dentist's response to patients who choose to reject treatment recommendations can be affirming for the patients and for their attitudes about dentistry, or it can be the reverse. In a popular monthly commentary in the *Journal of the American Dental Association*, Gordon Christensen expresses concerns about a growing loss of confidence in the dental profession.[6] He suggests that the dentists should present their recommendations for treatment from the standpoint of whether they are mandatory or elective. Furthermore, he suggests another category as well: "contested." This includes treatment choices that many other dentists might well disagree with. Such information would provide a helpful perspective to the patient and would help avoid the aggressive salesmanship that troubles patients and dentists alike. On the other hand, keep in mind that this view reflects some assumptions about whether an intervention can be objectively classified this way. There is a sense in which no treatment is mandatory and all can be contested if the patient's value preferences lead to rejecting the proposed treatment. With these comments in mind, what points of discussion should be included in the conversation between Dr Fogel and Mrs O'Brien?

The Duty to Benefit a Nonpatient

Thus far in this chapter we have explored cases in which the problem was determining what the benefits and harms were and what their relationship ought to be. The focus, however, has been on the benefits and harms for the patient. Classic Hippocratic health care ethics is unique in counting only the welfare of the patient as morally relevant. Often, however, the welfare of nonpatients may be at stake. Many people who do not happen to be the patient of any dentist have dental needs.

In Section 4.B of its Principles of Ethics and Code of Professional Conduct the ADA takes the position that dentists are obliged "to make reasonable arrangements for emergency care."[2] This obligation holds true both for patients of record and patients not of record.

Sometimes what constitutes "reasonable arrangements" can be debatable. How far a dentist should go in order to make sure that people with dental needs, but who do not have a professional relationship with a dentist, get dental services? Is there a special relationship with a former patient that creates an obligation for a dentist to take the patient back into a practice before taking someone equally in need who has never been in the dentist's practice?

The issue of providing care for nonpatients goes beyond the treatment of emergency patients. There can also be concerns about compromising patient interests for the good of others when one works for the good of the community. Similarly, there can be trade-offs between the welfare of individual patients and the good of others when one considers breaking confidence to report an infectious disease, risking a patient for a research project, or providing less-than-ideal dentistry to conserve resources—perhaps in a third-world country. In its broadest form, the issue also addresses the duties of dentists to their families when they conflict with patient welfare.

The cases in this section pose the question of whether it is only the good of one's present patients that is the obligation of the dentist or whether doing good for former patients and nonpatients counts as well.

Case 11: Saturday Afternoon Toothache

Dr Stuart Fine sees patients on Saturdays but closes his office at 2 PM. At 1:50 PM one Saturday, his office received a call from Mr Evan Kraft, who had a toothache and wanted to be seen. Mr Kraft was a former patient in the office. He had completed his initial course of treatment, which involved some routine restorative procedures, but had not responded to any of several attempts by the office to have him return for recall visits. Dr Fine had a policy that patients who did not return for recall visits were removed from his patient list and were so notified by mail. This policy was followed for Mr Kraft.

Mr Kraft was informed by the office staff that he was no longer a patient in that office, was reminded of his refusal to return for recalls, and was told he would have to look elsewhere for his care that Saturday afternoon. However, if his problem was something that could wait until Monday, the office would be happy to receive his call at that time.

DISCUSSION:

According to the classical Hippocratic ethical tradition, the duty of health professionals is to benefit the patient. What does that imply for the dentist's duty to former patients? Has Dr Fine conformed to the ADA's policy of making "reasonable arrangements" for emergency care? Can we conclude that the dentist has no duty to Mr Kraft beyond being willing to see him after the weekend is over?

Hippocratic ethics is consequentialistic: It focuses on producing good consequences and avoiding harmful ones, but it is special in focusing exclusively on the patient. By contrast, another kind of consequentialism, utilitarianism, insists on counting all consequences of one's actions, whether they apply to patients or not. A utilitarian would have no trouble concluding that the effects of Dr Fine's decisions on Mr Kraft count ethically. The only way a utilitarian would excuse Dr Fine for failing to help Mr Kraft on Saturday afternoon would be if he could do even more good spending that time some other way (with some patient, some other nonpatient, or even on interests of his own). When a dentist sets out to benefit people, do only his or her present patients count?

Case 12: A Neighbor's Toothache

Dr Daniel Edison spent many summer weekends with his family on his boat about 100 miles from the city where his practice was located. At 11 PM one such Saturday, his answering service informed him that a prospective patient was calling with a toothache.

The call turned out to be from Ms Patricia Harvey, who was a friend and neighbor, but not a patient of his. She was calling because she had an extremely painful toothache in a molar in which root canal treatment had been started by her own dentist. The tooth had been painful even before treatment was started and had become worse despite two treatments. It was now excruciating, and she was desperate to get the tooth removed. She had called her dentist, but he was not available, which seemed to be nothing new.

She did not know what else to do and called Dr Edison out of desperation. Because distance prevented his handling her problem personally, Ms Harvey requested that he give her the name of someone who could remove the tooth immediately.

Dr Edison hated to see his friend have her tooth removed when he thought there was a reasonable chance that it could still be saved. He knew that her dentist was not an endodontist and thought that a specialist might be able to get her out of trouble quickly without removing the tooth. On the other hand, he knew she was almost frantic with her pain and her wish was clearly to have the tooth removed. He thought about what he should do. One of his concerns was how her regular dentist would react if the new dentist he had in mind was successful in saving the tooth, as Dr Edison suspected he would be. What is Dr Edison's obligation to Ms Harvey? What is his obligation to the original dentist?

DISCUSSION:

In this case the ethics of friendship converges with the ethics of dentistry. Because Ms Harvey is not now and never has been a patient of Dr Edison's, the strict ethic of patient benefit does not apply here. Yet from the perspective of a more general utilitarian ethic, clearly Dr Edison can be of considerable help. Does he do this out of the duties of friendship, the duties of being a dentist, or just a general duty to help others in need? Would his obligation be any different if it were a casual acquaintance or a stranger who asked for his help?

A utilitarian considers the consequences to all affected parties. This would easily justify Dr Edison's efforts to help benefit Ms Harvey, but it would also justify considering the effect of referring Ms Harvey on Dr Edison himself. Specifically, it would justify Dr Edison's including the possible harm he himself would suffer if he alienates or annoys Ms Harvey's regular dentist. After all, Ms Harvey is not Dr Edison's patient.

Duties to friends are similar to duties to patients in that both are based on special relationships existing between two parties. They both rest on implied commitments of loyalty, an issue that will arise further in the cases discussed in the next chapter. The traditional Hippocratic form of the professional duty to benefit, which limits the dentist's attention to benefits accruing to the patient, would have the odd implication that the dentist as a dentist owes nothing to a nonpatient who happens to be a good friend. More modern versions of an ethic based on the principle that actions are right insofar as they do good for people would open the door to considering a special duty to benefit friends and family as well as patients.

Patient Welfare Versus Aggregate Welfare

Thus far the cases in this chapter have focused on the benefits and harms for individuals with dental problems. The tasks have been to determine how benefits relate to harms, how dental goods are determined, how dental goods relate to nondental goods, and whether former patients and nonpatients count within the framework of the dentist's duty to benefit the patient. The question still arises of whether we really have a duty to provide benefit to an individual with dental needs (regardless of whether the individual is a patient) even if doing so jeopardizes the welfare of others.

One of the classic problems in ethical theory is whether the benefits and harms for all parties must be taken into account, at least for health professionals, or whether the only welfare that counts is the patient's. Hippocratic health care ethics, as we have seen in several previous cases, is at odds with classic utilitarian ethics. In Hippocratic ethics, only the patient is morally relevant in deciding what a health professional ought to do. By contrast, in utilitarianism, all benefits and harms count, no matter to whom they pertain. According to utilitarian thinking it is the aggregate sum of net benefits for society that are relevant, not the welfare of the individual.

The following case poses the problem of whether the dentist should narrow his or her focus exclusively to the welfare of the individual or should broaden it to include benefits and harms for others as well. The case deals with conflict between the patient's welfare and the total welfare of all people who would be affected by the intervention. Should the dentist strive to maximize the aggregate net good that can be done (including perhaps his own welfare in the calculation), or should he limit the relevant benefits and harms to those of the patient?

Case 13: Why Not Restore the Incisors?

Dr Ken Goff had just finished an internship sponsored by the US Public Health Service and was assigned to the Indian Health Service (IHS) in New Mexico. On his first day, he saw a 4-year, 9-month-old girl with incipient-to-moderate caries on all of her maxillary incisors and most of her posterior teeth.

Dr Goff planned to restore all the teeth as he had been taught. He was starting to discuss the treatment plan with the child's parents when the dental assistant informed him that they did not usually restore teeth with only incipient or moderate caries in children of that age. There were too many children with similar or worse problems, and there just was not time to handle the smaller lesions considering the fact that the teeth would probably exfoliate before the lesions became abscessed. If the lesions were more advanced or if the child were 2 years old and had similar problems, they would treat them.

Dr Goff did not understand this policy as articulated by the dental assistant. He wondered if it was fully justified.

DISCUSSION:

The goal of the IHS is to raise the health of the American Indian people to the highest possible level; this is true for dental as well as general medical services. The problem in both areas is that the IHS receives inadequate funding. The end result is that only about 30% of the Indian population sees a dentist during a typical year as compared with almost 60% of the general population.

The dental resources of the IHS are strained. The level of dental caries is about twice as high as in the general population. In addition, the American Indian population is growing rapidly and the demand is massive. Merely handling the emergency needs uses a large portion of the resources. For this reason, care must be rationed. Decisions have been made about who gets care and what kinds of care can be delivered cost-effectively. Therefore, some individuals suffer.

To maximize the impact of its scarce resources, the IHS has established priorities for dental treatment. Ninety-three percent of all treatment that occurs is emergency care and primary prevention. The other 7% includes much of what dentistry comprises in private practice: routine restorative care, endodontics, prosthodontics, surgical periodontics, and elective oral surgery. This small fraction, although it does help the Indian population, mainly benefits the providers in that they keep their skill levels high in other areas of dentistry.

Dr Goff's options seem quite limited. If he really believes in the traditional Hippocratic ethic of doing whatever will benefit the individual patient, he might refuse to participate in the obviously less-than-ideal care. On the other hand, he might reflect on what would happen if the IHS adopted a policy of permitting dentists to provide the traditional level of restoration for patients such as the youngster he is examining.

Giving a full measure of restorative care under the present circumstances would clearly come at the expense of care for other patients. The care that would have to give way would come from emergencies, primary prevention, or other restorative care. Diverting resources from the potential beneficiaries of this care to the youngster needing the restorations would appear simply to shift the dental benefits from one patient to another. On what basis has the dental service established its priorities?

Emergency care normally deals with patients who have great, immediate need. It can be said that such emergency care offers great benefit for the amount of resources invested. Likewise, primary prevention is usually an efficient producer of benefits. For the resources invested, more dental problems are probably avoided with primary prevention than with restoration of incipient or moderate caries. Thus, for these interventions the rationale of the IHS is probably that the goal should be to do as much good as possible for the patient population as a whole with the resources that are available. That is probably their goal even if some individual patients with incipient-to-moderate caries have to go without the normal level of service. The moral question here is: Once Dr Goff understands this rationale, should he cooperate in a plan in which he must purposely sacrifice his patient "for the good of the community"?

The dentist seems to be forced on the horns of a dilemma. If he sticks to the traditional ethic of doing whatever will benefit his patient, he condemns other patients to even greater problems than those that would be faced by his young patient. On the other hand, if he adopts the utilitarian policy solution, he sacrifices his patient to the good of the aggregate.

Case 14: Inflicting Pain in Research

In 1981, Dr D.P. Lu published a paper in the *Journal of Dentistry for Children* entitled "Clinical Investigation of Relative Indifference to Pain Among Adolescent Mental Retardates."[7] The purpose of the study was to discover "whether the pain threshold of retardates is indeed higher, as commonly believed, than that of normal persons."

The study had two parts, both of which used children aged 11 to 16 years. Approximately 30 children with IQs above 85 served as control subjects; the other 105 were mentally retarded but had no other medical problems. The retarded children were divided into three groups: borderline (IQs from 84 to 70); moron (IQs from 69 to 55); and imbecile (IQs from 54 to 40).

Part I of the study measured the pain of an intraoral injection of a full carpule of a local anesthetic. The injection site was not stated. The injections were given "without forewarning to allow a spontaneous expression of pain." During the injections, the subjects were asked to *(1)* keep their heads still, and *(2)* "express pain by whining."

Part II measured the pain of cavity preparation. Each subject received a Class 1 cavity preparation and an amalgam restoration on a mandibular premolar. All caries had been previously diagnosed. The key feature was that the preparations were done without anesthesia. However, exceptions were made for those subjects whose pain was so great as to "not allow the procedure to continue without local anesthesia."

Two different four-point scales were used to evaluate the pain. One scale focused on behavior. A "4" was "excellent" and the subject neither whined nor moved. A "0" was "poor" and the subject "screamed and struggled enough to stop the injection" in Part I or, in Part II, to require that local anesthesia be given.

The other scale measured pain. Subjects were asked whether they experienced no pain (for which they scored 4 points); some, but slight, pain (3 points); relatively low pain (2 points); moderate pain (1 point); or great pain (0 points).

A number of subjects showed variations between the two scales. When the variation was more than two points, it was considered unreliable and was not included in the data. The two scales were combined and divided by two to give the "pain-threshold point." This number was then used for correlations with IQ. The result was a series of negative correlations that was statistically significant. This was interpreted to mean that retarded individuals have higher pain thresholds than do nonretarded individuals.

DISCUSSION:

To assess the ethics of this research, the envisioned benefits and harms must be estimated. This will have to be done in several stages. First, one might ask what would be the potential value of the knowledge. The study makes sense ethically only if it was unknown whether the typical pain threshold for retarded children was different from that for nonretarded children. At the time the study was published, the prevailing—though strictly speaking inconclusive— view was that there was no evidence to support any pain threshold difference between retarded and nonretarded people. More importantly, published standard tests for evaluating pain existed that should have been used as opposed to the dental model. Pain evaluation involving the oral cavity should never be used because it has so many variables that lead to obfuscation.

In addition, for research to be justifiable, it must be thought to have some value. Presumably in this case, this knowledge might be useful in developing more effective patient management approaches for retarded people. However, to assess the potential benefits of the research, we need to determine whether the methods will permit a valid conclusion. Is the choice of cavity preparations as a pain stimulus one that is likely to generate reliable data? How likely is it that the children's responses could be based on past dental experiences and not on the current stimulus? Will some children, especially handicapped children, feel uncomfortable in expressing the full extent of their pain?

Another question is the use of a pain scale based on verbal interpretation. Can individuals with IQs of 80 and lower distinguish between slight pain and relatively little pain? Should the investigator have used other published nonverbal scales that were available at the time?

Once we have estimated the potential benefit of answering the research question and determined whether the design can answer it, the next issue might be whether the risks to the control subjects were justified. What were the risks to the nonretarded adolescents from Part I? Did giving the carpule without forewarning to allow a spontaneous expression of pain constitute treatment without consent? Did it constitute a significant deviation from good dental practice? If so, this would constitute a burden to the mentally normal adolescent controls. Because they cannot benefit from the study, this burden would be solely for the purpose of the research.

While the standard codes of ethics of research insist that the burdens to subjects must be justified by the potential benefits, they do not make clear whether the burdens to the subjects can be justified by the benefits to the society as a whole. Some theorists insist that, in the case of minors, retarded people, and others who cannot give an informed consent, no risk is acceptable solely for the benefit of others. Other theorists are willing to tolerate modest risk, provided it is justified by the benefit to others. Can the use of the control subjects meet these tests? How much risk to control subjects is ethically acceptable?

Once the ethics of using the mentally normal children has been assessed, we can turn to the ethics of using the retarded patients. While it should be clear that their treatment, including the Class 1 cavity preparation without anesthesia, cannot be done for their immediate benefit, is there some sense in which, if the study were done using sound methodology, they might benefit from this study in the long run? Might they receive better treatment in the future if the general characteristics of the pain threshold of retarded adolescents were better understood? If so, would these specific burdens be justified? Would they be justified by the anticipated future benefits to these particular retarded youngsters? Would they be justified by the anticipated future benefits to retarded adolescents as a whole?

Case 15: Obligations of Care During Research

Late in the 1980s, a national research organization funded a collaborative study to investigate oral manifestations of AIDS in a military population. The study involved HIV-infected personnel who were asked to return for periodic examinations during the course of their infection. Oral mucosal pathology and HIV-related periodontal conditions were the primary emphasis of the study.

Because the project received a final review prior to implementation, the issue was raised whether routine dental care should be made available to the study subjects. It was anticipated that subjects would present with HIV-related oral conditions that required care, but the provision of care would have required resources far in excess of the available research funding. The research agency felt that dental care was the responsibility of the military, regardless of whether subjects were enrolled in a research project. However, it was apparent that it would be difficult for the military, without additional resources, to provide dental services to a large influx of HIV-positive patients.

DISCUSSION:

There seems to be little doubt that the research undertaken is worth pursuing. The investigation uses particularly vulnerable patients—HIV-infected personnel. On two counts these subjects are from a particularly vulnerable class: They are in the military, sometimes called a "total institution," where some have argued that true consent is difficult to obtain, and they are infected with HIV. There seems to be no doubt that they would benefit from clinical care if the investigator could provide it or arrange to have it provided.

Still, the research team has been assembled not to provide clinical care but to conduct research. Moreover, the organization that funded the research has access to public monies appropriated for the purpose of research, not clinical care. It could be argued that it would be unethical for the research team to use research funds to provide dental care.

What are the researchers' other options if they do not provide the care? Do they have a moral duty to find out why the subjects are not getting dental care through regular military channels?

If no provision is made for such care, to what extent is the research team obligated to make an effort to see that it is? Many investigators have found that they are able to recruit research subjects by offering some clinical services or at least decent conditions not available to those outside the project. Prisoners, patients in institutions for the mentally handicapped, and others who are in unpleasant conditions are often attracted to a research protocol because even though the risks may be of concern, the advantages offset the risks.

One problem that this creates is that if an investigator can find patients who are miserable enough, he or she can offer just enough clinical care and improvement in living conditions to make it rational for the patients to volunteer for the study. The effect is that when calculating projected benefits and harms, if these benefits are counted, people who are miserable enough will always find it prudent to become research subjects. Does offering clinical care in settings like those described in this case pose the problem of making needy people the best candidates for research, or does this concern simply provide a rationale for excluding clinical benefits from the investigator's agenda?

We should get further insights into these problems in discussions of principles of ethics that extend beyond calculating benefits and harms. In the chapters that follow we look at other ethical principles, including fidelity, autonomy, veracity, and justice.

References

1. Edelstein L. The Hippocratic Oath: Text, translation and interpretation. In: Temkin O, Temkin CL (eds). Ancient Medicine: Selected Papers of Ludwig Edelstein. Baltimore: Johns Hopkins University Press, 1967:6.

2. American Dental Association Council on Ethics, Bylaws and Judicial Affairs. Principles of Ethics and Code of Professional Conduct, with official advisory opinions revised to January 2004. Chicago: American Dental Association, 2004.

3. Sandulescu C. Primum non nocere: philological commentaries on medical aphorism. Acta Antiq Hung 1965;13:359–368.

4. Jonsen AR. Do no harm. Ann Intern Med 1978;88:827–832.

5. Beauchamp TL, Childress JF. Principles of Biomedical Ethics, ed 5. New York: Oxford University Press, 2001.

6. Christensen GJ. The perception of professionalism in dentistry: Further reflections on a lively topic. J Am Dent Assoc 2002;133:499–501.

7. Lu DP. Clinical investigation of relative indifference to pain among adolescent mental retardates. ASDC J Dent Child 1981;48:285–288.

chapter 7

Fidelity: Obligations of Trust and Confidentiality

In this chapter

- What Is Owed to the Patient
- Trust, Entrepreneurship, and Marketing
- Personal Relationships with Patients
- Loyalty to Colleagues

Cases

- Redo the Case?
- The Dentist's Obligations When the Patient Fails to Pay
- Confidentiality for a Pregnant Adolescent?
- A Wellness-Based Income Stream
- Style and Substance
- Advertising: An Outdated Issue?
- Corporate Funding of Orthodontic Programs
- Romantic Entanglement?
- The Dating Game
- Get Out of the Kitchen!
- Lack of Communication Between Dentists

In chapter 6 we opened our coverage of ethical principles with a discussion of benef-icence and nonmaleficence. These two principles represent important aspects of the service component in all professions, including dentistry. They emphasize the merits of the *consequences* of service. In this chapter, we discuss fidelity, a principle with a different emphasis—not on consequences but on its intrinsic rightness independent of consequences. Many ethical theories hold that morality is more than merely pro-ducing good outcomes and avoiding bad ones. They identify certain characteristics of actions that make them right or wrong regardless of the consequences. These characteristics are often labeled as *principles*. Among the principles that can be included are fidelity, respect for autonomy, truthfulness or veracity, and justice or equitable distribution of benefits and harms. Each of these principles identifies a fea-ture of behaviors that might make the behavior morally right or wrong. We will devote the next four chapters to these principles, starting with the principle of fidelity.

In chapter 2 we discussed the central importance of the fiduciary relationship between the patient and the professional. The ethical principle upon which the fidu-ciary relationship is based is fidelity. As such, fidelity can be viewed as the grounding principle for professions.

Fidelity, along with the principles of autonomy and honesty, which are covered in the next two chapters, embody three different aspects of respect for persons. It rests on a certain trust and confidence that commitments made between the parties will be honored.

The principle of fidelity is an important part of many ethical systems. In addition to its prominence in professional ethics, it is central to certain religious ethical systems (especially Judaism and Protestantism) that place emphasis on fidelity to covenant.*

The principle of fidelity can be understood to include the notion of keeping promises as well as more general obligations of loyalty and commitment-keeping. There are often good pragmatic reasons why once a promise is made it should be kept. One's reputation will certainly be injured if word gets around that one cannot be trusted to keep promises.

Even though there are often pragmatic reasons to keep promises, the ethically interesting situations are those special ones in which, on balance, more good is actu-ally done by failing to keep one's word. An example might be breaking the implicit promise of confidentiality in special instances, an option that Dr Davis faced in Case 1 (see Introduction) as he considered the disclosure of a patient's HIV status to her fiancé, also a patient. However, for those who believe that fidelity is a characteristic of actions that tends to make them right independent of outcome, breaking a promise is simply intrinsically wrong (even if the outcome is better if the promise is not kept).

Immanuel Kant was the most famous philosopher to hold that fidelity to promis-es is inherently one's moral duty regardless of the consequences.[2] Many other philosophers since Kant have reached a similar conclusion.[3] These are generally the same people who believe that respecting autonomy and telling the truth are moral-

---

*For an example of a Protestant theologian who worked extensively in health care ethics giving central position to the principle of fidelity, see Ramsey.[1]

ly right-making elements of an action independent of the consequences—the issues we face in the next two chapters.

As suggested previously, the three moral principles of fidelity, autonomy, and honesty are closely linked. Sometimes they are treated as aspects of a single, over-arching principle of *respect for persons*. Others view the principles of respecting autonomy, honesty, and fidelity (as well as the principle of the sacredness of life or the duty not to kill) as analytically separate principles of ethics, even though they are closely related. We treat them in three separate chapters. (The principle of the sacredness of life or the duty not to kill is important in ethics for physicians but is not normally critical for dentists.) The cases in this chapter all raise, in one way or another, problems of what is required for the dental professional to be faithful to commitments made to patients, colleagues, the profession, and the public.

Sometimes these commitments are made explicitly, as when a dentist promises a patient a certain type of restoration or promises a certain appointment time. When such a commitment is made explicitly, it is clear and uncomplicated. To break such a commitment is unmistakably wrong. In other cases, the promise is more implicit, as when the health professional implies a promise of confidentiality. Certain practices have come to be thought of as essential to the way professionals relate to each other and to their patients. Patients, for example, certainly expect that their dentist will be committed to treating them gently, not overcharging them, recommending only needed treatment, reducing their anxiety, acting with competence, and refraining from exploiting them for any reason. These commitments emphasize the scope and importance of professional relationships. The assumption of these responsibilities is also what makes professional relationships rewarding to the professional. Implicit promises such as these are believed to be as morally binding as the more explicit ones.

Among the commitments made to patients that might fall under the principle of fidelity are not only the general Hippocratic promise to work for the patient's benefit, but also more explicit promises to keep information confidential. Exactly what the nature of the promise is will be the subject of some of the cases in the first part of this chapter.

Commitments are also made to the profession and to fellow professionals. There are implied promises of loyalty and collegiality that can lead a dentist to want to protect a colleague who has made a mistake or lacks competence. There is also a commitment (in the words of the American Dental Association's [ADA's] Principles of Ethics and Code of Professional Conduct) to provide "competent and timely delivery of dental care within the bounds of the clinical circumstances presented by the patient."[4] The ADA goes on to say that "dentists shall be obligated to report to the appropriate reviewing agency as determined by the local component or constituent society instances of gross or continual faulty treatment by other dentists." Cases involving commitments both to patients and to colleagues are discussed in this chapter, and the issues of wayward colleagues are discussed in chapter 14.

What Is Owed to the Patient

The fiduciary relationship in professional ethics is sometimes referred to as a *contract*. It is part of the ethics of contracts that each party pledges something to the other. In legal contracts, when one party reneges, the other party is normally excused from any obligation to keep his or her part of the deal.

However, there is great controversy in professional ethics over the question of whether the relationship between the professional and the patient should be thought as a kind of contract.[5–7] It seems obvious that the relationship between dentist and patient cannot be interpreted minimalistically with the dentist giving exactly what the bargain calls for and no more. It cannot be reduced to a legalistic business deal.

For this reason, some have suggested that the more appropriate term for the fiduciary relationship is *covenant*. Drawing on religious metaphors, the professional and the patient can be seen as entering a covenant. The term can be used to emphasize the moral and social character of the bond. Others have responded by arguing that *covenant* does not convey the concrete obligations that each party owes the other. These defenders of the concept of *contract* point out that sometimes the term contract is used in a more ethical and less legalistic sense, as in references to the "marriage contract."

Working out the implications of this contract or covenant or fiduciary relationship with the patient is one of the most complex, but also one of the most important, parts of health professional ethics. One component is a general set of commitments to serve the patient or, to use the older language, to do what is best for the patient. This ethical commitment is so strongly represented in the tradition of health professional ethics that it can be said to be a promise made to the patient.

Exactly what is entailed, however, is sometimes difficult to determine. We have now learned that it makes little sense to promise to do what is literally best for the patient. That would mean always using the best procedures and best materials imaginable. Although patients would like to receive very high-quality care, they probably would not always want the best imaginable care when care that is almost as good costs much less in time, money, and effort. For instance, despite the view among many dentists that, in many situations, gold restorations would be better than amalgam restorations, most people, considering the lower cost and satisfactory performance of amalgam restorations, would not routinely choose gold. Similarly, patients probably should be willing to wait short periods of time for appointments. Even for emergency care, they probably should be willing to wait until morning for all but the most extreme emergencies. One reason why it makes little sense to promise the best possible care is that neither dentist nor patient believes it is reasonable to strive for what is literally the best.

Another reason is that doing what is best may come at the expense of the rights of patients—their right to refuse treatment or their right to otherwise act autonomously. For this reason, some are now saying that the proper promise for establishing a lay-professional relationship is for the professional to serve the *rights and wel-*

fare of the patient (recognizing that in some cases the welfare must be compromised to protect the rights).

How High Should the Standard of Care Be?

One set of problems growing out of our fiduciary relationship with patients is what should happen when the dentist recognizes that the care he or she delivered turned out to be less than ideal. When there are serious problems (such as a restoration that fractures), it seems obvious that the work must be redone. What, however, of restorations that pose only small problems? Who should bear the responsibility? When is care good enough? If the patient wants perfection, who pays? If the patient does not recognize the imperfection, should the dentist make a point of it? These are the issues addressed in the next group of cases.

Case 16: Redo the Case?

Dr Paul Goldman had been practicing prosthodontics for almost 15 years. Except for a 0.5-mm discrepancy, the treatment he had given Mrs Debbie Richards was of textbook quality. However, because of that minor problem, he was considering redoing the maxillary arch.

Mrs Richards was 55, and most of her teeth had been extracted. However, she very much wanted to keep the rest of them. Four mandibular incisors remained; her maxillary arch had only two central incisors, the left first premolar, both right premolars, and the right canine.

Dr Goldman made a mandibular partial denture and two maxillary fixed partial dentures. On the right side of the maxillary prosthesis, the remaining three teeth were crowned and the lateral incisor was cantilevered as a pontic. The fixed partial denture on the left side used the premolar and both central incisors as abutments and the lateral incisor and canine as pontics. Therefore there was no connection between right lateral and central incisors. This was done to reduce stress on the first premolar that was already vulnerable in its role as a single-rooted tooth used for a terminal abutment.

The provisional splints were cemented in as a single unit with all teeth connected. Twice the splint became loose because of the cement having washed out around the left first premolar. Dr Goldman thought that the loosening was caused by occlusal stress, which made him even more certain that he had done the correct thing in "breaking" the appliance between the maxillary lateral and central incisors.

Initially, both he and Mrs Richards were extremely pleased with the final result. The color was excellent and all margins were flawless. The occlusion against the mandibular partial denture was perfect. Three weeks later Mrs Richards returned with a complaint. During chewing the restorations separated between the maxillary lateral and central incisors, which caused significant food impaction. It was very disturbing to have food trapped there when she was in a social situation. Although Dr Goldman viewed Mrs Richards as an overly exacting person, his examination confirmed that what she was saying was absolutely true. The contacts between the right central and lateral incisors separated significantly during functional movements. He made some attempts to adjust the occlusion but nothing worked.

Dr Goldman had never seen this happen before. He thought that his judgment in design had been good. In retrospect, he felt he should have used precision attachments between the central and lateral incisors. He had avoided that because it would have required excessive bulk in that area.

Mrs Richards and her husband made an appointment with him to discuss the problem. He thought about whether to redo the prostheses. He wondered whether he should do so even though he believed that he had done nothing wrong. Furthermore, if he remade the maxillary appliances, who should pay?

DISCUSSION:

The fiduciary relationship between dentist and patient imposes an obligation for the dentist to be committed to the welfare of the patient. As long as the Hippocratic standard is unquestioned, this commits the dentist to doing what is in the patient's best interest. The exact meaning of this commitment often goes unexamined. This is a case that forces a more careful examination of this duty growing out of the fiduciary relationship.

When Dr Goldman accepts a patient into his practice, he certainly commits himself to do high-quality work. He might be said to commit to at least conforming to the professional standards of practice upheld by competent dentists in his community. But does he commit to doing literally what is best for the patient? In looking at the problem from the standpoint of promises or commitments made under the principle of fidelity, this is more a question of implicit, rather than explicit, promises. There is no evidence in this case that the problem should have been anticipated. He met his specific clinical commitment or promise and did it well, but an unexpected consequence occurred. However, did he meet the implicit promises that a prosthodontist makes to a patient?

Dr Goldman now recognizes that a modest problem exists. He would proceed differently were he to repeat the procedure, this time using precision attachments between the central and lateral incisors even if it would create additional bulk in the area. But how should he solve the problem of what to do for Mrs Richards?

Consider the following positions that he might take:

1. One possibility is that he could approach the problem by holding himself accountable to the standard of quality that his colleagues similarly situated would have provided. Then, if he judged himself deficient, he could redo the procedure at his expense. On the other hand, if he concluded that his colleagues would have found him faultless, he could feel free from the responsibility of remaking the appliance. However, he would still have to address Mrs Richards' concern about the food impaction.

   In reflecting on the first option, which calls into play the standards of one's colleagues, keep in mind that the collegial standard is usually invoked as a judgment on whether treatment was merely acceptable. Dr Goldman already thinks that what he did was acceptable. He is concerned that it wasn't excellent.

2. Dr Goldman could also ignore what his colleagues might have done and hold himself accountable to doing the best possible work. This would mean redoing the procedure at his expense, even though he felt that it would have been unreasonable to have expected him to have anticipated that particular problem. However, explaining all of that to Mrs Richards as a justification for having her pay for the retreatment would probably be impossible.

3. Dr Goldman could proceed according to options 1 or 2 but reduce his fee enough so that if, for some reason, the case must be redone, the financial consequences of charging a second time would be less onerous for Mrs Richards, while at the same time would reduce his losses to a more acceptable level.

4. In this era of informed consent, Dr Goldman could present the two plausible treatment alternatives to Mrs Richards together with a statement that she might not be completely satisfied with either option. If he chose that option, he would still have to decide what to do about the level of the fee in case she wanted a "second try."

Ethically, are there other options? Which one should Dr Goldman choose?

When the Patient Fails to Keep the Bargain

Determining exactly how high a standard a dentist should use in deciding whether the obligation to the patient has been fulfilled is just one of the issues raised by the question of what is owed to the patient. Ethical problems are also raised when the patient fails to fulfill his or her part of the contract. This question might arise if a patient fails to practice proper dental hygiene, persistently fails to keep appointments, or, as in the following case, does not pay his or her bill.

Case 17: The Dentist's Obligations When the Patient Fails to Pay

Mrs Sandra Lichter, who was in her late 50s, was a patient in the practice of Dr Ana Burt. Dr Burt's practice was primarily reconstructive, and she had performed that type of service for Mrs Lichter. Mrs Lichter had received full-mouth rehabilitation, consisting mostly of crowns along with one partial denture. Endodontic treatment and periodontal surgery had also been necessary.

The total bill was expected to be about $20,000. Dr Burt had been paid $2,000 by Mrs Lichter's insurance company, and she had asked her business manager to arrange a payment schedule with Mrs Lichter. The business manager was sure that a business agreement had been made, but every time Mrs Lichter came in she made some plausible excuse for not paying.

Finally, the case was completed. Dr Burt inserted all of the restorations on a trial basis and was pleased with the result. However, Mrs Lichter still had paid no part of her $18,000 bill.

Dr Burt wondered whether she should withhold final placement of all restorations until the bill was paid or insert the prostheses and continue to try to work things out with Mrs Lichter.

DISCUSSION:

Unlike in the previous case, Dr Burt is not worried about how high a standard she ought to use in deciding whether she had done her best work for her patient. Both she and her patient seem satisfied. The problem here is whether the "contract" should be fulfilled by Dr Burt when Mrs Lichter seems unwilling or unable to keep her part of the bargain.

The first issue here is whether it is ever acceptable for a dentist to withhold the completion of work until the patient keeps his or her end of the deal. Under the paternalistic ethic, the duty of the dentist was to do what was best for the patient. No conditions were attached pertaining to the responsibility of the patient. In fact, the patient was not seen as an active participant in the relationship, only as someone who was treated.

For those who accept in principle that a new relationship is emerging in which patients bear active responsibility and, therefore, have obligations as well as rights, the next question is what responsibility the patient bears. The ethic of contracts is that the parties bear mutual responsibility. Assuming both parties were competent and understood the nature of the agreement, if one party fails to fulfill her end of the bargain, the other party is not obligated to complete hers. That would seem to imply that Dr Burt would be justified in not completing the work until she is assured she will be paid.

It is hard to tell in this case whether Mrs Lichter could have begun paying her bill, but that may not make any difference morally. In a relationship that involves a contractual purchase of merchandise, if the bill is not paid, the merchandise is not delivered (or is repossessed). Is this the type of relationship between a dentist and a patient, or is the dental relationship one in which the dentist bears moral responsibility for improving the dental health of the patient even if she cannot pay, at least if the reason that she cannot pay is beyond her control? Suppose that Dr Burt decides not to cement the crowns permanently. If, at a later time, the cast crowns, which have been cemented temporarily, develop problems caused by the washing out of the temporary cement and the subsequent development of caries, is Dr Burt morally responsible? Would such actions constitute abandonment?

The ADA's position on abandonment[4] is that "[o]nce a dentist has undertaken a course of treatment, the dentist should not discontinue that treatment without giving the patient adequate notice and the opportunity to obtain the services of another dentist." It goes on to say that "[c]are should be taken that the patient's oral health is not jeopardized in the process." This suggests that the ADA is working with the more traditional model in which the fiduciary relationship with a patient requires completing the work regardless of the patient's willingness to pay. Those who view the dentist-patient relationship as more of an agreement between consenting parties would be more willing to support a dentist who withheld completion of the treatment.

We still need to decide what specific action Dr Burt ought to take. One view sides with the traditional model—sort of. Ultimately the potential long-term harms of not providing permanent cementation require that it be done. In addition, Dr Burt's office management system is at least partly at fault for the current predicament. No matter what Mrs Lichter's excuses were, the treatment should not have gone as far as it did without payment. So the cementation must take place, but not without considering two important caveats. One is that Dr Burt needs to have a significantly overdue talk with Mrs Lichter about the problem. We do not know much about Mrs Lichter's personality and attitudes, but hopefully the conversation can be done skillfully in a way that maintains, and perhaps strengthens, their relationship. (An important question to consider is what Dr Burt should say and how she should say it.) The second caveat is that even though the fiduciary relationship requires that the prosthesis be properly inserted, that does not mean that Dr Burt should not be paid. There is still a business contract between her and her patient. If Mrs Lichter absolutely refuses to pay for the treatment, it is time to take legal action.

Confidentiality

The fiduciary or contractual relationship may help to provide an understanding of another traditional element of health professional ethics: confidentiality. Health professionals have long recognized that they have a duty to their patients to keep confidential the information that they learn about the patient in the course of the professional relationship.

Only recently have we begun to realize how controversial this duty is. A close reading of the Hippocratic Oath reveals that, according to the Oath, the health professional should not disclose "those things that ought not to be spread abroad."[8] The implication is that there may be some things that are appropriately disclosed. Traditional paternalistic health care ethics determined what should be disclosed by the Hippocratic test: Always act so as to benefit the patient according to the provider's ability and judgment.

There are two problematic cases. First, should the professional disclose information when he or she believes disclosure would serve the patient's interest, even though the patient wants the information kept confidential? Second, should the professional disclose information when such disclosure may prevent a serious harm to third parties?

The following case raises the first question.

Case 18: Confidentiality for a Pregnant Adolescent?

Mary Smith, a 15-year-old girl, came into a dental clinic for a recall appointment. She had been a patient of Dr Virginia Jones in that clinic for many years. While waiting in the radiology area, she saw a sign instructing women to inform their dentist if they were pregnant. Mary became upset and asked Dr Jones why the sign was there. Eventually she confessed that she was pregnant and asked that Dr Jones not tell her mother.

Dr Jones knew Mary's mother quite well and felt she had an obligation to her as well as to Mary. Mary was not legally independent, and her parents had to give consent for any treatment that Dr Jones would propose. Knowing Mary's parents, Dr Jones was convinced that it would be beneficial to Mary if her parents knew and could provide care and support during this difficult time. Dr Jones wanted to respect Mary's confidentiality, but she was not sure that she should.

DISCUSSION:

There are several approaches one can take to the problem of confidentiality. This is an interesting and important case for dentistry, because different approaches will lead to very different conclusions about what Dr Jones should do.

The more paternalistic, traditional approach would resolve the problem by having Dr Jones ask what she believes would be best for her patient. In its most traditional form, this approach did not even hold the dentist to a standard of what his or her colleagues believed would be in the patient's interest. As long as the dentist really believed disclosure would be better in the long run, he or she had the right (maybe even the duty) to tell the patient's parents. A modified version would permit disclosure of the confidential information only if Dr Jones's colleagues would concur in her judgment about patient interest. In either case, there is no reciprocal set of commitments involved in confidentiality, only a judgment on the part of the professional about the patient's best interest.

The newer approach is to treat confidentiality as a duty that stems from the contract or covenant with the patient. The key is what is promised (or implied) to the patient at the time the relationship is established.

This approach derives the ethics of confidentiality from the ethics of promise-keeping. Whatever a dentist promises or implies as part of the commitment that establishes the relationship is what is owed to the patient. If, for example, Dr Jones believes that she can only promise to withhold information in cases when it would be consistent with the patient's interest to do so, she could make that offer to her patients. Of course, many patients who understood that she would disclose information when she believed that it would be in the patient's interest (even when the patient did not agree) would find that proposal unacceptable. It could be argued that making that policy clear to patients would be self-defeating; patients might refuse to disclose information to the dentist if she could not be trusted.

The alternative is to promise patients that information will be kept confidential—even when the dentist believes that the patient would benefit if it were disclosed. Increasingly, sister professions such as medicine are making such promises. The British Medical Association, for example, has adopted a policy that in such cases disclosure can take place only with the consent of the patient.[9]

The ADA's Principles of Ethics and Code of Professional Conduct addresses this issue in an interesting way: "Dentists shall maintain patient records in a manner consistent with the protection of the welfare of the patient."[4] That seems to place the ADA on the side of paternalism, which implies that Dr Jones not only may but also should break confidence to promote the patient's welfare.

The ADA goes on to say that "[u]pon request of a patient or another dental practitioner, dentists shall provide any information in accordance with applicable law that will be beneficial for the future treatment of that patient." This is somewhat ambiguous. Does it qualify the earlier statement meaning that dentists can break confidence for the welfare of the patient only when the patient or another dentist asks? Of course, if the patient asks, the ethical problem seems moot, but what if it is the dentist who thinks that confidence should be broken? What if it is another dentist who asks? Does the promise that the dentist makes permit disclosure in these conditions in order to do what Dr Jones believes will benefit Mary?

This raises problems of the second kind, however. In some medical situations a dentist may feel compelled morally to disclose information, not to benefit the patient, but to protect a third party.

This was the problem faced by Dr Davis, the dentist described in Case 1. He was caring for an HIV-infected patient whose fiancé apparently did not know that she was infected. The ethical issue posed by that patient, Andrea Armstrong, is different in important ways from those posed by the pregnant patient, Mary Smith. If Dr Jones broke confidence in Mary Smith's case, it would be for purely paternalistic reasons—to serve Mary's long-term interests (even though Mary might not understand or agree). Breaking confidence in this way is morally justified only to the extent to which paternalism is. In Andrea Armstrong's case, Dr Davis, if he is inclined to break confidence, is considering doing so not primarily for his patient's welfare but for the welfare of a third party, his patient's fiancé.

One of the attractive features of the Hippocratic ethical tradition is that it focuses solely on the welfare of the patient. As we have seen, however, that narrow focus can also be a problem, not only when patients like Mary Smith do not want their interests served, but also when third parties are put at serious risk if the patient's interest is served.

Twentieth-century ethics of organized physicians has supported breaking confidence in cases when there is a serious threat to the interest of third parties. The present American Medical Association (AMA) policy supports disclosure when there is a realistic threat of serious bodily harm.[10] By contrast, the ADA seems to permit no third-party interests to justify breaking confidence. With specific reference to HIV status (but focusing on disclosure to another dentist rather than a fiancé), the ADA says that the dentist should obtain permission from the patient before disclosing and should contemplate severing the relationship if the patient refuses. This, of course, would not warn Ms Armstrong's fiancé of his impending risk. Does it relieve Dr Davis of his moral responsibility?

Trust, Entrepreneurship, and Marketing

The previous section presented confidentiality as an integral part of the fiduciary relationship. The security felt by a patient that sensitive information disclosed in the course of treatment will be kept confidential by the dentist is a key feature of the professional trust relationship. Also of great importance is the patient's expectation that the dentist will act in his or her interests. Patients should be able to expect their dentist to deliver high-quality care, minimize pain or discomfort, honor their confidences, charge them fairly, and, in general, respect their integrity as people by not abusing their position. Patients have a right, and are almost forced, to trust that their dentist will act competently and compassionately on their behalf.

This expectation of trust is different from that developed with close friends. Trust with friends develops over time; it is earned. In contrast, patients should be able to expect trustworthiness in dentists by virtue of their training and their special role in society.

One reason that trust is so important in the relationship between patient and dentist is that there is usually a significant inequality in the relationship. The dentist has knowledge and skills not possessed by the patient. The possession of these characteristics places the dentist in a relative position of power and the patient in a relative position of vulnerability and dependency. With this inequality comes an obligation to act in ways that avoid the abuse of power.

In this and the following section, we present cases that deal with the implications of trust in the relationship between dentist and patient. This section's cases explore the delicate interplay between the professional role and entrepreneurship—functioning as a businessperson. The next deals with personal relations with patients that mix sexual interests with the professional relationship.

Case 19: A Wellness-Based Income Stream

Recently, Dr Louisa Sanchez, a general dentist, received a letter from a board-certified general surgeon inviting her to offer her patients "better health, more energy, and reduced cancer risk through custom vitamins and develop a lucrative wellness-based business." The claim for health benefits was accompanied by a *Journal of the American Medical Association* citation and a statement that two reputable pharmaceutical labs "are providing average Americans with a customized supplement program based on proven scientific testing."

The surgeon gave examples of four professionals who generated between $16,000 and $45,000 per month—an orthopedic surgeon, a podiatrist, an anesthesiologist, and an internist. Now, apparently, he and the company he was associated with wanted Dr Sanchez and other dentists to join the growing number of doctors who were selling these products to their patients in their offices. For some of them the additional "income stream" came to surpass that of their practices. The surgeon pointed out that, "with increasing overhead, increasing malpractice insurance, increasing regulations, and third-party payment hassles, many dentists are looking outside of their practices for additional income streams to secure their financial future."

All of this, the surgeon emphasized, could be accomplished by the dentist "while remaining true to the ideals of helping his/her fellow man."

Dr Sanchez had only to call the surgeon at a toll-free number to receive more information. And if her interest continued, the surgeon would visit Dr Sanchez personally "to fully explain the program."

Dr Sanchez was impressed with the opportunity to make extra money, even though she figured much of the letter was hype. On the other hand, she did not think she had gone to dental school to sell vitamins—custom or otherwise. But a colleague of hers said, "If you believe that what you are selling the patient is good even though it is not dentistry, what is the problem?"

Case 20: Style and Substance

In Dr Paul Homoly's book *Isn't It Wonderful When Patients Say "Yes": Case Acceptance for Complete Dentistry*, one chapter discusses problems he has with insurance, or as he puts it, "the contamination of dental insurance."[11] He contends that insurance interferes with one's ability to do "great dentistry."

In assessing the practices of "top practitioners," Dr Homoly differentiates between "style" and "substance." He says that the style of top practitioners includes "glamorous high-profile offices, in-office teaching institutes, celebrity patients, international travel, extraordinarily high fees, rigid financial arrangements, great affinity for new technology, and fancy marketing"—and it is all made possible by "substance."

"Substance," he asserts, is equated with the provision of "complete care." This is possible only when one excels in everything from diagnosis to advanced restorative techniques. However, one can provide "complete care" only if one has the sort of practice that permits the frequent use of one's sophisticated skills, whereupon one immediately goes head-to-head with the limitations of insurance. The main problem is the limitation of the maximum yearly benefit. He gives as an example a normal annual maximum benefit of $1,200. If the treatment plan is for $2,400, then insurance covers 50 percent of the fee. But if the treatment plan is $10,000, then the insurance covers only 12 percent. In Dr Homoly's words, "[w]hen you practice complete dentistry, dental insurance will not follow."

This means, Dr Homoly says, that dentists need to "minimize insurance"—convince patients "to deal with their insurance company on our terms, not the insurance company's." Patients need to be convinced that "pretreatment authorizations and assignment of benefits limit the range of care and lower the standards of care." This is much harder to do with established patients than with new patients, though it must be attempted. In addition, he says, "[y]our marketing efforts should be focused on attracting new patients who are at least fifty years old." These are the patients whose treatment needs are predictably more substantial. If one's new patients are mainly "young, with most of their teeth, the substance of your practice has little to offer them."

DISCUSSION:

These two cases depict one of the most important ethical issues facing dentists today: the commercialization of dentistry. Dr Sanchez in Case 19 is being urged to turn her practice into a lucrative business. Dr Homoly in Case 20 wants to convert the dentist's office into a high-income spa. Many dentists view these strategies as a major threat to the profession. Those who hold these views are concerned that dentists are thinking more about their own interests and less about their patients' interests. They fear that dental care is becoming more of a commodity than a health service and that dentistry is becoming more entrepreneurial—more like a business than a profession.

The erosion of professionalization has been going on for some time and for a variety of reasons. In 1997, *Reader's Digest* published an article called "How Honest Are Dentists?"[12] It described how a "professional patient" who consulted with several different dentists received estimates for proposed treatment that ranged from $500 to $30,000. The article outraged dentists, but it did not make dental patients very happy either.

In addition, because of major advances in materials technology, cosmetic dentistry has become an important part of the profession. However, the salesmanship associated with discretionary treatment has become the source of much concern. The more dentists view their services as optional and elective, the faster they descend the slippery slope of believing that salesmanship is a key value in dentistry.

There is evidence that dentistry's enviable high ranking as a trusted profession is beginning to weaken. For decades, dentistry was ranked second or third in the Gallup Poll's list of most trusted occupations. By the mid 1990s, it was fifth, and in 2000 it had dropped to eighth[13]—a respectable ranking, of course, but perhaps on the decline. In a 2001 *Journal of the American Dental Association* column,[14] Dr Gordon Christensen attributed the weakening of public trust to, among other things, the view of dentists as preoccupied with greed and their own interests. At the end of the slippery slope mentioned previously are an increasing number of patients who have adopted the protective attitude of "let the buyer beware." Some members of the profession believe that what is at stake is nothing less than the transformation of dentistry from a profession to a business. In this context, the sale of products in dental offices greases the slippery slope even more.

Not everyone is concerned. People who sell such products take the view that, "If I can help my patients, I should be rewarded for it." Or, as Dr Sanchez's colleague suggested, if you believe what you are selling is good—dentistry or not—what is the problem? They also feel that patients are entitled to buy these products from them, and that many patients like the idea of being able to make a convenient purchase while they are at the dental office. Finally, there is the feeling that they are autonomous practitioners, with the right to practice dentistry as they wish.

Furthermore, the ADA Code does not exactly reject the idea of office sales of commercial products out of hand.[4] Advisory Opinion 5.D.2 says that if dentists choose to sell such products to their patients, they "must take care not to exploit the trust inherent in the dentist-patient relationship for their own financial gain." They also "should not induce their patients to purchase products or undergo procedures by misrepresenting the product's value." The point is also made that dentists should not take the manufacturer's word on face value regarding safety and efficacy. Dentists have "an independent obligation to inquire into the truth and accuracy of such claims and verify that they are founded on accepted scientific knowledge or research." Finally, the Code cautions dentists to "disclose to their patients all relevant information the patient needs to make an informed purchase decision, including whether the product is available elsewhere and whether there are any financial incentives for the dentist to recommend the product that would not be evident to the patient."

Considering these conflicting views about selling commercial products in the dental office, what would you recommend that Dr Sanchez do? If the product were not related to general health, but to oral health—such as electric toothbrushes—would it make any difference? What about products such as tooth-whiteners, whose contributions to oral health are questionable? Finally, does the ADA's position adequately deal with any ethical problems that might exist?

Dr Homoly's strategy for improving income in Case 20 is more ambitious. He is not merely urging dentists to sell a product like a vitamin line; he is advising that, by adopting sophisticated marketing techniques to control the image and style of the office, one can significantly increase sales. He is offering entrepreneurship in its most developed form.

The dominant view within the profession, especially among those focusing on ethics, is sure to be suspicion of those who would convert the profession into a business, even an elegant business. But is there anything to be said for entrepreneurship? Even the business model is not without its ethics. Dishonest practices are condemned just as they are within a profession. Businesses also talk about social responsibility. The AMA confronted the tension between business and professional models in the early 1990s when it found that many physicians were entering business arrangements with entrepreneurs to own the laboratories and imaging centers to which they would refer their patients—in effect, engaging in self-referral.[15] In examining how to respond, the AMA found that many members supported ownership arrangements. They also discovered that some ethicists even found virtue in the fact that acknowledging that some physicians saw themselves as business-people might prompt health care professionals to admit to interests other than serving the patient, and that this might make patients have more realistic expectations of what can be expected in the relationship. Can a similar case be made for dentistry, or should the practices promoted by Dr Homoly and to Dr Sanchez be condemned as destroying the profession?

Another dimension of the tension between professionalism and entrepreneurship arises in advertising, as is illustrated by the following case.

Case 21: Advertising: An Outdated Issue?

Your Beautiful Smile . . .

The Wonders of Cosmetic Dentistry

Do you feel self-conscious about your smile?

Do you have . . .

- spaces between your teeth?
- stains?
- chipped teeth?
- silver fillings?
- crowded teeth?

Do you want to improve your smile? Modern dentistry can work wonders. For example, now you can close spaces between teeth and fix crooked or chipped teeth to provide a nicer, less self-conscious smile. You can whiten teeth for a more youthful and healthy look. Cosmetic dentistry doesn't only make you *look* better, it makes you *feel* better.

DISCUSSION:

In 1975, the US Supreme Court decided that certain professions were no longer exempt from antitrust laws. A direct consequence of that judgment was the Federal Trade Commission's (FTC's) subsequent ruling that restrictions on advertising by any profession constituted an unfair monopoly that obstructed free competition.

Instantaneously, the practice of advertising deemed unethical by dentists became ethical, or at least legal in the eyes of the FTC. The response from dentistry and other professions was a grassroots outcry that advertising denigrated their professions and sent signals to the public that professionals were more interested in selling than service. It has been many years since the FTC's decision, however, and the attitudes of younger members of professions are not the same as those of their predecessors. Advertising is now an established fact of life, and many practitioners take it in stride. Still, the ADA, in its Principles of Ethics and Code of Professional Conduct, devotes several pages to the issues of advertising. It accepts the FTC's view and now focuses on condemning advertising that is false and misleading—a morally uncontroversial application of the principle of veracity that is consistent with FTC views.

Despite the ADA's expressed uneasiness about lack of truthfulness, it is our observation that the issue does not excite most members of the profession. Nevertheless, concerns continue to be expressed. For example, Welie et al state that

> [a]dvertising is morally problematic because it assumes a commercial rather than professional model of dentistry. The client seeking the best bargain knows that he must beware; he knows the seller will try to maximize her own profits. This is part of the game of free market trading. Advertising is one of the tricks used by sellers to lure buyers, preferably away from other sellers. Advertising by dentists likewise fosters competition among dentists rather than a sense of joint responsibility for the quality of professional dental care.[16]

Thus, there is a conflict between the FTC's assertion that patients are well served by having greater choices and Welie et al's concern that commercialization is overriding professionalization. Part of what is at stake is perhaps a conflict over how we will understand the role of the dentist in the future. For those who accept the idea that the dentist is an entrepreneur and that patients are served by this more realistic, businesslike image of a dentist, the FTC position will be attractive. For those who want to retain the ideals of a profession, including the claim that its members are altruistic, devoted to patient welfare, and above the world of business, adopting the business mentality will seem counterproductive.

Many practitioners seem not to be concerned about advertising. Is this simply because its critics are wrong—there is no harm? Would patients be better off if dentists openly acknowledged they had become businesspeople adopting business practices, including advertising, or is there so much commercialization of dentistry that advertising and the change in status it implies are just not recognized as problems? If you had it in your power to reverse the FTC ruling, would you do so?

The commercialization of dentistry finds expression in another form, the close cooperation between business corporations and dental education, of which the next case is an example.

Case 22: Corporate Funding of Orthodontic Programs

In 2003 the ADA Commission on Dental Accreditation gave initial accreditation to a new program in orthodontics and dentofacial orthopedics at Jacksonville University in Florida. A complaint filed by the American Association of Orthodontists based on a possible conflict of interest caused by the program's corporate funding was rejected. As a result, Jacksonville was permitted to proceed with the process of developing its program, including the recruitment of students. A similar proposal is being considered at the University of Colorado, where, as of this writing, an application for initial accreditation is being prepared.

Both programs would be funded by the same organization, the Orthodontic Education Company (OEC), the managing partner of which is a dentist, Dr Gasper Lazzara. In the case of the Colorado program, for example, OEC would commit $92.7 million over a period of 30 years, along with a $3 million donation that would support a new section of the dental school named after Dr Lazzara. The OEC would provide stipends and scholarships for most of the trainees (in Colorado's case, 12 of 16) in return for the funding. After graduation, these individuals would be committed to practice for 7 years at one of the various OEC locations around the country.

The stated rationale is to help meet the national shortage of orthodontists, certainly an important issue given the current acute shortage of funding for dental education in general. In addition, it will offer orthodontic treatment to low-income children at reduced fees. This is the first example of corporate funding for a dental specialty program.

Several concerns have been expressed about the programs. Despite the ability of the professionals at Jacksonville and Colorado to plan a program that meets the standards of the Commission on Dental Accreditation, many people are still worried about what the unforeseen effect of a for-profit organization might be on specialty education, including the selection of residents.

DISCUSSION:

Here the entrepreneurship of a dentist, Dr Gasper Lazzara, and his company, the OEC, penetrates not merely the dentist's office, as in the previous cases, but dental academia as well. The benefits to both the company and the schools seem apparent, assuming that ultimate performance matches stated expectations, the benefit to those patients who will eventually need orthodontics also seems evident. From one school alone, 16 new specialists a year will become available. Arrangements have even been made to ensure that the needy are treated at reduced fees.

So where is the moral controversy? Discussion could focus on at least three levels. First, it stands to reason that the students in this program will not be learning to use any particular manufacturer's equipment and supplies. Presumably, however, they will be training to participate in the OEC's programs and will undoubtedly be oriented to them. After 7 years of service to the company, they will be free to practice wherever they wish and in whatever manner they choose.

Second, with its investment, the OEC will buy image and advertising that are priceless. The company will be closely associated in the eyes of students, practicing dentists, and the public with academic dentistry and the credibility it brings.

Third, the relationship raises more abstract issues about the compatibility of a profession and a business. If the cases in this section are any indication, dentistry is blurring the boundaries between business and professional roles. This case seems to escalate that integration at the institutional level. On balance, is this good or bad for dentistry?

Personal Relationships with Patients

In addition to relationships with business, dentistry also encounters ethical controversy at a more personal level. Inevitably, dental professionals will have opportunities to develop personal relationships with patients, sometimes with trepidation and uncertainty, as in the following case and in Case 25, and sometimes with the dental professional's support, as in Case 24.

Case 23: Romantic Entanglement?

Dr Stephanie Meadows had graduated from dental school almost 5 years earlier and was earnestly building her solo practice and her reputation as an excellent dentist who was active in her community of 75,000 people. Her profession was very important to her, and she took its responsibilities very seriously. She had little time left over for anything else, including the development of personal relationships with men.

Thus, she was surprised when she found herself becoming attracted to one of her long-time patients, John Anderson. They talked about little other than the usual patient-dentist topics, but she sensed that they had common interests and similar viewpoints. He, too, was unmarried.

Dr Meadows began to think that she would like to get to know him better—perhaps have dinner with him—and she sensed that he had the same feeling. However, she believed strongly that dentists should avoid romantic entanglements with their patients. She wondered how to handle her unexpected interest, or if it would be better to ignore it completely.

Case 24: The Dating Game

Dr Jack Draper is a general dentist in a large group practice. He went to Dr Alan Madison, his friend and one of the other partners, for some confidential advice. Dr Draper said that he was currently dating one of his patients and wanted to marry her. The problem was that he had previously been involved with a different patient who was now threatening to "make a stink" if he did not marry her instead. During the course of their conversation, Dr Draper acknowledged dating and having sexual relations with a number of his patients, including the one who was making a fuss. He was upset by the mess he was in but thought that he had done nothing wrong. He felt that because he was an eligible bachelor, there was nothing wrong in having "looked everywhere" for a suitable spouse.

Dr Madison was troubled by his friend's predicament and considered what he should do.

DISCUSSION:

These cases involve several important issues, both with respect to relationships with patients and, in Case 24, loyalty toward colleagues. In the first of these cases, Dr Meadows wonders whether to take the initiative to start a personal relationship. The case would end gracefully if she decided not to pursue her interest in her patient but would become more problematic if she decided to try to further her relationship with him. Dr Draper's case is even more complicated. He has dated several patients, and at least two of the relationships have become quite serious. What happens as a result of the discussion between Dr Draper and Dr Madison could affect many people, including other dentists in the practice.

Problems involving interactions among members of the profession are considered in the next section and in chapter 14. The primary focus for discussion here is whether Dr Draper's social activities have moral implications for patients.

Quite apart from any moral reasons why dentists should not date their patients, there are practical reasons for not doing so. What happens if the relationship breaks up? Can the dentist and patient then continue with their formal professional relationship? One way some dentists handle the situation is to refer a patient who he or she intends to date to another dentist.

If these dentists referred all such patients, would it then eliminate any ethical problems in these cases? Health professionals who have relationships with patients, like professors who have relationships with students, stand in positions of authority. The patient is almost inevitably vulnerable. The one in authority risks abusing his or her position of authority to gain social and sexual benefits. This has led to a traditional consensus that such personal relationships with patients must be avoided. If these dentists' actions become known, as Dr Draper's would-be fiancée has threatened, other patients in the practice might be adversely affected. Patients, both men and women, might view the dentist's behavior not as an expression of normal behavior in young people, but rather as a pattern of risk-taking and disregard for others. They might wonder whether these dentists might be disposed to take advantage of them in other ways. In addition, there is a possibility that the objects of their attentions themselves might be harmed. At least one other patient in Dr Draper's case, previously similarly situated, views herself as maligned. Even from the clinical standpoint, the lack of objectivity that comes with intimacy could affect the doctors' judgment. All of these concerns stand behind the widely held view that such relationships should be avoided.

In its 2004 revision of its Principles of Ethics and Code of Professional Conduct,[4] the ADA stated that, "[d]entists should avoid interpersonal relationships that could impair their professional judgment or risk the possibility of exploiting the confidence placed in them by a patient." This was the first revision of the ADA document that contained such an admonition, and even this version was not very explicit. However, even when the ADA had no provision in its Code, state boards of dentistry repeatedly sanctioned dentists for having sexual relationships with their patients.

The movement toward greater equality of status between health professionals and their patients has begun to provide a basis for raising doubts about this traditional prohibition. If the moral problem stems from the authority a professional holds over a patient who is vulnerable, then leveling the status of the parties might mitigate the risks. One of the authors of this text, for example, knows two professionals (a physician and a professor) who had relationships with their counterparts and ended up marrying them. Both professionals handled the matter in a way that earned the author's respect. However, even those who reject the consensus recognize that there are serious dangers.

A significantly different problem in personal relations with patients arises in the following case.

Case 25: Get Out of the Kitchen!

Dr Barbara Sanderini graduated from dental school, completed a general practice residency, and became an associate in an urban practice owned by Dr Tamara Baker. Everyone in the practice was female, including the support staff and the two other associates.

The salary was good, but after about 6 months, Dr Sanderini concluded that it was a mistake to have joined the practice. Dr Baker was a gruff woman in her 50s with poor social skills that affected both patients and employees. An atmosphere of tension and hostility permeated the office, and the associates responded by becoming increasingly isolated. In addition, the support staff was poorly supervised and patient records were a mess. One of the hygienists, Dawn Davis, was a young, attractive woman whose most noteworthy characteristic was her success in finding ways to avoid work—unless it involved opportunities to flirt with young, attractive male patients. Dr Sanderini found Ms Davis's behavior repulsive.

By chance, however, Dr Sanderini and Ms Davis found something about which they agreed. Ms Davis was walking past Dr Sanderini's operatory at the moment a male patient made provocative observations about Dr Sanderini's sexuality. Later, Ms Davis told Dr Sanderini that she had had the same experience with that patient repeatedly over several years. Furthermore, during the last visit, his transgressions had involved some touching. This patient was notorious for the same behavior with other members of the staff.

The patient's sexual innuendoes continued during his next visit to Dr Sanderini. By this point, Dr Sanderini was very annoyed. She spoke with Ms Davis, and they both agreed that the patient's behavior had to stop.

Together they went to see Dr Baker, who listened to them unsympathetically and did not take them seriously despite their complaints about how the patient affected the entire office. Instead, Dr Baker clearly believed that Ms Davis had deserved what she got because of her provocative behavior, and she implied that Dr Sanderini belonged in the same category. Dr Baker saw no reason to confront the patient and refused to say anything to him; if

Dr Sanderini and Ms Davis had a problem with a patient, they needed to deal with it themselves. She summed up her reaction to their complaints by saying, "If you can't stand the heat, get out of the kitchen!"

DISCUSSION:

This case presents two levels of moral dilemma. First, what should Dr Sanderini and Ms Davis do and what would be a proper response from Dr Baker, their employer? And, second, what should happen when the dentist-employer gives an entirely inappropriate response?

The dental hygienist and the dentist have developed an appropriate first response. After diverting the patient's undesired attention, they present the issue to their employer. The most obvious, proper response would be to remove the patient from the practice. His pattern of totally unacceptable behavior is persistent and involves at least two members of the office staff. The only issue is whether Dr Baker owes the patient the normal courtesy of referring him to a colleague. Of course, if she does refer and the colleague has female staff, she is simply setting them up for comparable abuse.

The easiest strategy might be to attempt to identify a colleague with a male hygienist if one is available, but that may simply divert the patient's attention to other office staff, who will almost certainly be women. This raises the question of whether, if there is no referral possible without imposing an offensive patient on the staff of a colleague, dismissing the patient without referral would be morally acceptable. Of course, the dentist retains the right to terminate relationships with patients for various reasons. This is certainly an appropriate reason, but normally the ethics of such terminations at the dentist's initiative includes a requirement for an appropriate referral. A strong case can be made that grounds such as sexual harassment of staff would justify an exception to the duty to make a referral, but that may not turn out to be satisfactory. The patient seems to understand the value of dental hygiene and would probably seek out another dentist on his own, leaving the staff of some unknowing dentist vulnerable to similar abuse.

One issue here is whether—given the seriousness of the patient's actions—the dentist's general duty to work for the good of a patient applies under those circumstances. If it does, a properly motivated dentist might consider an alternative—having a stern and specific conversation with the patient. She might also consider taking the dental hygiene task on herself, presenting perhaps a less attractive target for the patient. However, that might simply leave other staff vulnerable if the patient continues to return to the office.

In this case, however, the dentist was not motivated to take her employees' complaint seriously. That is a serious failure, probably a violation of the law. In such a case, the employees would be well within their rights to quit and seek employment elsewhere, but that may not be feasible. They may need to work in this location or may fear they will be unable to find another position. In that case, they will need to consider the avenues available to respond to a dentist whose behavior is grossly inadequate. They might explore options with the other sympathetic staff, call the dentist on the inappropriateness of her behavior, seek support from their respective professional associations, or, if the matter is not resolved, take legal action. These options are explored further in the cases in chapter 14.

Loyalty to Colleagues

The previous case involved problems of trust in relationships between a dental professional and a patient and also between two dental professionals. Fidelity also raises questions in relationships between dentists. There has long been a sense of a professional bond between members of a profession. In the days when health professionals were exclusively men, the image of a brotherhood was used. In fact, oaths such as those attributed to Hippocrates are sometimes interpreted as oaths of initiation into a brotherhood.

It is important to ask exactly what this bond of loyalty to colleagues implies ethically, especially when it comes at the expense of patients. For example, dentists have sometimes felt obligated to protect colleagues who are incompetent, impaired, or otherwise substandard in their practice. Over and against this tendency, however, is a sense of professional duty to protect patients by reporting colleagues who provide substandard care.

In addition, problems involving loyalty to colleagues are made worse by the lack of communication. The following case demonstrates such a predicament.

Case 26: Lack of Communication Between Dentists

A general practitioner referred a patient who required molar endodontics to Dr Roger Green, an endodontist. Dr Green treated the tooth without complication and sent the patient back to the generalist.

Six months later Dr Green heard that the treatment on the tooth had failed and that the general practitioner had recommended that the tooth be extracted. The patient agreed and the tooth was removed.

Dr Green was disturbed by what had happened. When endodontic treatment fails, as it occasionally does, the tooth usually can be retreated. He wondered why the generalist had not contacted him about retreatment and why the generalist had recommended extraction. Dr Green considered calling the generalist to see what had happened.

DISCUSSION:

The general practitioner has left the impression in Dr Green's mind that he was dissatisfied with Dr Green's work. Moreover, the generalist went ahead and recommended extraction without further consultation. One can imagine why Dr Green would be distressed by these events. His competence has been challenged both by the generalist's recommendation to have the tooth extracted without further consultation and the patient's decision to do so. In the context of professional collegial relations, the issues are what the generalist owes Dr Green and what Dr Green should do.

In analyzing the case, it is important to keep in mind the other party in the relationship: the patient. Given the discussion of the morality of confidentiality, the generalist may discover that the patient wants nothing further to do with Dr Green, if, for example, the patient feels Dr Green's approach was inappropriate or that Dr Green was incompetent.

The principle of fidelity requires loyalty in this case to the patient as well as to Dr Green. This suggests that before the generalist says anything about the patient's dissatisfaction, he should discuss with the patient whether to communicate the failure to Dr Green. On the other hand, communication of the generalist's own views may not involve the patient. This suggests that the generalist could call Dr Green. And if that were to happen, what should the generalist say to Dr Green?

In addition, Dr Green could, of course, take the initiative to call and ask about the patient and the report that he had heard. This possibility brings up a related confidentiality issue. Someone apparently told Dr Green about the patient's outcome. Was there a violation of confidentiality that led to Dr Green's learning about the problem in the first place?

Although the endodontic failure may have been completely unrelated to inadequate treatment, there is a possibility in this case that the endodontist lacked competence or at least that the generalist believed this to be true. We looked at the case, in part, from the point of view of the endodontist and asked whether he had a right to be told about the failure. More often the problem arises from the point of view of the dentist who is convinced that a colleague is not practicing adequate dentistry. In chapter 14 we discuss in detail cases in which dentists are suspected of lacking competence, being dishonest, or being impaired. Many of these cases, like those presented in this chapter, focus primarily on the principle of fidelity.

Conclusion

This chapter and the three chapters that follow discuss four ethical principles—fidelity, autonomy, veracity, and justice—that are believed by many people to help determine whether actions or practices are morally right or wrong. Defenders of these principles see them as morally relevant regardless of consequences. These principles signal elements of actions or practices that would make them right "if other things were equal." Thus, according to their defenders, they are prima facie right-making characteristics of actions. By contrast, a pure consequentialist would treat only the consequences of an action or practice (the principles of beneficence and non-maleficence) as relevant to determining whether an action or practice is right.

References

1. Ramsey P. The Patient as Person: Explorations in Medical Ethics. New Haven, CT: Yale University Press, 1970.
2. Kant I. Groundwork of the Metaphysic of Morals. Paton HJ (trans). New York: Harper and Row; 1964.
3. Ross WD. The Right and the Good. Oxford, England: Oxford Press, 1939.
4. American Dental Association Council on Ethics, Bylaws and Judicial Affairs. Principles of Ethics and Code of Professional Conduct, with advisory opinions revised to January 2004. Chicago: American Dental Association, 2004.
5. May WF. Code, covenant, contract, or philanthropy. Hastings Cent Rep 1975;5:29–38.
6. Veatch RM. The case for contract in medical ethics. In: Shelp EE (ed). The Clinical Encounter: The Moral Fabric of the Patient-Physician Relationship. Dordrecht, Holland: D. Reidel, 1983:105–112.
7. Masters RD. Is contract an adequate basis for medical ethics? Hastings Cent Rep 1975;5:24–28.
8. Edelstein L. The Hippocratic Oath: Text, translation and interpretation. In: Temkin O, Temkin CL (eds). Ancient Medicine: Selected papers of Ludwig Edelstein. Baltimore: Johns Hopkins University Press, 1967:6.
9. British Medical Association. Confidentiality & Disclosure of Health Information, 14 October 1999. Available at: http://www.bma.org.uk/ap.nsf/Content/Confidentiality+and+disclosure+of+health+information#Disclosurewithoutconsentinthe. Accessed 13 Apr 2004.
10. American Medical Association Judicial Council. Current Opinions of the Council on Ethical and Judicial Affairs of the American Medical Association: Including the Principles of Medical Ethics and Rules of the Council on Ethical and Judicial Affairs. Chicago: American Medical Association, 2002.
11. Homoly P. Look before you leap: Minimizing dental insurance. In: Isn't It Wonderful When Patients Say "Yes": Case Acceptance for Complete Dentistry. Charlotte, NC: PennWell, 2001: 329–340.
12. Ecenbarger W. How honest are dentists? Reader's Digest 1997;50–56.
13. Gallup G (ed). Gallup Poll: Public Opinion 2001. Wilmington, DE: Scholarly Resources, 2002.
14. Christensen GJ. The credibility of dentists. J Am Dent Assoc 2001;132:1163–1165.
15. Conflicts of interest. Physician ownership of medical facilities. Council on Ethical and Judicial Affairs, American Medical Association. JAMA. 1992;267:2366-2369.
16. Welie JVM, Simpson M, Westerman GH. The troubled history of dental advertising. Part 4: Ethical reflections. Bull Int Dent Ethics Law Soc 2002;2.2:8–11.

chapter 8

Autonomy and Informed Consent

In this chapter

- The Critical Concepts
- Consent and Competent Patients

- Autonomous Choices and Incompetent Patients
- Provider Autonomy

Cases

The cases in chapter 6 involved disputes over what constitutes the good of the patient, how that good relates to possible harms for the patient, and how the good of the patient relates to the good of others. Chapter 7 added the principle of fidelity—the first of the principles that identifies right-making characteristics of actions other than consequences. In this chapter we consider an additional principle, the principle of autonomy.

In contemporary health professional ethics, it is often debated whether the patient (and sometimes other parties) should have a right of action grounded in self-determination or autonomy.

The Critical Concepts

The Concept of Autonomy

Autonomy is an important term in contemporary professional ethics. It is both a psychological and moral term. From the psychological standpoint, people are said to be autonomous if they live according to their own freely chosen life plans. However, as discussed in chapter 4, virtually no one is either entirely autonomous or completely without autonomy all of the time. It is therefore preferable to speak of "substantially autonomous" or "substantially nonautonomous" people who function along a continuum of capability in the performance of autonomous acts.

From the moral standpoint, we can also make moral judgments about whether it is right or wrong for people to act autonomously. In chapter 4 we discussed the view that it is morally right to respect the choices or actions made by people who are generally psychologically autonomous. Those who hold this view are, at least to some degree, committed to the moral principle of respect for autonomy. However, it is also possible to hold that even if a person's action is autonomous, there is no moral obligation to respect that autonomy

One reason we might espouse the principle of autonomy is the belief that people often know how to maximize their own welfare better than anyone else. In situations where the patient and dentist disagree about what is best for the patient, if we wanted to maximize patient welfare and believed that the patient knew his or her interests better than anyone else, then we might want to respect the patient's autonomous choices.

It seems unreasonable to assume, however, that substantially autonomous people always make choices that maximize their own welfare; surely, even they make some mistakes. They may be confused about the facts, miscalculate the implications of their choices, or even be uncertain about what they really value. Moreover, substantially autonomous people may sometimes purposely subordinate their own good for the good of others. They may sacrifice their interests for those of their children, spouse, or friends or even for strangers. They may even act on impulse.

It is here that the principle of autonomy emerges as a truly independent moral principle separate from a device to maximize patient welfare. As we saw in chapter 7, many people believe that there are independent determinants of morally right and wrong actions other than considerations of maximizing benefits and minimizing harms. Individuals with these views hold that principles such as respect for autonomy can sometimes make an action right even if it produces less than the best possible outcome. In the cases presented in this chapter, dentists face the problem of whether they should respect the autonomy of patients and other decision-makers even if they are convinced that a substantially autonomous person is making a choice that will not produce the best possible consequences. Those who believe there is some moral reason to respect autonomy, even when doing so will not lead to the best possible consequences, are in one way or another defenders of a truly independent principle of autonomy.

Paternalism

Paternalism is often presented as the opposite of respect for autonomy. There are, however, many reasons why we might attempt to override autonomy. For example, we might force treatment on a person with an infectious disease. The moral claims of other parties might supersede that person's autonomy. Almost everyone believes that, at least in extreme cases, it is sometimes morally acceptable to compel behavior in order to protect others. This reveals that respecting autonomy is not automatically the right thing to do.

What, however, of cases in which we think that by compelling the behavior of a substantially autonomous person we can improve that person's welfare? Paternalism is the view that it is sometimes ethically acceptable to engage in such an act for the good of the individual who is being compelled. The philosophical literature attempts to delineate the criteria for more or less acceptable paternalism.[1,2] For an action to be labeled paternalistic, it must be against the wishes of the person being compelled but for his or her welfare. Even staunch paternalists would concede that, for paternalism to be justified, it must be expected to do more good for the one being compelled than if the person were permitted to act on his or her own. This must be true even taking into account the psychological harm of the compulsion.

Much of the current literature on justifiable paternalism stops at this point. There is an additional minimal criterion, however, that would seem to be necessary even from the point of view of a defender of paternalism. It could be called the *due process criterion of paternalism*, and it is especially important in the clinical professions. We can imagine a clinician who becomes convinced that his or her patient would be better off by being coerced into having a dental procedure rather than autonomously refusing the procedure. Despite the dentist's conviction (even taking into account the psychological harm of the coercion), there is still a serious risk that the dentist has miscalculated. He may, as we saw in chapter 6, overvalue certain dental goods or certain kinds of dental goods. He may simply have a strange or unusual set of values. For these reasons, the due process criterion would seem to be applicable. Under this criterion, the one doing the coercing must be publicly authorized to coerce and must undertake careful procedures to ensure that the calculation of the patient's good is not biased. For this reason, it could be argued that no private citizen, even a health professional, has the right to act paternalistically.

But what about paternalistic intervention for individuals who are not substantially autonomous? Some would hold that such interventions are not truly paternalistic because there is no autonomy to violate. Thus, they would say, we cannot act paternalistically against small children, the severely retarded, or the mentally incompetent.

However, individuals may have conditions such as serious illness or depression that compromise their autonomy. When treatment is provided for these individuals against their wishes, we sometimes use the term *weak paternalism* to describe that action. The term is also used to refer to a temporary paternalistic action to hold an individual long enough to determine whether he or she is acting in a substantially autonomous manner[3,4]—such as temporarily restraining someone who is attempting suicide but who appears not to be acting autonomously. Weak paternalism is usually easier to justify than is *strong paternalism,* that is, paternalism against an individual who is known to be substantially autonomous.

Informed Consent

Informed consent is closely linked in medical morality to the principle of respect for autonomy. Informed consent results from giving a patient the relevant information needed to authorize or refuse a proposed course of therapy (or research) and enabling him or her to make a choice about the intervention.[5–8] Informed consent may be advocated as a way of maximizing the welfare of the patient. If the patient is more likely than anyone else to know his or her own interests, informed consent could be a strategy for maximizing benefit.

Yet the principle of respect for autonomy provides a more powerful foundation for the practice of obtaining consent. If the principle of autonomy requires that people be given a chance to be self-determining, then informed consent would be morally required, even if it turns out not to be necessary to maximize the patient's welfare. The following cases all pose problems related to respecting autonomy and obtaining an adequately informed consent. In the first cases, we explore issues involving patients who are arguably competent to consent or refuse consent. Then we look at cases involving surrogate consent for incompetent patients. Finally, we examine the question of whether the dental professional also is entitled to respect for his or her autonomy when the patient asks for a treatment that the professional does not want to provide.

Consent and Competent Patients

Questions of informed consent arise in a most straightforward way with patients who are substantially autonomous. In legal terms, we look first at patients who are, or at least may be, competent to make their own decisions. Dentist Allen Hirsch and philosopher Bernard Gert have provided a framework for assessing the competence of patients.[9] They point out that competence should not be regarded as a "global characteristic"; that is, people may be competent for some decisions and not for others. Even in dentistry, a patient may be capable of understanding some choices— whether to use local anesthesia for a restoration—but incompetent to understand others, such as whether full-mouth extraction is necessary. The criterion for competence suggested by Hirsch and Gert is whether the patient is capable of understanding and appreciating the information that is being conveyed during the consent process. This means that competence cannot be assessed solely on the basis of the plausibility of the patient's decision. A patient's decision may be unusual, but nevertheless one that he or she understands and that fits with his or her life patterns. On the other hand, a decision by a patient that in the dentist's view is the best one may be made without real understanding. The first decision would be made competently; the second would not.

Determining the Competency of Patients

Hirsch and Gert distinguish between what they call fully competent, partially competent, and incompetent patients. However, no human, no matter how well informed and how intelligent, will "fully" understand all choices, whereas people we call incompetent can nevertheless understand some choices.

The first case poses the problem of how the dentist should assess the patient's capacity to make choices.

Case 27: How Far Do Obligations Go?

The Jones family had been patients of Dr Marianne Foster for many years. Mr Jones was now deceased, and the two children, Thomas and Nancy Jones (ages 27 and 24), still received their dental care from Dr Foster. On their mother's behalf they asked Dr Foster to see their mother for pain in the mandibular left quadrant. Mainly, however, they wanted Dr Foster to know that their 54-year old mother had a problem with alcohol and drug abuse.

At the time of the appointment, Mrs Jones said that the pain continued. Dr Foster examined her but found no conclusive source of the pain. The only dubious possibility was a molar with a defective restoration. Dr Foster replaced the restoration and prescribed 15 tablets of Darvocet for the pain.

After a few days, Mrs Jones called to say that the pain persisted and requested more Darvocet. Dr Foster refused and referred her to an oral surgeon for further diagnosis.

The oral surgeon essentially found nothing except the possibility of alveolitis associated with a small idiopathic bone cyst. The surgeon recommended no treatment. Mrs Jones requested more Darvocet from Dr Foster, who continued to refuse.

A referral to a second oral surgeon resulted in the removal of the idiopathic bone cyst. Mrs Jones's pain persisted, and she again called Dr Foster, who again refused to prescribe more Darvocet.

Dr Foster had been in contact with Mrs Jones's family throughout this entire disturbing episode. They were extremely concerned about Mrs Jones because she had steadfastly refused to get treatment for her alcohol and drug abuse. Dr Foster wondered what else she could do and how far her obligations to Mrs Jones should go.

DISCUSSION:

Assuming for the moment that Mrs Jones is mentally competent, are there any ethical problems raised by Mrs Jones's actions? For example, if she is competent and acting autonomously, is there any argument against her right to refuse the recommendation for substance abuse treatment? Likewise, assuming she is autonomous, does her autonomy give her any right of access to Darvocet? The principle of autonomy, as used in informed consent, normally is seen as giving a right of refusal. It cannot give people the right to demand that health professionals grant access. There is no possible basis for arguing that ethically Mrs Jones has a right to have Dr Foster prescribe a drug that Dr Foster believes is not in Mrs Jones's interest.

If Mrs Jones is assumed to be mentally competent to make her own decisions, what does this imply about Dr Foster's involvement of the family in the case? Her conversations with the family imply that she believes that Mrs Jones is not competent to make her own decisions. Otherwise, Mrs Jones's right of confidentiality would be violated by Dr Foster's discussion of sensitive aspects of the case (such as drug abuse and alcoholism) with her family.

Now we should ask whether Mrs Jones is really a substantially autonomous person. Some people are legally incompetent to consent and refuse consent because they are members of classes legally presumed to be incompetent (such as children). Other people are declared incompetent by the courts. Mrs Jones appears to belong in neither of these groups. While in most cases patients should be presumed competent until it is established that they are not, health professionals have a moral duty, perhaps even a legal one, to assess patients' capacity to make autonomous decisions.[10,11]

If Dr Foster believes that Mrs Jones really lacks the capacity to make autonomous decisions, she cannot rely on Mrs Jones's consent for or refusal of treatment. In some cases, a health professional can obtain such a patient's permission to have a family member act as a surrogate. For instance, a patient in extreme pain may willingly admit he or she is in no condition to deliberate rationally about the risks and benefits of a procedure and may readily authorize the dentist to get consent from a family member. Mrs Jones is not likely to accept such an approach, however. If Dr Foster really believes Mrs Jones is not competent but is unwilling to admit it, then she may have to seek to have Mrs Jones declared such—admittedly an extreme action. The alternative is to treat her as competent. If the principle of autonomy prevails, then Mrs Jones's refusal of treatment would have to be accepted.

The Standards for Consent

Once we determine whether a patient is to be treated as competent, we must establish what we have to tell the patient (or surrogate decision-maker for the incompetent patient) for a consent to be adequately informed. To do this, we need a standard of reference. Previously the assumed standard was what is called the *professional standard*. Health professionals, according to the professional standard, had a duty to disclose all information that their professional colleagues similarly situated would have disclosed about the proposed procedure. The problem with the professional standard is that it does not necessarily give patients adequate information that they need to make an informed consent decision. It is possible that for a patient to make a substantially autonomous choice, he or she would need information about treatment alternatives that many dentists normally do not provide. For example, dentists who do not like to use posterior composite resin restorations may not mention them as alternatives to amalgam restorations.

To avoid problems like this, many are now advocating what is called the *reasonable person standard*. According to this standard, the dentist must disclose all information that a reasonable person would find "material" or meaningful in deciding whether to consent to a proposed treatment. The following case illustrates the problem of choosing a standard of reference for deciding what to disclose to patients in the consent process.

Case 28: Informed Consent in Kotzebue

The Indian Health Service operates a two-chair dental clinic in Kotzebue, Alaska, a native village about 30 miles north of the Arctic Circle. One day Dr Eric Walton saw Bobby Yant and his mother, who lived an hour and a half from Kotzebue by plane. The picture was a familiar one. Bobby was 3 years,

7 months old, had nursing-bottle tooth decay, and was in pain. He needed eight pulpotomies and 10 stainless steel crowns. Dr Walton considered what to suggest to Mrs Yant. Ideally, Bobby should have been treated under general anesthesia, but there was no hospital in Kotzebue. Furthermore, it would have been impractical and very expensive to send Bobby hundreds of miles to a larger community that had a hospital. Dr Walton thought that he might be able to treat Bobby without sedation over the course of several visits. However, he knew that Mrs Yant, who had a low-paying job, could not afford to stay in Kotzebue for several days.

Dr Walton had done hundreds of sedation cases, during which he had monitored the patients with a pulse oximeter. His patients had not had any significant problems. However, although he had had some formal training in sedation, it was less than that which was required under current guidelines for the use of deep sedation. Dr Walton knew that with the drugs he must use and their dosage levels, the sedation often entered deeper levels. He called two dentists practicing in Anchorage and Seattle who had served in the Kotzebue clinic prior to his arrival and discussed his dilemma.

All things considered, with the concurrence of his colleagues, and feeling pressure to help Bobby and his mother out of a difficult situation, Dr Walton decided to tell Mrs Yant only about treating Bobby in one visit using sedation.

DISCUSSION:

The first issue here is whether the requirements for informed consent are different in remote areas like Kotzebue, where the combined circumstances of limited resources and problems of geography, weather, and transportation limit treatment options. Is Dr Walton justified in presenting only one option to Mrs Yant? Does the concurrence of Dr Walton's colleagues provide support for his position?

In this case, three major treatment options exist: *(1)* expensive transport to another community, *(2)* treatment locally without sedation, and *(3)* treatment with sedation in a local setting that does not conform to accepted standards for such treatment. Dr Walton could have told Bobby's mother about these options and then, after recommending one course or another, asked her to consent to the recommended one or to propose another. Instead, Dr Walton, with the concurrence of all of the colleagues who knew the situation, decided to present only one option—local, one-visit sedation.

Dr Walton probably contemplated the legal implications of performing the sedation under circumstances that did not conform to current guidelines. That is a matter for him and his lawyer to discuss. He also faces the question of what constitutes an adequate consent in these unusual circumstances. Is it acceptable to present only the course believed by the dentist to be the best, all things considered?

Under the professional standard, Dr Walton should disclose the information (including treatment options) that his colleagues would have disclosed under similar circumstances. He is going to be able to show that his two colleagues who knew the circumstances would have disclosed only the one option. He could probably show that other dentists would have done as he did if they were in such a position. This means he probably could show that, based on the professional standard, he had provided adequate information.

The reasonable person standard requires that he present all of the options that patients in this situation would want to know about before making a choice. It is difficult to speculate how many choices Bobby's mother would have wanted to consider. It is also difficult to demonstrate that Dr Walton would have known in advance that Mrs Yant would have ruled out transport to a community with a hospital that could provide general anesthesia. Mrs Yant may have been contemplating such a trip for other purposes; she may have relatives who could receive Bobby for the therapy and pay his expenses; or she may place great value on that kind of treatment and be willing to go to unusual lengths to get it. It is difficult for Dr Walton or his colleagues to know that Mrs Yant would not have wanted to be informed of that option.

The two local options may not involve significant differences in cost. The choice involves a trade-off of the pain and inconvenience of several visits with the risk of sedation under less-than-ideal circumstances. Even if Mrs Yant would, in the end, have chosen local sedation by Dr Walton, she might have wanted the opportunity to consider the other two options. Under the reasonable person standard, Dr Walton would have to present all three options if reasonable patients similarly situated would have wanted them presented.

The only qualification would be if Dr Walton had reason to believe that Mrs Yant would want a different amount of information than most people would under these circumstances. If he knew that she would, without a doubt, rule out some options (or want to know about other options) then, according to what is called the *subjective standard*, he would have had to give her the information she wanted rather than what the typical reasonable person would want. The reasonable person (adjusted to take into account the subjective, unique interests of the patient) is increasingly seen as the accepted standard for determining if a consent is adequately informed.

The Elements of Consent

After we determine whether the patient is capable of consenting or refusing consent and decide which standard to use in determining what should be disclosed, we then must employ what can be called the *elements of consent*—the specific pieces of information that must be disclosed or discussed with the patient. The recommended procedures for obtaining informed consent are covered in all dental schools as part of clinical competency requirements and will not be discussed in this chapter; they can be found in appendix 2. However, several important ethical issues arise in relation to what the dentist needs to disclose to the patient. These are discussed in the remainder of the chapter and include the following:

1. Treatment alternatives and their risks and benefits
2. Who will perform the treatment and what the charges will be
3. Differing views of treatment options held by other dentists
4. Special interests of the provider or other parties
5. What procedures, if any, are for research purposes

Treatment Alternatives and Their Risks and Benefits

The following cases present consent situations in which dentists must decide what to disclose. Using the professional, reasonable person, and subjective standards discussed in the previous section, what information should these dentists disclose to their patients?

Case 29: What Counts as a Risk?

Ever since the safety of amalgam became a public controversy in the 1990s, a good number of Dr Barnes's patients had raised concerns about the amalgam restorations that he had put in their teeth. They feared that mercury from the restorations might precipitate any number of immunologic disturbances, including multiple sclerosis. Dr Barnes had read as much as he could about this controversy and had concluded that the American Dental Association (ADA) was correct: There was no objective evidence to substantiate these concerns. On the other hand, he personally felt that there might well be a reasonable basis for concern and that there was insufficient evidence to absolutely rule out the possibility that the mercury was a problem.

Dr Barnes was not happy about the prospect of removing the amalgam restorations that he had placed over the years. Amalgam had been in use for more than 100 years and was being improved upon all the time. Furthermore, he felt that the alternative materials, despite significant improvements, were often still less satisfactory than amalgam. He decided to take the position recommended by the ADA. He would remove the amalgam restorations if requested by his patients, but only after a thorough discussion about the problems of the alternatives. He also decided that if a patient raised no concerns, he would not discuss the issue at all. However, the latter decision bothered him. He felt that the absence of definitive evidence of harm did not necessarily certify that the amalgam restorations were completely harmless, either. Dr Barnes began to wonder if he should inform his "quiet" patients about his concerns.

DISCUSSION:

One of the elements of informed consent is an explanation of the treatment options. Thus, Dr Barnes must decide whether to present the alternatives to the use of amalgam. To resolve his dilemma, Dr Barnes can decide whether to follow the professional standard or the reasonable person standard. If he uses the professional standard, it is clear that he could follow the path recommended by the ADA and taken by the great majority of his colleagues.

If he uses the reasonable person standard, it is not as clear what he should do. The question is whether a reasonable person would need to know that: *(1)* there has been recent widespread public discussion about the safety of amalgam restorations, *(2)* the ADA has responded by reaffirming amalgam's safety, and *(3)* while Dr Barnes basically agrees with the profession, he is not totally satisfied that all of the evidence is yet available. Should Dr Barnes discuss the amalgam controversy with his patients, even if they do not mention it? If he relies on the professional standard, he will need to explain only the treatment options that were mentioned by his colleagues. If, however, he adopts the now-preferred reasonable person standard, he will need to determine whether reasonable patients would want the additional information about the treatment options and to provide it if they do.

Who Will Perform the Treatment and What Will the Charges Be

Case 30: Informing Patients About Who Will Perform Procedures

Mrs Dorothy Wolfe was 40 years old, lived in a wealthy suburb of a large midwestern city, and knew that she needed periodontal care. Because she was insured by a major insurance company, she checked her roster of participating periodontists and selected Dr Margaret Wozniack from a list of three.

On her first visit, Dr Wozniack explained that Mrs Wolfe needed extensive scaling and curettage. This would be accomplished in two more visits. The cost would be $75 for the diagnostic visit and $450 for each of the other two visits, for a total of $975. After each visit, Mrs Wolfe paid $225; her insurance would cover the rest.

The treatment went well. However, Mrs Wolfe never saw Dr Wozniack after the initial consultation; the entire treatment was done by the hygienist. This bothered Mrs Wolfe, but she was unsure about the standards of treatment and never complained.

While paying after the last visit, the receptionist said that Dr Wozniack wanted to see Mrs Wolfe in a month for a follow-up visit. Mrs Wolfe agreed. On her return she was pleased that Dr Wozniack actually examined her, checking both her periodontium and her occlusion. As Mrs Wolfe was leaving, the receptionist informed her that she owed $125 for the visit. Mrs Wolfe angrily refused to pay, saying that it was not part of the original treatment plan. She discussed her complaint with the peer review committee of the dental society. The committee chair then called Dr Wozniack to try to arrive at an equitable settlement.

DISCUSSION:

This case raises issues involving the first three elements of an informed consent. Consider first the treatment alternatives. The treatments involved in this case are not terribly unusual. Dr Wozniack may even consider this to be a case where no consent is required. In fact, she did give Mrs Wolfe some information about her proposed treatment plan. She told her she wanted to do scaling and curettage and that it could be accomplished in two visits. She also quoted her a $975 fee. Should Dr Wozniack approach this interaction as one in which she is telling her patient what she is going to do, or as one in which she is proposing a treatment plan to which the patient may or may not consent?

The answer will depend, in part, on whether she perceives the situation as one in which there are alternatives. Are there any alternatives in this case? Could the treatment have been done in a different number of visits? Could additional procedures be done or some omitted? Could Mrs Wolfe have simply decided against the entire plan? Were there significant variations in the technique that would have involved different risks, benefits, discomfort, or costs? Keeping in mind that one possible option for Mrs Wolfe would be to decline all treatment, an argument can be made that the assumption of only one possible course of action is probably unreasonable. If so, Dr Wozniack could propose what she thinks is the best course and attempt to obtain Mrs Wolfe's consent.

There is another option, which Donald Sadowsky calls "multiple prescription dentistry."[12] Dentists can present a number of treatment plans that are within the range of plausibility, each of which might make sense for some patients but not others. The approach is built on the assumption that there is no single, definitive treatment plan that is objectively the best for patients. It might also be used when a dentist recognizes that, even if there is a single "best" course, that course may not be rational for a patient given his or her economic, social, and psychological situation.

Under multiple prescription dentistry, the concept of informed consent as practiced by many dentists does not really apply. To these individuals, informed consent implies that the dentist will first make a choice and then ask the patient to approve it. With the multiple prescription concept, however, if the dentist realizes that there are several possible options or suboptions within reason, he or she may feel compelled to refrain from presuming to know which is best for a particular patient.

Under the professional standard, Dr Wozniack would need to determine what her colleagues would have told Mrs Wolfe. She would need to decide whether they would have mentioned the cost, the follow-up visit, the fact that the hygienist would perform all of the treatment proposed, and any variations in what could be done for Mrs Wolfe. Under the reasonable person standard, Dr Wozniack would have to determine what a reasonable person in Mrs Wolfe's situation would want to know about each of these items.

This case also introduces a second element of informed consent: an explanation of who will perform the procedures. When Mrs Wolfe agreed to the proposed treatment plan, she apparently assumed that Dr Wozniack would perform the procedures and may well have based her judgment about the reasonableness of the cost on that assumption. If someone other than the dentist will perform any of the procedures, the patient has a right to understand that fact. Sometimes it may be obvious, as when a hygienist provides routine scaling and cleaning, but in other cases a patient would have no basis for knowing. An informed consent must include adequate understanding of who will perform all aspects of the care.

Finally, the case introduces a third element of an adequately informed consent: accurate information about the charges. It seems clear that if Dr Wozniack planned to include a follow-up examination in the treatment plan, it should have been disclosed to Mrs Wolfe as part of the overall proposal with the cost included so that she could agree to the total anticipated fee. Only those elements that legitimately could not be anticipated in advance should be added to the treatment plan at a later time. If Dr Wozniack intentionally left out the follow-up visit in order to make the cost seem lower than what was actually expected, consent was surely inadequate.

Differing Views of Treatment Options Held by Other Dentists

Case 31: Should the Sealants Be Done, Too?

Tammy Williams, an 8-year-old patient of Dr Bob Zarnecki, was referred to Dr Joe Corbin, a pediatric dentist, for removal of an abscessed mandibular primary molar. Tammy had become very upset when Dr Zarnecki had attempted local anesthesia. At first he referred her to an oral surgeon for extraction under general anesthesia. However, Tammy's mother, Mrs Williams, refused because her sister had almost died while having extractions under general anesthesia. Dr Zarnecki then referred Tammy to Dr Corbin for the extraction with nitrous oxide conscious sedation, no other treatment being necessary.

Dr Corbin's examination confirmed the presence of a draining abscess. He explained the risks of nitrous oxide and how it differed from general anesthesia. Mrs Williams was still apprehensive and authorized its use only if absolutely necessary.

On the day of the procedure, nitrous oxide was, in fact, necessary. However, the extraction occurred without significant incident. During the treatment Dr Corbin noted that the first permanent molars were deeply grooved and somewhat hypoplastic. They needed sealants. Dr Corbin knew that Dr Zarnecki did not use sealants because he did not think that they worked.

Dr Corbin wondered whether he should tell Mrs Williams that he thought that sealants were highly indicated for Tammy. He knew that if he did, he would most likely offend Dr Zarnecki. Dr Corbin decided to state his views. He explained that sealants have been proven to prevent decay but that not all dentists used them. However, because Tammy was quite fearful of injections, he advised that she have the sealants applied.

DISCUSSION:

Here two different consent issues could be singled out for special attention. First, Dr Corbin needs to determine what information to transmit in regard to treatment alternatives—what he should say about local anesthesia, nitrous oxide, and general anesthesia options. There may be risks that Dr Corbin's colleagues generally do not discuss with patients but that reasonable patients would nevertheless wish to know about. There may be other treatment options or variations on these options that might be disclosed under any of the three standards. It is clear that the risks of general anesthesia and nitrous oxide need to be discussed, but, given Mrs Williams' level of concern, Dr Corbin probably should discuss the use of local anesthesia as well. Local anesthesia for dental procedures is familiar to most people and its successful use is so widespread that it is generally considered safe by the public. Yet, as with any agent, it can cause problems that include toxic effects, allergic reactions, and even death. On the other hand, the toxic effects only occur when local anesthesia is used in excessive quantities; the frequency of any kind of allergic effect is less than 0.0001% and the frequency of death is approximately one death per trillion injections.

How can dentists decide upon the minimal criteria for the discussion of risks? The answer, as suggested by Hirsch and Gert,[9] lies in a combination of the frequency and intensity of the problem. Judgments are made starting with the idea that problems that are rare and inconsequential need not be disclosed. Somewhere on an ascending scale, a possible outcome will be sufficiently frequent and serious that reasonable people need to know about it. In the case of local anesthesia, it is generally agreed that patients who have not had it before should be told that their soft tissues will feel numb for a couple of hours. At the same time, most dentists feel that because the frequency of serious side effects is very rare, specific discussions of the risks are not necessary. Thus, relying on the professional standard, Dr Corbin probably does not need to disclose them. However, it is still an open question whether the typical patient would want to know about them. Even rare side effects may need to be discussed, especially if the effect is very serious, such as death. A dentist might conclude that a risk of one per trillion is so remote that reasonable patients would not find the information relevant to their decision to consent. Still, Mrs Williams's unusual concern may require disclosure based on the subjective standard.

The second consent issue concerns the sealants. Under the professional standard, the appropriate question is whether other pediatric dentists receiving such referrals would raise the sealant option. Knowing that the referring dentist does not use sealants might dissuade dentists from raising the issue. However, the problem here is that the usual practice does not seem to be the appropriate basis for deciding whether to bring up the sealant topic with Mrs Williams.

Under a reasonable person standard the key question is whether it is likely that a typical reasonable patient (or in this case, reasonable parent) would want to know about the sealants. If so, what would she want to know? It seems quite likely that Mrs Williams would want to know Dr Corbin's opinion that they are "highly indicated." She probably would also want to know that the family's primary dentist disagrees. If Dr Corbin decides that Mrs Williams would want to know about the sealant option, bringing it up could involve an apparent conflict with the ADA's Principles of Ethics and Code of Professional Conduct, which states that only the treatment that is requested by the referring dentist should be performed on referred patients. Because the ADA Code also commits the dentist to working for the patient's welfare, this may be a case in which Dr Corbin must violate one or the other of the Code's provisions. If Dr Corbin thinks the sealants are in Tammy's interest and that Mrs Williams would want to know about the option, he seems duty-bound to bring the subject up.

Special Interests of the Provider or Other Parties

The fourth element of an adequately informed consent is information about special interests that the provider or others might have that might not be apparent to the patient. These might include special financial interests that the dentist has in products or services that he or she is recommending to a patient. A case that involves a decision faced by a dentist about whether to sell "custom vitamins" in her practice is presented in chapter 7 as an issue of fidelity (Case 19). However, it is also relevant to the issues of this chapter with respect to disclosure.

These special—and conflicting—interests include the subtle daily interactions of practicing dentists with their patients, in which recommendations to patients are made under the obligation of beneficence but also materially benefit the dentists. In addition, they include the special interests of dentists who sell commercial products to their patients for profit, own dental laboratories, consult with dental products manufacturers, or invest in pharmaceutical companies.

Increasingly, health professionals are asked to find patients to serve as potential subjects for research projects. Sometimes they are paid "finder's fees" as compensation. The norms of research with human subjects now require that the dentist disclose that he or she is being compensated in these situations.

What Procedures, if Any, Are for Research Purposes

If a dentist is involved in clinical research—either formally, as part of a funded investigation, or informally, to satisfy the dentist's curiosity—informing the patient of which procedures are undertaken for research purposes constitutes an additional element of an informed consent. Some additional problems arise when the consent is for systematic research. In addition to the problems encountered in the previous cases in this chapter, there are special problems of undue influence and conflict of interest. The cases that follow raise some of these issues.

Case 32: The Casa Pia Study of Dental Amalgam Health Effects on Children*

The University of Washington collaborated with the University of Lisbon in Portugal to do a study funded by the National Institute for Dental and Craniofacial Research (NIDCR). The topic of the study was the safety of dental amalgam, a longstanding problem that still had no definitive resolution. Although government panels still recommended the use of amalgam in the absence of good evidence of harmful health effects, they also pointed out that more research on health effects was necessary.

The study was to involve 500 children, ages 8 to 10, in the Casa Pia school system in Lisbon. Eligible children would have dental caries and no previous exposure to amalgam. The children would be randomly assigned to two groups, one of which would receive amalgam for the restoration of large posterior lesions, with alternative materials (mainly composites) used elsewhere. The other group would receive alternative materials for all lesions. Each year, all of the participants would undergo a number of neurobehavioral and neurological tests as well as urinary mercury analyses.

The study was ready to begin when an ethicist on the Data Safety and Monitoring Board expressed concern about the consent process. About 20

*Case provided by Timothy A. DeRouen, PhD, executive associate dean for research and academic affairs and director, Comprehensive Center for Oral Health Research, School of Dentistry, University of Washington.

percent of the Casa Pia students were wards of the state, either because of their status as orphans or because of unstable family situations. For these students, the director of the Casa Pia school system was authorized to give consent—one person for about 170 children!

At first, the investigators considered finding an alternative way to obtain consent for the 20 percent in question. However, the director was a highly respected member of the Lisbon community and to risk insulting his ability to meet this responsibility adequately might have been damaging, both to the director and to the study. Furthermore, the director previously had, in fact, been designated as the children's legal guardian.

The investigators saw this as an important issue because they felt it dealt with the balance between expecting benefits in research on the one hand and the need to protect a potentially vulnerable population on the other.

DISCUSSION:

This case poses several important consent issues. The first is determining which elements of this intervention are research and how to explain that to the parties responsible for the consent. One may view the use of amalgam materials as a current standard practice, so the mere fact that the children in the experimental group would receive amalgam does not constitute research. Alternatively, if the concerns about amalgam were so great that they were no longer classified as standard practice, then they would have to be described as research interventions. Of course, even if the amalgam restorations were considered standard practice, the treatments would still require consent just like any other therapy and the controversy over the risks of amalgam would have to be presented. Determining how to obtain that consent is, as we shall see below, rather complicated in this case. Likewise, the same issue arises with respect to the use of composites, which, like the use of amalgam, also constitutes a standard practice and therefore does not have to be presented as research.

At least two features of these interventions appear to be research—that is, undertaken for the purpose of producing generalizable knowledge. The randomization of children to receive amalgam or composite for their posterior lesions is the first. The subjects and their surrogate, the director of the Casa Pia school system, need to know that they are being assigned at random to a treatment group. This is something that would never be done in routine therapy; it potentially undercuts the clinician's judgment about which of the two materials is preferred in individual cases.

Presenting the risks of these two options is also complex. If amalgam had been questioned (which is the premise that led to the study), then its suspected risks must be presented, but any potential risks of the composite must be presented as well. Labeling any of these risks as "research risks" will depend on whether one considers one or the other treatment a deviation from standard practice.

The second major intervention that is research and must be identified as such is the neurobehavioral and neurological tests and urinary mercury analyses that will occur once the restorations have been placed. Both the students and their surrogate need to know that these procedures are not required for regular therapy.

Even if the investigators can properly identify those interventions that constitute research, they still need to determine whether they have an adequate consent process. Since this study is taking place in Portugal, it must meet all Portuguese requirements. But because the research is being conducted by the University of Washington and is funded by the NIDCR, it must also meet American standards, including approval by the University of Washington institutional review board, which governs all of its research, and by the NIDCR.

The subjects of this study are children between 8 and 10 years of age. They cannot themselves give an adequately informed consent, but they can be expected to give their assent and should be excluded from the study if they refuse. The concepts of consent and assent from minors is discussed in Case 36.

In addition to meeting Portuguese and American standards for consent or assent from the children, adequate consent must also be obtained from the children's parents or surrogate. That is what led to the controversy over the involvement of the director of the Casa Pia school system. As the legal guardian for a portion of the children, he would be the one to give the consent if anyone could. Because the study involves research procedures on patients who cannot themselves give consent and because it involves some potential risks (including the risk of exposure to mercury from the amalgam when other treatment options were available), there is controversy over whether parents or guardians can give consent or permission for their children to enter the study, The American norm is that parents can give permission provided that the risk is related to treatment for a condition from which the children suffer and is only a minor increment above the risks of ordinary life. Because the children have caries lesions and the risk of the amalgam is, at most, minor, the study seems to meet this standard; the parents could give permission if they wanted to.

The problem is more complex for the children in the Casa Pia school system who belong to a particularly vulnerable group—orphans or children otherwise separated from their families. Relying on a surrogate, even a legal guardian, to approve the children's entry into a research project is controversial. Some hold that it is only permissible if the study could not be done on children from intact families. Others hold that it can include vulnerable subjects, provided that other children from intact families are included as well. The safest course would have been to exclude those Casa Pia children who were wards of the state and any others who do not have parental involvement in the consent process.

The Response to Consent and Refusal of Consent

Informing a patient and asking for consent to treat implies that the patient has a right to accept or refuse the suggested treatment plan. Sometimes patients may respond in an unexpected manner; they may refuse to consent to the recommended treatment plan. The following case raises the question of how the dentist should respond to a patient's refusal of treatment.

Case 33: Surgery for a Jehovah's Witness

Mrs Wilma Allen, a 42-year-old single black woman with no dependents who was employed as a secretary, consulted Dr Richard Jaeger, an oral and maxillofacial surgeon, about a large swelling in her left cheek. A panoramic radiograph showed that the sinuses were cloudy. Examination of a biopsy specimen revealed a large amount of dysplastic fibrous tissue, and the lesion was diagnosed as reparative giant cell granuloma. The indicated treatment was surgical removal.

Two complicating factors existed. One was that Mrs Allen had sickle cell disease; her hematocrit was 15, and her hemoglobin was 5.

The other factor was that Mrs Allen was a Jehovah's Witness. Although she had no objection to the surgery, under no circumstances would she consent to receive blood products. Her position was absolutely firm.

Dr Jaeger talked with Mrs Allen about what would happen if nothing was done—the lesion would grow larger and become more disfiguring. He also told her that removing the lesion without her authorization for a transfusion, considering her serious involvement with sickle cell disease, could result in grave consequences, even her death. Even so, Mrs Allen refused to change her mind. Dr Jaeger discussed the matter with members of her church and they all agreed with Mrs Allen.

Mrs Allen was willing to have the surgery done, but Dr Jaeger was extremely reluctant to do it. What should Dr Jaeger do?

DISCUSSION:

The problem with this consent conversation is not in determining what the patient should be told, but in how to respond once the patient has refused what seems to be the treatment that is in her best interest.

The case illustrates a problem we encountered in chapter 6; it may turn out to be very difficult for the dentist to determine exactly what is in the patient's best interest. Here it seems that a blood transfusion would serve Mrs Allen's medical interest, but even that is not obvious. Dr Jaeger does not know in advance how important a transfusion may be. He does know he is dealing with an unusual hematocrit and that, if the worst should occur, he certainly would want to have the transfusion option available.

On the other hand, Mrs Allen's interest may not be exclusively in survival in this world. Jehovah's Witnesses believe, based on scriptural interpretation, that receiving foreign blood excludes them from eternal salvation.[13,14(pp91-105)] Moreover, in some cases, the receipt of blood can lead to terrible psychological sequelae and sometimes social ostracism. From Mrs Allen's point of view, the transfusion really may not be in her best interest.

Even if it were, the case raises the question of whether a substantially autonomous person has the moral and legal right to refuse to consent even if refusal means a risk of death. The law seems clear by now that mentally competent adults, at least those without dependents, have a legal right to refuse lifesaving blood transfusions.[14(pp91-105)] Morally, the matter is more complex. Within her moral framework Mrs Allen surely believes she has the right—indeed the moral duty—to refuse the transfusion.

What about Dr Jaeger's point of view, however? We have seen that from the traditional patient-benefiting perspective, one might argue either way. From the standpoint of autonomy, however, Dr Jaeger should respect Mrs Allen's right of refusal. This respect for autonomy is required by law and widely accepted as the ethically appropriate choice.

What are his options if he decides to honor Mrs Allen's refusal of a transfusion? He could do the surgery and be prepared to use blood substitutes if necessary, a position acceptable to most Jehovah's Witnesses. He could consider obtaining some of Mrs Allen's blood in advance for use in autologous transfusion. In this case, however, he would need to find out if Mrs Allen considered this acceptable. The more difficult question is whether Dr Jaeger could, on grounds of conscience, send her away if she refuses to accept his recommendation for surgery with transfusion if necessary. This issue of provider autonomy is taken up later in this chapter.

Autonomous Choices and Incompetent Patients

The previous case dealt with refusal of treatment by an adult who was presumed to be mentally competent. In other situations the patient is clearly not competent, but someone must still decide what should be done for the patient. The dentist is in a good position to identify a range of plausible options, but as we have seen in previous cases, choices must often be made in which there is more than one acceptable option. In such cases, different people, including different dentists, will choose differently. Other cases involve trade-offs between the dental well-being of the patient and other competing goods. When the patient is clearly incompetent, someone must speak for him or her.

Adults, while they are competent, often designate surrogates through a mechanism called the *durable power of attorney*.[10,15] If the patient has designated a surrogate, that person clearly seems to be the best choice. In extreme cases courts will review the surrogate's choices and overrule them if necessary, but normally the decision of the one so designated for medical choices will prevail.

If no one has been designated, the pattern has increasingly been to assume that the next of kin should make these choices for the incompetent person. For decades, pediatric dentists have assumed that a parent can and should choose among plausible treatment options. Likewise, for senile patients and others who are mentally incompetent, the next of kin assumes the decision-making role. If the next of kin or other surrogate makes a plausible choice, usually no one will question it. However, what if he or she makes an unexpected choice? That issue is raised in the next two cases.

Case 34: The Case of the Vacillating Parent

Dr Joan Smith, a pediatric dentist, was examining Joey Daniels, who at age 2½ was a heavy 31 pounds. Joey had no medical problems, but he had a history of nursing-bottle caries. He was brought in because of continued problems related to that diagnosis. Joey was also proving to be a severe behavior management problem. Examination showed that two maxillary incisors were abscessed, and the caries on the other two were so extensive as to make them virtually unrestorable. Radiographs were impossible to obtain because of Joey's behavior. Dr Smith's customary policy was to orally present a proposed treatment plan, including explanations of risks and alternatives. When she was satisfied that the parent understood and agreed to the proposed treatment, she then proceeded without obtaining written approval.

Dr Smith followed this policy with Joey's mother. She explained to Mrs Daniels that the best choice was the extraction of all four incisors. Although two of the incisors might be saved, it was very unlikely that the restorations would hold up over time. Dr Smith told Mrs Daniels that it would be necessary to give Joey a sedative and prescribed chloral hydrate (60 mg/kg) and Vistaril (1 mg/lb, maximum of 25 mg). She also explained that the effectiveness of the sedative was quite unpredictable and that it only worked well approximately half the time. In any case, it would be necessary to use nitrous oxide to supplement the sedation. Finally, Dr Smith explained that some physical restraint was necessary and that Joey would be wrapped in a blanket (Pedi-Wrap) to keep him from moving. Mrs Daniels seemed to understand the procedures and verbally agreed to the treatment plan. Dr Smith scheduled Joey for an early-morning appointment the following week.

At that appointment, Dr. Smith administered the sedative agents. Then, just as she was ready to anesthetize the teeth, Mrs Daniels said she could only afford the extraction of two teeth and that Dr Smith should remove only the two worst ones. Dr Smith could not believe what she was hearing. Everything was ready, and Mrs Daniels was saying to do only half the treatment. Dr Smith quickly explained the situation and told Mrs Daniels not to worry about the money at this point; something could be worked out. The important thing, Dr Smith said, was that Joey was sedated and should not have to undergo multiple sedations. Mrs Daniels responded by questioning whether all four teeth really needed to be removed, but she finally agreed, and Dr Smith proceeded.

Joey screamed, kicked, moved his head back and forth, and sweated profusely. Even after the Pedi-Wrap was put on, Joey required restraint. Dr Smith administered nitrous oxide and increased it to 50% but saw that it was not helping. She therefore gave 100% oxygen to flush out the nitrous oxide and decided to go ahead as best she could. Mrs Daniels and the dental assistant were also needed to help hold Joey down. Dr Smith anesthetized the teeth, inserted the Molt mouth prop, and extracted all four teeth. The procedure was without incident except that bleeding was difficult to control at first.

Joey was exhausted, and Mrs Daniels was visibly upset, apparently shaken by having witnessed what Joey had to endure. Surprisingly, she paid the entire fee.

Later that morning, Dr Smith received a call from the office manager of a pediatric dental practice located in the general vicinity. Mrs Daniels had called them with a request to be seen because her child was bleeding. She had also told them that Dr Smith had extracted some teeth that did not need to be removed, and she requested a second opinion.

Dr Smith called Mrs Daniels at 1 PM to discuss the situation, including the bleeding problem. She offered to see Joey but explained that some oozing from tooth sockets was normal. During the conversation Mrs Daniels accused Dr Smith of extracting good teeth, while Dr Smith tried to explain that, in fact, they all needed to be removed.

DISCUSSION:

This case raises several related issues: what Mrs Daniels should be told for a consent to be informed, whether there was a valid consent, and, if not, whether Mrs Daniels had a right to insist on a less-than-ideal plan to extract only two teeth.

The first issue is whether Dr Smith told Mrs Daniels what she really needed to know: Even if removing all four incisors was dentally best for Joey, did Dr Smith realistically convey all the options? Two teeth were virtually unrestorable but might have been saved. Mrs Daniels appears to believe that that was a possible dental option. Given her finances, she might have elected that option even though it would leave her son with a questionable outcome. General anesthesia was also a possibility that could have been discussed.

The next problem, assuming there was an adequate disclosure, is whether there was a valid consent. There was no written consent; legally, Dr Smith might have difficulty proving what the understanding was. Legally as well as ethically, what is critical is whether Mrs Daniels really understood her options and agreed to the plan Dr Smith followed. Whether the agreement is in writing may be important for legal purposes, but the meeting of the minds, not the written document, is what is important ethically.

Suppose Mrs Daniels had insisted on the removal of only two teeth and the restoration of the others. Should Dr Smith have insisted on what she thought was the best course dentally? Here the issue is whether Mrs Daniels, as Joey's surrogate, should have the autonomy to make choices comparable to those of competent patients like the Jehovah's Witness who refused a blood transfusion in the previous case. It seems clear that both legally and ethically there is some moral limit on the discretion that a surrogate can have in estimating what is best for incompetent patients. Courts can and do routinely override surrogates in medical cases such as those in which parents attempt to refuse lifesaving blood transfusions for the children.[14(pp129-130)] The issue is whether Mrs Daniels is being unreasonable in the way that we consider the Jehovah's Witness parent is. If so, she could be overridden by a court. Alternatively, we might decide that even though Mrs Daniels's choice does not seem to be what is really best, it is not as questionable as that of parents who risk their children's lives based on religious principle. In many cases parents are permitted to make somewhat unexpected choices that are less than what seems best; the courts do not intervene unless the surrogate's decision is beyond reason.[16,17] Dr Smith, thus, must decide whether she thinks Mrs Daniels's choice is within tolerable discretion or is beyond reason. If she thinks Mrs Daniels is going beyond reason and cannot persuade her to change her mind, Dr Smith's only option would be to seek court intervention to attempt to get Mrs Daniel's decision overruled. Dr Smith still may be left with a situation in which the patient's mother can't pay the bill, but at least she would have done the morally correct thing.

Sometimes, as in the next case, the problem is not one of the limits of the surrogate's discretion, but of who the valid surrogate ought to be.

Case 35: Consent in a Problem of Legal Guardianship

Barbara Fulsome was a 20-year-old woman who was moderately retarded, partially deaf (requiring a hearing aid), and capable only of limited speech. She was otherwise in good health. Barbara had been visiting the hospital dental clinic for many years. Because of a question of neglect, she was often accompanied, as she was in this case, by an assigned social worker.

Dr Brian Jones was newly in charge of the hospital dental clinic. He noticed that the consent form had been signed by Barbara's stepfather. When questioned, the social worker admitted that the stepfather was not Barbara's legal guardian. Legal guardianship was being sought by the state Department of Social Services because of inadequate home care and the fact that Barbara's mother's whereabouts were unknown.

Dr Jones decided to at least perform an examination. It showed an intact permanent dentition with severe periodontal disease. Several posterior teeth had furcation involvement. In addition, the third molars were incompletely erupted, periodontally compromised, and in need of extraction. There was a complete lack of home care, as shown by heavy plaque deposits.

Previous chart entries showed that intramuscular narcotic sedation had been used because of uncooperative behavior. Dr Jones felt its use now would be inappropriate because of the lack of proper consent. The intramuscular sedation had not been very successful anyway.

Another problem was that Barbara would soon turn 21, at which time the social worker's involvement would end. The dental benefits Barbara received through medical assistance would also end, thereafter limiting her to emergency dental care. At that point it was uncertain what her living arrangements would be.

Dr Jones thought that the best plan would be to complete all treatment under general anesthesia in the hospital in one $2\frac{1}{2}$-hour procedure. The treatment would involve the extraction of all periodontally compromised teeth, including the third molars, as well as root planing and the sealing of all other teeth. The social worker assured Dr Jones that the guardianship question would be resolved before Barbara's 21st birthday, a prediction that proved overly optimistic. The social worker therefore suggested that Dr Jones begin the treatment and said that she would accept legal responsibility for Barbara's dental care.

Dr Jones had to decide what to do. He knew that general anesthesia was out of the question because of the consent problem. However, he felt that he could justifiably perform the treatment using a different approach, mainly because if he waited much longer, Barbara would only be eligible for emergency care. Also, without treatment, her periodontal status would worsen and possibly cause acute pain.

DISCUSSION:

Here the problem is whether Barabara's stepfather—or anyone else—has the authority to give consent for her. At age 20, Barbara would be considered an adult capable of offering her own consent, but for her retardation. Had she been declared legally incompetent and a guardian appointed for her, Dr Jones could approach her as an adult who has never been adjudicated to be incompetent in the present case. It is customary to presume incompetence in the case of someone who is clearly incapable of consenting—an unconscious patient or a severely retarded one, for example. This patient is not clearly incompetent, however.

Assuming Barbara's own consent is not acceptable, Dr Jones could decide to go to her next of kin, even though in this case, that person (Barbara's mother) is accused of providing inadequate care. Legally, Barbara's mother is probably still the one with authority to consent or refuse consent for the treatment. Excluding her without court authorization is questionable. Another possibility is that the social worker could assume responsibility. In some jurisdictions, social workers employed by the government's welfare department have the authority to take temporary custody of a minor for purposes of obtaining emergency medical care without the involvement of a neglectful parent. Invoking that authority would give the social worker a basis for consenting on Barbara's behalf. Classifying the intervention as an emergency is a bit of a stretch in this case, but it may be the only way to obtain the needed treatment. Another option would be to attempt to have Barbara's stepfather appointed as her guardian.

This case and the preceding one involved parental decisions about therapy. The issues are more complex when a nonautonomous person—a child or a mentally incapacitated adult—is a potential subject for dental research. The issue arose in Case 32 about the study of amalgam on the children in the Casa Pia school system in Portugal, and it arises again in the next case.

Case 36: Voice Control in Research

Dr Louise Jackman was a pediatric dentist who was working with a periodontist on a project designed to evaluate systemic factors in prepubertal periodontitis, a specific genetic form of early-onset periodontal disease. The subjects were children 4 years of age through adolescence who had bone loss on any location of their primary molars or on the mesial aspects of their permanent first molars and/or central incisors. The protocol called for drawing 25 mL of blood to evaluate certain characteristics of the white cells. Payment of $50 was to be made for the child's participation in the study.

Predictably, some of the children, especially the younger children, did not want their blood drawn and resisted the procedure. However, some of the parents wanted their children to remain in the study and authorized the project personnel to proceed despite the child's protests. Dr Jackman determined that she could gain compliance in almost every case if she used the same behavior management approaches that she would use in a treatment situation, namely, voice control and some restraint. However, she debated whether she was justified in using therapeutic behavior management techniques in a research situation, even when the parent had given permission to do so.

DISCUSSION:

Dr Jackman and her colleague need to obtain some blood for what appears to be an important study. At minimum, Dr Jackman needs to make clear to the parents that the blood is being drawn for research purposes rather than as part of therapy. The parents' consent to have their children participate in the study is an essential requirement, but research also introduces additional complexities.

At least in studies that are unrelated to therapy, the general rule is that in addition to permission from parents, the assent of the child is required. (This same assent would be required in Case 32 about the children from the Casa Pia school system who were part of a study of the risks of amalgam restorations.) Assent is contrasted with consent. Consent implies the capacity of the person giving it to process information and to adequately understand the nature of the choice being made. Assent implies simple approval or disapproval without necessarily having the capacity to make an informed choice. Thus, assent does not require substantially autonomous approval the way consent does. Refusal of assent from a child is common in therapeutic dentistry, but we recognize that if the patient is not autonomous, patient welfare may require that the parent or surrogate override the patient's objection. In research, however, by definition the procedure is not undertaken for the welfare of the patient. In this case, the blood is being drawn for research, not for therapy, so the child's objection cannot be overridden on patient welfare grounds. Normally, the refusal of a child or other incompetent patient is considered sufficient to block participation in such a study.

One central issue in this case is whether the importance of the knowledge to be gained ever justifies overriding a lack of consent or assent. It seems plausible that the knowledge gained from this study will be important, but we normally would not force someone to be a research subject just because the knowledge gained would be of great value. Likewise, we would normally accept an incompetent person's refusal to give assent if the intervention was for research rather than therapy.

Another issue is whether there are alternative ways of conducting this study without overriding the child's refusal. Sometimes investigators can obtain children's blood in a less invasive and troublesome manner, such as by drawing extra blood during a routine clinical blood drawing. That would certainly be preferable to subjecting a child to a needle stick solely for research purposes.

Still another problem raised by this case is whether the parents have a sufficient conflict of interest to justify excluding them from the consent process. Normally we assume that parents can give consent for therapy because they will have the child's welfare in mind. Parental consent is more problematic in research because research is not conducted for the benefit of the child. Still, we assume parents would at least not seriously compromise their child's welfare. In this case, however, the parents seem to have a real conflict of interest because of the potential compensation being offered. Moreover, if that conflict were to disqualify the parents in the case of the children who object, it would seem to disqualify them even in the case in which the child does not refuse to assent.

Assuming that it is ethically legitimate to involve the children against their wills, Dr Jackman faces the problem of the ethics of using her behavior management approaches. She assumes that they are ethical in a therapeutic setting, but it is not as clear that they are ethical for research. Even if she is correct in assuming that for therapy, restraint and voice control would be acceptable, there is a significant difference in using such approaches in a research setting, where the objective is not the benefit of the patient.

Provider Autonomy

The principle of autonomy requires that freely made, substantially autonomous choices be respected, even if overriding those decisions would produce more good for the decision-maker. So far we have considered the autonomy of the competent patient and of the surrogate for the incompetent patient. A third and final question raised by the principle of autonomy is whether health care professionals also have moral rights grounded in autonomy to refuse to provide care requested by patients. In cases in which the health care provider feels his or her conscience would be violated, can he or she simply exercise autonomy and refuse to consent to continuing a professional-patient relationship? Professional autonomy in decision making is an issue in the cases that follow.

Case 37: How Many Alternatives?

Dr Ed Van Sciver had a patient with a mandibular second molar with a large mesial, occlusal, and distal (MOD) amalgam restoration. The mesiobuccal cusp had completely broken off. The tooth was certainly restorable, and there were no endodontic complications. However, Dr Van Sciver wondered how far to go in presenting alternatives to the patient in his pursuit of an informed consent. To mention all possible alternatives sometimes seemed pointless. In this case, Dr Van Sciver thought the full range of choices included:

1. Cast gold crown
2. Cast gold crown with porcelain facing
3. Gold onlay
4. Replacement of the MOD amalgam, including the fractured cusp
5. Repair of the amalgam without replacement
6. Composite resin
7. Porcelain onlay
8. Extraction

Some of these choices were very low on his list of favorites—for example, the composite resin restoration, the porcelain onlay, and the extraction. He did not see these as reasonable alternatives, although some people, depending on their circumstances and values, might choose them.

Dr Van Sciver was also skeptical about the repair of the amalgam as a reasonable alternative. He did not view it as quality treatment, and he would not have chosen it himself. On the other hand, he had to admit that he had had a similar repair in his own mouth. It had been placed as a temporary, expedient restoration but had lasted for years. The problem was its unpredictability.

The MOD amalgam replacement with a rebuilt cusp was certainly an alternative for the patient to consider. It was not the choice Dr Van Sciver would make, but it would be quite an acceptable restoration.

The crown was obviously the best choice—either with or without the porcelain facing. It was more trouble-free than was the gold onlay, and it should last longer. That was what Dr Van Sciver had been taught, what he believed, and what he would choose for himself. The problem he, like all dentists, was faced with was that he could not provide patients with objective data that would allow them to make a reasonable and informed choice. For example, there are no studies comparing crowns versus four- or five-surface amalgam restorations over periods of 5 or 10 years. Outcome data such as these are lacking in many treatment situations in dentistry.

DISCUSSION:

This case begins with what seems like the problem of how much information should be transmitted for consent to be adequately informed. Given that Dr Van Sciver admits that some people would choose even those options that he finds least attractive, there is reason to believe that patients should be informed of these options. The next issue is what Dr Van Sciver would have to tell the patient about each option. Surely, the information would have to include costs, likely length of benefit, and side effects. He would also have to tell the patient that even though he does not approve of some of these options, other dentists might choose them.

Suppose that the patient, after being adequately informed, opts for the composite resin restoration, the porcelain onlay, or the extraction. Then the problem of respecting patient autonomy changes considerably. On what basis does Dr Van Sciver believe that the cast gold crown is the best choice? It is possible that those reasons do not necessarily make it the most rational choice for the patient. For example, Dr Van Sciver's opinion that he would choose it for himself undoubtedly takes into account his own economic means, which may not be the same as those of the patient. The issue here is whether, if the patient insists on one of the less acceptable options from Dr Van Sciver's point of view, the dentist is obligated to provide the care.

Keep in mind that the principle of autonomy gives one the right to act on one's own plan. This is what philosophers call a *liberty right*—the right to avoid acting, to walk away, to cancel any relationship that exists between professional and layperson. If the patient has the right to cancel the doctor-patient contract, does the dentist have the same right when the patient insists on a treatment that violates the dentist's sense of professional standards?

To answer, we may have to ask what the dentist has promised, explicitly or implicitly, when accepting licensure by the public. If the profession jointly or the dentist individually has promised to provide certain services—for example, those that responsible colleagues would provide under similar circumstances or those considered by the public to be basic or fundamental—then the professional's obligations may not be revokable unilaterally. On the other hand, if Dr Van Sciver can refer his patient to another competent dentist more willing to provide the controversial service and such referral does not jeopardize the patient's welfare, then referral may be the best plan all around.

Case 38: The Patient Is in the Middle

Dr Samuel Pitts was a general dentist who had practiced for many years in an older house located on a busy suburban street close to a large city. He had a part-time associate, Dr Cathy Gerber, who was a graduate student in the orthodontics program of a nearby dental school.

Late one Saturday, a 6-year-old boy came into the office with his father and without an appointment. The child was an occasional patient in Dr Pitts's practice, and the family was known to be on medical assistance. The boy had a toothache and a slight fever and appeared very apprehensive. Dr Pitts was busy with another patient and had two more waiting, so Dr Gerber saw the child. Her examination showed a deep caries lesion on a mandibular second primary molar accompanied by swelling of the buccal gingiva. The first permanent molar was not yet erupted. The child's father wanted the tooth removed.

Dr Gerber disagreed. She knew that when second primary molars are removed before the first permanent molars erupt, significant loss of dental arch space almost always occurs. She believed that the clinical and radiographic picture indicated that root canal treatment should be done. Dr Gerber wanted to refer the patient to a specialist, with the child to be seen on Monday, and made that suggestion to Dr Pitts.

Dr Pitts did not believe in root canal treatment for primary teeth and thought the tooth should be removed. Furthermore, something needed to be done immediately because of the boy's pain and infection. He also believed the parent's wishes for the tooth to be removed needed to be considered. Dr Gerber's concern about space loss could be managed with a space maintainer.

Dr Pitts told Dr Gerber to remove the tooth. He felt quite strongly about it, both because he thought it was the right thing to do clinically and because it was his practice and he felt that he had the right to control the treatment that was conducted there. He would have done it himself except for the fact that he was so busy.

Dr Gerber felt just as strongly that the tooth should not be removed and told Dr Pitts to remove the tooth if he wanted to, but she refused to do it herself.

DISCUSSION:

Dr Gerber is in a moral bind. Should she not be permitted to practice dentistry as she sees fit and to make the referral she thinks is best? On the other hand, her role as an associate in Dr Pitts's practice might be seen as obligating her to practice as Dr Pitts sees fit. Does Dr Gerber have a right grounded in her own autonomy to insist on the referral, or can the patient's father insist on the extraction?

If Dr Pitts were available to perform the extraction, transferring the patient to him might be best for everyone. On the other hand, if Dr Gerber really is convinced that extraction is not in the young patient's best interest, she might have to ask herself whether the father's choice is so wrong that it is intolerable. Getting a court order to block the extraction and refer seems inconceivable. Yet if Dr Gerber believes the father is intolerably in error in his choice, getting a court order would seem to be her only choice. Although the boy would have to wait, when one considers Dr Pitts's willingness to perform the extraction and the implausibility of seeking judicial intervention to overrule the father, a good case can be made to transfer the case to him. This both respects Dr Gerber's professional integrity and fits with the standards of Dr Pitts's practice. When one takes into account the implied commitments to Dr Pitts's other patients and the fact that the boy came without an appointment, the best strategy seems to be for Dr Pitts to offer to take the case himself as soon as he can.

Conclusion

These cases depict a head-on clash between the dentist's autonomy to practice dentistry as he or she sees fit and the patient's (or surrogate's) right to choose a legal professional service that is acceptable to some competent dentists. Patients' autonomy in and of itself does not give them the right to demand a service of a professional. However, some of the commitments made by professionals at the time of licensure possibly obligate them to provide some desired services in those cases in which patients cannot get them from other competent dentists who are willing to provide them. Now we turn to the third ethical principle that recognizes moral duties beyond maximizing good consequences. The ethics of dealing honestly with patients, another part of the ethical obligation to show respect for persons, is the focus of the cases in the following chapter.

References

1. Gert B, Culver CM. The justification of paternalism. Ethics 1979;89:199–210.
2. Dworkin C. Paternalism. In: Wasserstrom R (ed). Morality and the Law. Belmont, CA: Wadsworth, 1972:107–126.
3. Feinberg J. Social Philosophy. Englewood Cliffs, NJ: Prentice Hall; 1973:33.

4. Beauchamp TL, Childress JF. Principles of Biomedical Ethics, ed 5. New York: Oxford University Press, 2001:181.

5. Lidz CW, Meisel A, Zerubavel E, Carter M, Sestak RM, Roth LH. Informed Consent: A Study of Decisionmaking in Psychiatry. New York: Guilford Press, 1984.

6. President's Commission for the Study of Ethical Problems in Medicine and Biomedical and Behavioral Research. Making Health Care Decisions: A Report on the Ethical and Legal Implications of Informed Consent in the Patient-Practitioner Relationship, vol. 1. Washington, DC: US Government Printing Office, 1982.

7. Faden RR, Beauchamp TL, in collaboration with King NMP. A History and Theory of Informed Consent. New York: Oxford University Press, 1986.

8. Appelbaum PS, Lidz CW, Meisel A. Informed Consent: Legal Theory and Clinical Practice. New York: Oxford University Press, 1987.

9. Hirsch AC, Gert B. Ethics in dental practice. J Am Dent Assoc 1986;113:599–603.

10. President's Commission for the Study of Ethical Problems in Medicine and Biomedical and Behavioral Research. Deciding to Forego Life-Sustaining Treatment: Ethical, Medical, and Legal Issues in Treatment Decisions. Washington, DC: US Government Printing Office, 1983:125,126.

11. The Hastings Center. Guidelines on the Termination of Life-Sustaining Treatment and the Care of the Dying. Briarcliff Manor, NY: The Hastings Center, 1987:123–127.

12. Sadowsky D. Moral dilemmas of the multiple prescription in dentistry. J Am Coll Dent 1979;46:245–248.

13. Moore ML. Their life is in the blood: Jehovah's Witnesses, blood transfusions and the courts. North KY Law Rev 1983;10:281–304.

14. Veatch RM. Death, Dying, and the Biological Revolution, revised ed. New Haven, CT: Yale University Press, 1989.

15. Martyn SR, Jacobs LB. Legislating advance directives for the terminally ill: Living will and durable power of attorney. Nebraska Law Rev 1984;63:786.

16. Veatch RM. Limits of guardian treatment refusal: A reasonableness standard. Am J Law Med 1984;9:427–468.

17. Areen J. The legal status of consent obtained from families of adult patients to withhold or withdraw treatment. J Am Med Assoc 1987;258:229–235.

chapter 9

Dealing Honestly with Patients

In this chapter

- Bold-faced Lies
- Misleading and Limited Disclosure

Cases

- Lying to a Child to Avoid Producing Anxiety
- A Patient's Request to Stretch the Truth
- A Complicated and Controversial Man
- Dentists Deceived
- Obligations When the Patient Fails to Disclose HIV Status
- Nondisclosure of Hepatitis
- The Wrong Prosthesis

In the cases in chapter 8, dentists faced the problem of whether to respect the autonomous choices of patients, especially when the dentists had reason to believe that their patients would be better off if patient autonomy was violated. Informed consent is increasingly grounded on the moral principle of autonomy. While autonomy is a significant part of the notion of respect for persons, there are other dimensions as well. One is the ethical principle of veracity, or truth-telling. The cases in this chapter examine the ethics of dealing honestly with patients.

Often dishonesty turns out to make no sense for the dishonest person or for anyone else. The liar destroys his or her reputation; the lie is self-defeating. The dentist who consistently lies to his or her own advantage will be found out. There are special cases, however, when it is morally debatable whether an exception might be made in situations where a lie or a shading of the truth could be justified because of the benefits to the patient. In these cases the question is whether the clinician should continue to pursue the patient's welfare or should deal honestly with the patient even if the patient will be worse off.

Ethical approaches that focus on maximizing net welfare—the ethics of the Hippocratic Oath and utilitarianism—hold that the only morally relevant feature of behavior is the outcome: the benefits and harms. By contrast, some ethical systems go beyond consequences to recognize other relevant features of actions. Fidelity and respect for autonomy are examples we encountered in the two previous chapters. Telling the truth might be another. The philosopher Immanuel Kant, for example, said that "[t]o be truthful (honest) in all declarations is . . . a sacred and unconditional command of reason, and not to be limited by any expediency."[1]

Until about 1975, most health care professionals, at least most physicians, were Hippocratic. They believed it was ethically acceptable—indeed ethically required—to lie to patients when they thought it would benefit them.[2] Since that time, attitudes have shifted dramatically. Now many health care professionals are questioning the ethics of lying to patients for their own good or for the good of others. The changes in attitudes have been so significant that there is currently a much greater inclination to disclose information to patients.[3]

Bold-faced Lies

In relatively few instances, dentists may feel that they are justified ethically in telling outright lies to patients or to others. More often the ethics of honesty raises questions of not completely disclosing the truth. The first cases in this chapter involve lies—statements made by dentists that they know are false. Some lies seem clearly indefensible. Others are more debatable because the dentist could offer some moral defense of the lie.

Case 39: Lying to a Child to Avoid Producing Anxiety

Luke Braddock was a 9-year-old child with a long history of dental experience. He had recently moved to a small midwestern community and in the process his family had delayed establishing a relationship with a new dentist. When Luke's father brought him to Dr Hansen, Luke had serious problems, the worst of which was an unsalvageable permanent mandibular first molar that was causing serious pain. Although Dr Hansen did not like to contemplate extraction on a patient's first visit, she determined that the extraction was necessary and needed to be done immediately to give the boy some relief.

Luke was moderately apprehensive about seeing a new dentist. He was trying to show courage. Finally, after the area was anesthetized, he asked Dr Hansen point-blank what she was going to do.

Dr Hansen had never been confronted so directly. She did not want to upset the child. After a short pause she said, "I'm just going to look in your mouth." At that point she was already approaching carefully from behind Luke's head so the boy could not see the forceps. The tooth was extracted before Luke knew what was happening.

DISCUSSION:

There is no question that Dr Hansen meant well. She did not want to upset the boy by answering in a straightforward way that she was about to pull his tooth. On the spur of the moment, she could come up with nothing better than to tell what is sometimes called a "white" lie—that is, a lie that seems well intentioned.

If Dr Hansen were challenged to defend her lie, she probably would claim that she did what she believed was for the benefit of her patient. This, in fact, is exactly what the Hippocratic ethic would require. She was, no doubt, convinced that the boy would be terribly upset if told in advance about the extraction. Assuming that Dr Hansen really believed that the lie was the best thing for the boy in this awkward situation, an ethic of patient benefit would support the lie. The question is whether there are any reasons why it would be morally wrong to say that she was just going to look when, in fact, she was going to extract.

In this case, it turned out that the patient was so upset with the surprise that he was horrified at the thought of returning to Dr Hansen and was never able to see her again. Even for a dentist motivated solely by doing what was best for the boy, the possibility of such psychological trauma should have been factored into the calculation of expected benefits and harms. Suppose that Dr Hansen carefully takes into account the risk of long-term trauma and still concludes that more good than harm is done by the lie. Is there then any reason why it would be wrong to tell this kind of lie? If you believe it would be wrong to lie, it could be for two different reasons: either because of the long-term bad consequences or because it is simply wrong for a dentist to lie, even for a good cause. Dr Hansen may not have adequately considered the long-term consequences of lying. In this case, she may not have realized that Luke would be so traumatized that a long-term fear of dentists could cause serious harm for many years. The other possibility is that it is simply immoral to tell a lie even if the consequences would be better than those of telling the truth. This is the position that Kant and many others have taken. Recently, the American Medical Association (AMA) has adopted this view as well. Lying to someone, according to those who hold this view, shows disrespect. It is wrong in the same way that breaking a promise or violating someone's autonomy is wrong—regardless of the consequences. Those who hold this view may add the principle of veracity to their list of principles that make actions right. The principle of veracity is sometimes considered along with the principles of fidelity and autonomy as part of the general ethic of respect for persons. Others treat it as a separate principle. In either case, the fact that one is intentionally speaking dishonestly counts as a moral wrong even if doing so produces better consequences.

In Case 39, the patient was clearly the beneficiary, but no one (other than possibly the patient or the dentist) really would be harmed. Some argue that the health professional's duty to do what will benefit the patient could even encompass lying for the patient when others (who are perhaps less deserving) would be harmed. The next case illustrates that situation.

Case 40: A Patient's Request to Stretch the Truth

Ms Mary Weiner, age 20, was a patient of Dr Sonya Hale, as were her brother and other family members. Mary had a history of seizures and had been taking Dilantin for a long time. Her seizures were controlled, but she had significant Dilantin hyperplasia. Dr Hale had planned to refer Mary to a periodontist to have the hyperplastic gingiva removed. However, the referral was delayed when Mary was in an automobile accident. She suffered facial fractures and significant trauma to other areas of her body. Multiple surgeries were necessary, and she was in the hospital for almost 8 weeks. In addition, at least one more surgery would be required.

When Mary next spoke to Dr Hale about the referral for gingival surgery, she asked if there was any way that Dr Hale could say that Mary's facial trauma made the Dilantin hyperplasia worse so that the procedure could be covered under Mary's general health insurance policy. If the hyperplasia had been caused simply by the Dilantin, her general health insurance would not cover the surgery, but if the trauma had been a contributing factor, the treatment would be covered. Mary obviously felt that she had been through so much that she deserved some kind of consideration from Dr Hale.

Dr Hale was troubled by the request. Although Mary was wearing arch bars because of the facial surgery, the resulting increased oral hygiene problems could have caused only a very minor increase in the already-existing hyperplasia. On the other hand, she sympathized with Mary and also did not want to lose the rest of the family as patients. Dr Hale thought about what she should do.

DISCUSSION:

Two new issues are introduced in this case as compared with the previous one. First, there is a slight basis for saying that the accident caused at least some of the hyperplasia. Sometimes people distinguish between lying and merely withholding the full truth. The dentist could argue that because the accident could have caused some of the hyperplasia, she was dealing honestly with the insurance company, but that surely would be distorting the situation.

Even if Dr Hale concluded that the connection between the accident and the hyperplasia was tenuous at best, she might see the advantages to Mary in deceiving the insurance company as much more than the financial benefits alone. Deceiving the insurance company might also make it possible to combine the difficult hyperplasia surgery with the final facial surgery during a single general anesthetic. If that were done, Mary's risks and discomfort would be considerably reduced. The question becomes one of whether the additional benefits for Mary would help Dr Hale justify stretching the truth in her dealings with the insurance company.

Second, the lie would cause injury to another party—the insurance company (and ultimately other subscribers to the insurance coverage). If the dentist is Hippocratic, she is devoted to doing what she believes will benefit the patient and protect the patient from harm. There seems to be no doubt that lying to the insurance company would benefit Mary. If the harm is done to other parties but not to Mary, there seems to be nothing wrong with the lie from the Hippocratic (patient-benefiting) perspective. However, there still may be other reasons why the lie or even the deception is ethically unacceptable. Two additional reasons to object to the lie can be considered: the harm done to others and the mere fact of telling a lie. A social utilitarian would consider the benefits and harms to other parties in addition to the patient. The harm to the insurance company and to fellow subscribers would then be included as a reason not to lie. The problem with social utilitarianism, however, is that it would require Dr Hale to compromise the patient's interests whenever society would be better off, something most dentists would find unethical. That would leave the principle of honesty—that it is simply wrong to tell a lie or distort the truth as the basis for opposing Mary's request. Defenders of the principle would conclude that it is unacceptable for Dr Hale to deceive the insurance company simply because it is dishonest, even if Mary would be better off.

Both of the previous cases present lies for the benefit of the patient, but one also might sometimes consider lying for the benefit of other parties. Lies in the interests of obtaining accurate information, as in the next case, can be told in order to obtain important information from respondents who otherwise might not answer questions honestly.

Case 41: A Complicated and Controversial Man

From his earliest days, Dr Dan Barney was the sort of person who believed in treating people fairly. It was the way that everyone in his family felt about life— and they were vocal about it. Everyone knew where the Barneys stood on public matters: It was always on the side of the underdog.

When Dr Barney graduated from dental school, he became a pediatric dentist and opened a practice in his hometown. When Medicaid patients called for appointments, he accepted them. He knew that other dentists in town refused to treat them, but his view was, "They're kids! How can you turn a kid down? That's what I'm there for!" Soon his practice was 30 percent Medicaid, and after 10 years, it was half Medicaid. Dr Barney was largely oblivious to these trends in his practice, but his office manager pointed out that he could make a lot more money if he cut back on his Medicaid patients.

Dr Barney wouldn't do it. He thought his income was not too bad as it was. Furthermore, these were the kids who needed care the most. However, his office manager's concerns about Medicaid made him aware of two very different issues. One was just how bad the Medicaid fees were. As a result, Dr Barney initiated a decade-long campaign to raise the Medicaid fees in his state, which had some of the lowest fees in the country. He worked tirelessly to provide his state with documentation that low-income children were being denied access to dental care. Because of that documentation and his persistence in acquiring the support of elected state officials, including the attorney general and finally the governor, his campaign prevailed and the fees were raised.

The second by-product of Dr Barney's newly acquired awareness about Medicaid was his realization that very few dentists were caring for these patients. He would see children who traveled 60 miles to get to his office and in so doing, passed by the offices of 20 or 30 dentists who would not accept Medicaid patients. This realization gnawed at him, and the more he thought about it, the angrier he became. That anger influenced the way that he acquired data for his campaign to raise Medicaid fees. Between patents, he began personally calling the offices of a large sample of the dentists in the state, including both pediatric and general dentists. He would tell the receptionist who answered that he was the father of a young child with dental pain and swelling and would ask for an appointment. The office staff would begin the appointment process, but when they discovered the child was on Medicaid, the door was usually shut. The results of Dr Barney's survey were quite discouraging.

At a meeting of the state's pediatric dentists, Dr Barney disclosed what he had been doing. Although some of his colleagues congratulated him, many others were disturbed by his actions.

Case 42: Dentists Deceived

In 1989, Dr H.M. Hazelkorn published an account of research designed to describe the attitudes and behaviors of dentists toward men who were in high-risk groups for HIV infection.[4] Fearing that dentists would not reveal their true attitudes when conventional questionnaire or interview techniques were used, Dr Hazelkorn hired a male actor to portray either a homosexual, a heterosexual, or an intravenous drug user.

The actor had a number of carious teeth and appeared at the dentists' offices with radiographs and a role-related story. Following an examination, the actor paid for the service and attempted to schedule another visit for treatment. If that was successfully accomplished, he left the office but returned a few minutes later to ask for his radiographs back so that he could get a second opinion. Following this exchange with the dentists, or earlier if a second appointment was denied, Dr Hazelkorn entered the dental office with a request to conduct an interview. During this interview the dentists were told that the patient was an actor and were also asked about their attitudes about homosexuality and patients who are HIV positive or who have AIDS. The focus of the subsequent data analysis was to reveal to what extent dentists discriminate against people who are in high-risk categories for HIV infection.

DISCUSSION:

Using deception or outright lies in survey research is so common that some people might assume that it is standard practice. Many researchers might not even realize that the research techniques in these two cases were examples of dishonest communication. Nevertheless, in a chapter on truth-telling, it is important to consider the ethical justification of the practice. Dr Barney called colleagues claiming to be the father of a child on Medicaid. Dr Hazelkorn hired an actor who misrepresented himself and failed to disclose the true nature of his visit to the dentist. The statements these dentists made were knowingly false, although arguably for a good cause and perhaps hurting no one. The question here is whether the good cause and the fact that no one was hurt justify the dishonesty. It may well be the case that the dentists being called would not have answered honestly if Dr Barney had simply identified himself and asked them if they took Medicaid patients. If Dr Barney defended himself by saying his lie was necessary to avoid dishonest responses from fellow dentists, he would seem to be claiming that one lie justifies another—a controversial position.

Similarly, in Dr Hazelkorn's project, if dentists knew that the actor was testing their views about patients in high-risk categories, he might not have been able to get reliable responses.

It is possible that the information in the two cases could have been obtained by using people who actually fit the categories the researchers wanted to present. Dr Barney could have used real Medicaid patients who needed dentists. Had parents of prospective Medicaid patients called, their statements would have been true. Those who find violations of the principle of veracity unacceptable would say that it would have been ethically (as well as scientifically) preferable to have parents of real Medicaid patients place the calls. Assuming that conducting the study that way would have been more inconvenient and time-consuming, the truth-telling principle suggests that there is still a moral reason for Dr Barney to have done so.

Similarly, Dr Hazelkorn could have attempted his study using real patients who could truthfully present themselves as homosexual, heterosexual, or intravenous drug users. However, because they would have been different patients with at least somewhat different dental problems, he might argue that the data would not have been as reliable. In both cases, even if the dentists had used real patients, they still would have had to face the problem that they were conducting research using dentists as subjects and deceiving their subjects about their entry into a research project.

Those who are utilitarian (who limit their ethics to the principles of beneficence and nonmaleficence) would point out that there certainly are good reasons why Dr Barney and Dr Hazelkorn needed the information they were gathering. It could be argued that the total good done by lying and deceit far exceeds any harm done. A utilitarian ethic holds that an action is morally right if the net consequences are as good or better than any alternative action. Nevertheless, those who see ethics as more than just doing good and avoiding harm would deny that this would be sufficient to justify the lies and deception in these cases.

Nonutilitarians hold that there are right-making and wrong-making characteristics of actions other than their consequences. For example, some nonutilitarians hold that a lie tends to make a statement morally wrong. Even a nonutilitarian might find a reason to justify the lie, however. They might accept the principle of truth-telling but recognize that sometimes it conflicts with other moral principles. In such cases the principles may have to be balanced against each other and one will have to lose out. In this case the principle of justice might be cited as a basis for justifying the lie.

Justice is a principle that will be examined in more detail in chapter 10. It holds that one right-making characteristic of actions is that they arrange benefits and harms in equitable patterns. In these cases, the dishonest phone calls and misrepresentation by an actor may be major factors in more equitably distributing dental care. According to those who consider justice a right-making characteristic of actions, the principle of justice might justify the lie even if predicted good consequences by themselves do not.

A nonutilitarian might be in an awkward position of maintaining that the principle of veracity is a right-making characteristic and that the principle of justice is another. We could then say that Dr Barney's phone calls and the actor's deception contain one dimension that makes them wrong (the lie) and another that makes them right (that they promote more equitable dental care). When we analyze individual moral dimensions of actions in this way, we can say that the principles are prima facie principles (or principles considering only one moral dimension). The concept of prima facie moral principles is an important one in ethical analysis. We say that an action is prima facie right when we are considering only one moral dimension of the action such as the fact that it promotes equity or that it is honest. Analyzing individual moral dimensions of actions in this way helps to show exactly what it is about an action that we think would tend to make it right or wrong. In fact, if there were no other moral dimensions, we would conclude that the act itself is wrong. However, if other dimensions are involved as well, it is possible to say that an action (such as the lie told to these dentists) was prima facie wrong (because it violated the principle of honesty or veracity), but was nevertheless the right thing to do when considering other moral principles, such as beneficence or justice. One could say it is prima facie wrong to lie and prima facie right to promote benefits and to distribute them justly. At this point one still would not know whether, on balance, the dishonest statement to the dentists in the survey was right or wrong.

When two or more prima facie principles conflict, some method must be used to resolve the conflict. One approach is to rank principles in order of priority. We might always rank one principle higher than the other (we can say that the higher-ranking principle "trumps" the other), or we might attempt an intuitive balancing of the competing claims. For years, the AMA, the professional association of physicians, ranked beneficence as the highest principle, thus justifying lies for a good cause, but in 1980, it changed its stance to call for honesty as the physician's duty in such cases. As of 2002, the American Dental Association (ADA) has also taken the position on this issue that dentists' "obligations include respecting the position of trust inherent in the dentist-patient relationship, communicating truthfully and without deception, and maintaining intellectual integrity."[5]

Misleading and Limited Disclosure

Many of the ethical problems involving truth-telling that are faced by dentists do not really involve outright lies. Dentists can often avoid lying. Simply by their silence, they can frequently mislead patients or fail to disclose something of potential interest to patients that the patients could in no way anticipate.

Although we might argue that every instance of a lie is morally wrong (at least prima facie), no one can hold that there is a moral duty to speak all of the truth in every situation. There are many things one might say that are simply too trivial, irrelevant, or offensive to express. Presumably, if one has a friend who is ugly, there is no moral duty to say so, at least if one is not asked. In fact, there may even be a duty to avoid saying so.

Sometimes, however, there may be a duty to speak the truth even if not asked. In the consent process, we saw that many people believe that dentists have a duty to disclose what the reasonable person would want to know. Much of that information deals with issues about which the patient would have no way of knowing. He or she would not even know which questions to ask. It is precisely because the patient would not know what to ask that there seems to be a duty to disclose the truth.

A key may be found in the nature of the relationship, if any, that exists between the parties. Strangers meeting on the street have a very limited duty to each other when it comes to disclosure. A health professional who has an ongoing relationship with a patient, however, has a more stringent duty that may require disclosing all of those things that reasonable patients would want to know about their situations. Whether that duty is part of the principle of veracity or the principle of fidelity (which we discussed in chapter 7) can be debated. Once a formal doctor-patient relationship is created, there is an implied promise of truthful disclosure that binds the parties.

The duty to disclose potentially meaningful information in the dentist-patient relationship can be seen as a two-way street. Although we might most often think of honesty as a duty of the health professional, it can also be thought of as a duty of the patient. Before turning to a series of cases dealing with the dentist's duty to disclose, we first look at a case where it is the patient who has some potentially relevant information about which he is not asked.

Case 43: Obligations When the Patient Fails to Disclose HIV Status

Mr Charles Yount had been a patient in Dr Sara McKenna's practice for more than 5 years. Dr McKenna had always suspected that Mr Yount was gay. Recently, Mr Yount came to the office for an emergency visit and a preliminary diagnosis of oral candidiasis was made. Dr McKenna referred Mr Yount to an oral surgeon for a second opinion and a biopsy. Dr McKenna learned from the oral surgeon that Mr Yount had told the oral surgeon that he had been HIV positive for several years. Although Dr McKenna had reviewed Mr Yount's medical history at each visit for the past 5 years, Mr Yount had not mentioned any changes in his health even while being monitored by a physician for the last 2 to 3 years. Dr McKenna discussed the issue with Mr Yount, who finally admitted that he was HIV positive.

Dr McKenna was angry with her patient for not telling her of his seroconversion but freely admitting it to the oral surgeon. She felt that Mr Yount had deceived her and considered not treating him in the future, but perhaps referring him to a clinic for treatment instead.

DISCUSSION:

Mr Yount never told an outright lie to Dr McKenna; he simply failed to disclose a piece of information that most dentists would perceive to be very relevant to the care of the patient. Mr Yount either thought that his HIV status was not important information for the dentist to have or that it was none of her business. He may also have been concerned—with some basis in collective experience—that if he told the truth, the dentist might have found some excuse to get rid of him as a patient. Dentists, on the other hand, are advised to use universal precautions and to treat each patient as if he or she might be seropositive. But there are other reasons why a dentist might find this information important (such as needing to take into account possible compromise in the patient's immune status). Did Mr Yount have a moral duty not only to avoid lying but also to take the initiative in deducing that Dr McKenna should have this information?

It seems clear that Mr Yount would be under no such obligation to tell strangers or even casual acquaintances. Regardless of whether he has a moral obligation to avoid lying if asked specifically by an acquaintance about his HIV status, he surely is under no obligation to go out of his way to bring up the subject.

There are, however, certain people with whom Mr Yount might have a special relationship that imposes additional obligations of disclosure—for example, a spouse or sexual partner. If Mr Yount had consented to be in a research survey that asked about HIV status, he might have such a relationship with the investigator as well.

Here the question is whether establishing a relationship with a health professional imposes an obligation to disclose what the professional needs to know or would find important in providing professional services. By establishing a patient-dentist relationship, did Mr Yount, in effect, promise to disclose to Dr McKenna information that he would expect she would need to know to practice good dentistry? If so, that obligation cannot be limited to avoiding outright lies. It includes an extra duty on the patient's part to ensure that potentially important information is transmitted even if the dentist fails to ask for it.

If the patient has a special duty not only to be honest with the dentist, but also to initiate conversations to ensure that the dentist is informed about things that the patient perceives would be important to the dentist, the dentist, in turn, has a duty, as part of the lay-professional relationship, to go beyond avoiding lies and initiate conversations about information that the patient would reasonably want to have. The next group of cases poses this problem.

Case 44: Nondisclosure of Hepatitis

Ms Cheryl Grady was a dental hygienist who worked full time in a large office. Her employer, Dr Donald Hollinger, became ill with hepatitis and was hospitalized for almost a week. Ms Grady did not know what form of hepatitis Dr Hollinger had. However, she became concerned about the risk of transmission when the office manager told her that, per Dr Hollinger's orders, under no circumstances should she tell the rest of the staff about Dr Hollinger's illness.

Ms Grady was quite concerned. In addition to all of the patients with whom Dr Hollinger had contact, he also had a staff of 12 people. Furthermore, he worked as an associate in two other offices. Ms Grady thought that Dr Hollinger should inform his patients and staff about his illness.

Ms Grady called the city health department anonymously and without mentioning Dr Hollinger's name. Their opinion was that the dentist should not be working with patients. Ms Grady discussed the situation with Dr Hollinger, but he said that he had just been married, badly needed money, and could not risk disclosing his illness.

DISCUSSION:

Unless some curious patient asks Dr Hollinger or Ms Grady whether anyone in the office has hepatitis, no one will be telling an active lie. In that sense this case differs from those in the first part of this chapter. Still, questions of the ethics of communication arise. First, should Dr Hollinger inform his staff and/or patients about his hepatitis? The staff is at risk. The problem could be viewed as one of the duty of an employer to inform his or her staff about risks in the workplace. To the extent that an employer generally has a duty to notify employees about significant risks, Dr Hollinger's duty is no different from that of any other employer.

Dr Hollinger also faces the question of his duty to his patients. In chapter 8 we discussed the standards of informed consent. The dentist is obligated to disclose to patients the information they would find material in deciding to consent to treatment. In this case, the issue is whether reasonable patients would find Dr Hollinger's hepatitis status relevant to their decision to agree to have Dr Hollinger treat them. Some forms of hepatitis, particularly hepatitis B and C, are transmitted through blood contamination. A dentist who cut himself could bleed into the patient, who would then be exposed to the hepatitis virus. Although dentist-to-patient transmission is very rare, it can occur. Because patients probably have a choice of comparably competent dentists in the community, they may wish to take the hepatitis status into account when deciding to remain in Dr Hollinger's practice.

The Centers for Disease Control and Prevention (CDC) has considered the issue of viral transmission of bloodborne HIV and has concluded that health professionals who ordinarily face no real risk of exposing patients need not disclose their HIV status, but that those performing high-risk procedures must disclose if they are HIV positive. Certain surgeons who face a high risk of scalpel or needle sticks are specifically mentioned, as are dentists. While the CDC has not made the same point with regard to bloodborne hepatitis, the issues are identical. If there is a duty to inform patients in the case of HIV, the same reasons would support a duty to warn if the dentist is carrying a hepatitis virus that could be transmitted through blood contamination.

Case 45: The Wrong Prosthesis

Ms Hope Lazzaro was a new patient of Dr Madeline Wexler. Another dentist had made Ms Lazzaro a resin-bonded prosthesis to replace a maxillary central incisor. It was now loose, and she wanted Dr Wexler to recement it. Dr Wexler explained that this involved removing the prosthesis and having it re-etched before insertion. However, she cautioned that there might be decay under the loosened prosthesis that could require a new prosthesis. Ms Lazzaro understood the situation and the two different fees that might be charged and authorized the treatment.

As Dr Lazzaro had feared, caries was found when the prosthesis was removed. It turned out to be deep enough to jeopardize the stability of the prosthesis, and Ms Lazzaro agreed to have a new prosthesis made. Dr Wexler took an impression and sent it to the laboratory. The old prosthesis was included so that the shade could be copied.

When Ms Lazzaro returned for the try-in, both she and Dr Wexler were extremely pleased with the results. Dr Wexler said she would have the new bridge etched and would insert it at the next appointment.

The prosthesis came back from the laboratory in a bag with the standard admonition: "Etched Bridge—Do Not Touch." Because Dr Wexler was confident of the fit, she and her dental assistant proceeded to cement it in. However, it did not seem to have the same firm fit as before, and it was unexpectedly difficult to seat. In addition, Dr Wexler thought it did not look quite as good. However, Ms Lazzaro was thrilled with the new prosthesis.

While the cement was setting, the assistant took the casts out of the laboratory box. In it was another, smaller box which she opened. Inside was the new prosthesis that was supposed to have been inserted. Ms Lazzaro's old prosthesis had been re-etched mistakenly by the laboratory instead of the new one.

Dr Wexler considered what to do. Ms Lazzaro loved her "new" prosthesis. Dr Wexler was not sure that she could remove the recemented prosthesis without fracturing the compromised abutment tooth. Should she tell Ms Lazzaro what happened? How should she handle the fee?

DISCUSSION:

In this case the dentist can probably get out of her predicament gracefully by simply saying nothing. She probably does not need to actively lie; she simply could avoid telling the full story. What reasons are there to disclose what actually happened?

The first question is whether there are actions that the patient or dentist might reasonably want to take that would require the patient to be informed. One action involves the billing. We must also consider whether Ms Lazzaro should be expected to pay for the new prosthesis, and, if not, how Dr Wexler can explain why without telling her patient what happened. Another is whether, under the circumstances, the patient might want to consider switching to a different dentist.

Assume for purposes of discussion that these problems could be solved without informing the patient of the errors. Is there any remaining reason why the dentist simply owes it to the patient to tell about the mistakes?

Many people hold that the duties of the doctor-patient relationship are radically different from those of strangers or casual acquaintances. If so, it may have something to do with the fiduciary relationship. Fidelity, or faithfulness to a relationship, may be the basis for special expectations in the doctor-patient relationship. One of the obligations of fidelity might be the duty to inform the other party of information that they can reasonably be expected to want or need to know to fulfill their part of the relationship.

References

1. Kant I. On the supposed right to tell lies from benevolent motives. In: Critique of Practical Reason and Other Works on the Theory of Ethics. Abbott TK (trans). London: Longman's, 1909:363.
2. Oken D. What to tell cancer patients. A study of medical attitudes. JAMA 1961;175:1120–1128.
3. Novack DH, Plumer R, Smith RL, Ochitill H, Morrow GR, Bennett JM. Changes in physicians' attitudes toward telling the cancer patient. JAMA 1979;241:897–900.
4. Hazelkorn HM. The reaction of dentists to members of groups at risk of AIDS. J Am Dent Assoc 1989;119:611–619.
5. American Dental Association Council on Ethics, Bylaws and Judicial Affairs. Principles of Ethics and Code of Professional Conduct, with official advisory opinions revised to January 2002. Chicago: American Dental Association, 2002.

Justice in Dentistry

In this chapter

Cases

The cases in the previous three chapters posed problems in which a dentist faced a conflict between following the principle of beneficence (doing what would appear to do the most good) and following a principle such as remaining faithful to a commitment or promise, respecting autonomy, or telling the truth. These conflicts have generally arisen between individual dentists and their patients.

A similar moral tension arises at the social and public policy level. The principle of beneficence is often applied in an attempt to resolve such conflicts. As we saw in chapter 6, utilitarian ethics strives to do as much good as possible. When more than one person's welfare is involved, this means producing the greatest good in aggregate—taking into account the welfare of everyone affected.

However, just as there is sometimes a moral doubt that it is always ethical to do what will produce the most good when one patient is involved, at the societal level there is sometimes doubt that the morally right allocation of resources is to arrange them so that they produce as much good in aggregate as possible. Those who do not automatically accept that the aggregate good should be maximized believe that an additional moral principle must come into play—the principle of justice.

Justice is a moral notion with a very long history. According to Aristotle, justice means giving everyone his or her due.[1] Equals are to be treated equally, and unequals are to be treated unequally. Aristotle recognized, however, that it can be very difficult to determine what counts as morally relevant. The need for dental restorations normally would seem to be relevant when the distribution of dental services is being decided; race and sex seem irrelevant. Between these obvious extremes are differences that may be much more controversial: income, age, location of residence, and whether dental needs are brought on by patients' voluntary lifestyle choices. Whether these are morally legitimate grounds for deciding who gets care is the problem explored in the cases in this chapter.

The general problem posed by the principle of justice is what should happen when there are not enough resources for everyone—not enough dentists, dental equipment, or funds to pay for dentistry, for example. One possibility would be to give every patient an equal amount, but that would mean giving equal amounts of dental service to those who need extensive services and those who need none. Surely that is not the right answer. A pure utilitarian would arrange the distribution so that the greatest amount of good is done in aggregate. That also can be controversial. The amount of good is usually measured by multiplying the intensity of the benefit by the length of time that it will last. This could mean that very old people would get low priority because, for example, even if they could benefit greatly from a dental restoration, the length of time the restoration lasts would be limited by the time the patient lives. Likewise, if some dental services are costly and time-consuming and other services (in other patients) can produce the same amount of good for less money and time, trying to maximize the amount of good done would mean purposely concentrating on those patients who could be benefited cheaply.

The principle of justice holds that sometimes the way in which the benefit is distributed counts morally. "To each according to his or her need" is an example of a justice-based way of distributing scarce resources. To each according to merit, ability to pay, or any other criterion would be other versions of justice-based allocations.

The cases in this chapter pose problems of how dentists, as individuals or collectively, should allocate their services, time, and benefits. The cases in the first section deal with societal allocation questions, which are sometimes called macroallocations. Those in the second section will look at allocation questions facing individual dentists, or microallocations.

Macroallocation: Allocating Dental Benefit at the Societal Level

The most general allocation questions involve what portion of total societal resources should be devoted to dentistry. One of the more intriguing problems in professional ethics has to do with what role members of a profession ought to play in deciding what portion of a society's resources should go to services in their field. They are obviously the real experts in dentistry; however, they might well place uniquely high value on the good that their field can provide. Dentists probably place unusually high value on caries-free teeth and well-functioning dentitions, just as lawyers might place high value on legal protection, accountants on impeccable account books, and the clergy on the spiritual life. In a world of scarce resources where no one can have all of every good thing in life, we can assume that a less-than-ideal level in each area makes sense. If the experts in each sphere uniquely value their own area, they can be expected to make somewhat biased decisions about how much of society's resources should be spent in their sphere. Thus it would not be surprising if dentists as a group believed more resources should go to dentistry, physicians believed that more should go to medicine, and so forth.

At the societal level, then, decisions must be made about how to spread the resources available to dentistry among the many dental needs. Dentists with different agendas are likely to disagree. Pediatric dentists may make a case for protecting children's teeth; geriatric dentists may likewise make a case for the needs of the elderly. Public health dentists may advocate prevention while restorative dentists may emphasize relieving the suffering of patients who already need interventions. The first case in this section looks at how public health dentistry might allocate a limited budget for dental sealants.

Case 46: Dental Sealants on a Limited Budget

In 1983 the National Institutes of Health created a consensus development panel on dental sealants as part of its ongoing project to assemble panels of experts to review matters of important public scientific controversy. The panel was made up of some of the country's leading academic and clinical dentists, as well as a dental technologist, a lawyer who was a children's health advocate, and a bioethicist. They were to assess the safety and effectiveness of the use of dental sealants and to make recommendations about their use.[2]

The panel had no difficulty concluding that sealants were generally safe and effective and that they were best used on children soon after the eruption of the permanent teeth. A controversy emerged, however, at an unexpected point in the panel's deliberations.

After recommending that public health dental officers give high priority to ensuring that the children in their communities had their teeth sealed, the question arose about what should be done when not enough funds were available to seal the teeth of all of the children in a given county. In particular, some county dental health programs served a number of communities, some of which had publicly fluoridated water while others did not.

For technical reasons, children growing up in communities with a fluoridated water supply can make more efficient use of dental sealants. Because fluoride is especially effective in reducing caries on proximal surfaces, fewer Class 2 restorations will have to be placed and consequently fewer sealants will be destroyed. Thus, if a county public health dental officer wanted to use a limited preventive dentistry budget with maximum effficiency, he or she would target communities where children drink fluoridated water.

The panel at this point faced a serious moral dilemma. Would it be fair to purposely give the advantage of sealants preferentially to children in communities where the water supply was fluoridated? It is surely not the fault of the children in the communities without fluoridated water that their teeth do not get fluoride protection. Moreover, some of those children actually get fluoride through application by their dentist. Still, it would be terribly inefficient for a school-based program to identify those children who are treated privately and to seal only their teeth.

Should the dental sealant panel recommend that limited funds for public sealant programs go to the children who can be treated most efficiently? Should these children get the funds even though they are already better protected (for proximal caries) and even though it is not the fault of the other children that they do not have fluoridated water supplies? Or do all children under the jurisdiction of the county public health dental officer have rights of access that should not depend on their parents' decisions about their water? If so, because it is impossible to seal all of the children's teeth, which children should get priority: those with the greatest economic need, those with the worst teeth, or those selected at random?

DISCUSSION:

The panel faced an interesting problem. If they wanted to prevent the most decay per dollar invested—if they wanted the limited funds used as efficiently as possible—they would purposely discriminate against patients without community-fluoridated water supplies. A similar problem arises in many other health allocation decisions. For example, it is often more efficient to treat middle-class patients than low-income patients. Sometimes it might be more efficient to treat a certain gender, race, ethnic group, or age group. When the specific facts of the situation make discrimination more efficient in terms of improving overall community health statistics, those who accept social utilitarianism—that is, those who apply only the principles of beneficence and nonmaleficence—will intentionally choose the most efficient allocation, even though it is discriminatory. The dentists on the panel who were utilitarian favored giving priority to the children in the community-based fluoridation programs. Other members of the panel, including the patient's rights–oriented attorney and the bioethicist, insisted that the principle of justice had to be considered. They argued that the principle of justice would require a policy in which all children had an equal chance at getting the sealants—even though it was less efficient and fewer caries would be prevented.

The problem of allocating scarce dental resources among patients with a need for services often arises in community dental programs designed for low-income patients. In the following case, there is an increasing number of needy patients. The only way to serve them is to scale back the services. The alternative is to refuse to accept new patients.

Case 47: Scale Back the Services?

The dental health director of a large western city is in charge of several programs that provide dental service to low-income people. Although his programs cannot offer complete comprehensive care, they provide emergency service to anyone in need; in many cases, basic restorative care also can be given. In addition, for some patients with substantial needs, treatment beyond the basic requirements is available.

The demand for dental services has been increasing because there are more patients who cannot afford to pay for care in the private sector. The director wonders what to do about the increased demand for services. Should he turn some people away to maintain his previous policy? Or should he scale back the scope of services offered to serve more people?

DISCUSSION:

In this case, as in Case 46, there are not enough funds to provide the care that the dental health director desires. Unless more money becomes available, something must suffer. In this case, presumably all of the people who qualify for the program are financially needy (if they are not, then better screening probably is in order). One of the strategies that is contemplated is a time-tested principle of allocation: First come, first served. Those who entered the program early enough will continue to receive the full range of presently covered services. This is a principle that is often used when the scarce resources cannot be divided among those who need them. For example, it has been used for allocating scarce organs for transplant. Obviously, it accomplishes nothing to give each worthy heart transplant candidate half of a heart.

In the present case, however, it is possible to distribute the scarce resources so that all patients, existing and latecomers, could have part of their needs met. In one way or another, the city dental health director could limit the services so that those with the strongest claim receive the care.

If that strategy is chosen, someone must decide on what basis the care would be limited or what counts as a strong claim. The choice could be made on straight efficiency grounds—providing the services, whether basic restorative care or more complex procedures, that result in the largest benefits. That approach would most efficiently maximize the total good done, but some patients—for instance, the elderly—might not even get basic restoration if such treatment turned out to be inefficient in their cases.

Another approach would be to develop a list of services that all patients would receive regardless of when they entered the system and how efficient the service is in particular cases. For instance, the program could cover basic restorative procedures and extractions but not endodontics, periodontics, or fixed prosthodontics. Some people with considerable needs and perhaps even in severe pain who could be relieved efficiently with these more complex procedures might not get served. If some limits must be imposed, the basis could be first come, first served; maximum aggregate good; preference for basic over higher-tech care; or most acute, severe pain (even if the patient is inefficient to treat). Choosing to maximize the aggregate good based on social utility would be chosen by utilitarians; those who give priority to the principle of justice would either serve those who come into the program first or attempt to reduce the list of covered procedures to focus even more on the needs of the worst-off patients.

One of the factors often taken into account when deciding who should receive resources is age. In the medical literature, there is much debate about whether elderly patients should get lower priority.[3,4] While one interpretation of the principle of justice would insist that the elderly receive equal treatment regardless of their age and the shorter time they will benefit from it, another interpretation of justice would permit treating the elderly differently on the grounds that they have already had a long life. The latter view is sometimes used to justify lowering the priority for elderly patients to receive major organ transplants. (Many people believe that a 90-year-old should not have the same priority as a younger person for a heart transplant.) On the other hand, most people believe that all individuals, regardless of age, have an equal claim to the relief of severe pain and discomfort, which is likely to be the objective of the limited list of services that is likely to survive the health director's priority setting. If age is to be the basis for giving one of these groups preference over the other, we need to determine whether it is because of efficiency or because of fairness. The following case poses the problem of choosing between children and adults.

Case 48: Children Versus Adults

An eastern state has an annual dental Medicaid budget of $7.6 million. Of that amount, $5.1 million is allocated for children and $2.5 million is allocated for adults. Currently, comprehensive care is mandated for children, whereas funding for adults is almost exclusively for emergencies. A major problem of the Medicaid program is that access to care for children is very difficult despite the mandate for comprehensive care. This is because the state's Medicaid fees are so low that it is difficult to find providers. In fact, this state's fees are among the lowest in the country.

The program's dental director was considering a way to get more providers for children. He could eliminate the adult program and transfer the money to the children's program to raise the fees, making it easier to attract providers. He figured that he could probably get approval for the proposal if he decided to put it through. He considered the pros and cons of making this move.

DISCUSSION:

The ideal solution to this problem for those specially committed to dentistry would be to appropriate more money for the dental Medicaid budget. In the real world, however, that might not be possible. Other people have other priorities. Whether or not those priorities are ethically defensible, the funds allocated for dentistry are likely to remain at less-than-ideal levels.

Assuming that additional funds are not forthcoming, what would be a fair solution to the problem? Some arguments for increasing the proportion allocated to children are based on efficiency, or maximizing the amount of good that can be done. Perhaps interventions done early enough will prevent greater harm in later years. They may establish beneficial patterns that would make the benefits of childhood dentistry large in comparison to the costs. Along this line of reasoning, if the $2.5 million spent on adults could do more good if it were spent on children, then the switch should be made.

However, some interventions done for children may not be that efficient. Especially for interventions that affect primary teeth, the length of the benefit will be much shorter. Sealing primary teeth, for example, is not as efficient as sealing permanent teeth. If we opt for the straightforward effort to maximize the good, some children may actually lose.

Another basis for deciding this question is to ask what is fair, regardless of whether the maximum possible good is done. There are several possible answers to that question. Some would argue that fairness requires treating the worst-off patients regardless of whether they are children or adults and then readjusting the allocation based on what it takes to achieve that goal. If so, keep in mind that sometimes treating the worst-off patients may not be the most efficient use of resources. This would be a case of a direct conflict between efficiency and equity.

Some people have begun to calculate fair or equitable allocations by looking at how well off a person is over his or her lifetime rather than how well off he or she is at a given moment. From this perspective, an elderly person who has had good dentition all her life but is now experiencing moderate tooth mobility related to bone loss might be thought to be better off than a child whose immediate problem with caries is less severe, but who will have to live a long life with the problem. Regardless of how the question of age is settled, those committed to the principle of justice want to determine which patients are worst off and use the limited Medicaid funds to meet those needs.

Age is one category that raises questions of justice; income is another. One place where this issue has arisen recently is in the use of live patients during the licensing board examinations for dental school graduates. The problem raised is that of exploitation. Is the use of health services to entice people to use their bodies for the good of society exploitative, or is it merely another way they can get needed dental care? The next case involves the use of live subjects for licensing exams.

Case 49: The Ethics of Licensure

In recent years, opposition to the current system of dental licensure in the United States has grown significantly. A special point of contention has been the use of live patients. As dentistry is the only health profession to perform invasive, irreversible procedures on live patients for licensure, resolutions for the elimination of live patients have been passed by the American Dental Association (ADA), several state dental associations, the American Dental Education Association, and the American Student Dental Association. At least one state has granted licensure simply upon completion of a program in general dentistry. In addition, opponents have challenged the very idea that any state or regional testing board ought to pass judgment on clinical competence; they believe that graduation from an accredited dental school should be sufficient.

Those calling for change say that the use of live patients has several problems. To begin with, focusing on isolated procedures out of the context of a treatment plan suggests that patients are only a means to an end, not people needing health care. Furthermore, there is a widespread view that during board exams ethical constraints appear to be suspended. Stories abound about taking multiple radiographs until the potential "board lesion" looks just right. Despite the usual practice of not requiring patients to pay for procedures, it is a widespread practice for candidates to unofficially pay their patients for their time and inconvenience. The price varies, but payments of $100 or $200 are probably fairly common. The word gets out to patients about the opportunity to make money, and sometimes students feel forced by their patients to provide payment to ensure that patients keep their appointments. In addition, every time a board exam is given, it seems that one or two students fail simply because their patient broke an appointment. Furthermore, opponents say, the system does not really serve to keep incompetent dentists from practicing. People who fail the exam just retake it until they pass. Finally, some skeptics say that the use of live patients is no longer necessary. Modern patient simulators have been available for some time and are used in many dental schools, even though their usefulness may be mainly to test manual dexterity. Others say that what might work is a method where live patients are used only in the context of an educational program that better ensures patient safety, follow-up care, and the appropriate sequence of treatment.

The current system is supported by the American Association of Dental Examiners, which believes that the safeguards to the public offered by the current structure of dental education are inadequate, that there needs to be an independent system for monitoring the product of dental education and accreditation, and that the existing system is an essential prerogative of state government. As to the use of patient simulators, the association says that portions of the exams are already performed on mannequins and to expand their use would endanger the public at large. Furthermore, the association's statistical analyses show more variation for mannequin procedures than for procedures performed on patients. In addition, although students do fail because of broken appointments, it only amounts to 1% of all who take the exams. The association also challenges the notion that eventually everyone passes. In one subset of their analyses, 7% of the candidates who took the exam never passed it. Finally, with respect to the view that graduation alone is enough to ensure competence, the association invokes the many anecdotal failures of dental schools to weed out incompetent students.

With several issues at stake, foremost of which is whether live patients should participate in the licensure process and how to best safeguard those who do, what is the answer?

DISCUSSION:

The use of live patients in the licensure process raises many issues. Some of them could potentially be addressed without eliminating the use of live patients in the exam. Abuses in retaking radiographs, for example, might be prohibited. Failing students because a patient misses an appointment seems to be an excess that could be addressed. Some issues, however, are of fundamental importance. They pit the interests of the broader community in having competent dentists against the interests of the particular members of the society who end up as the patients for the examinations. Presumably, these patients have significant dental needs that are met, but they pay an unusual cost in terms of time, inconvenience, exposure to unneeded procedures, and potentially incompetent dentistry. No reasonable person would choose this method to have their dental needs met if they didn't feel they had to. Thus, if good-quality universal dental insurance were available for all citizens, it would be very difficult to get these patients to volunteer. It is a version of the classic problem in health care ethics of how care for the poor should be provided: Should it be charity care, or should the costs be assumed by society in general? It is compounded by the frequent payment of money to get patients to agree to suffer unusual risks and procedures that take unusual amounts of time. Because the burdens may be unusually great and the extra time involved extensive, payment for these services combines the charity model with a commercial model.

Paying members of the community to provide needed services involving medical procedures to the society has a long history. In the United States, paying blood donors has generated controversy, both because the quality of the blood is suspect and because some believe it is offensive to turn medical procedures into commercial transactions. Richard Titmuss wrote a blistering attack on commercialization defending the British system requiring that donations be a gift, free from compensation.[5] A similar controversy has arisen over the payment of human research subjects and donors of organs for transplant.[6]

Much of the controversy over paying people to use their bodies for the good of society stems from the claim that it exploits the poor, who are likely to be the only ones willing to take money to use their bodies this way. It has even been compared to prostitution. The question here is whether providing free care and, in many cases, paying live patients to be part of the licensing exam is similar to these other examples of paying people for the use of their bodies and, if so, whether it constitutes exploitation of the poor.

The defenders of the practice claim that no poor person is forced to become a patient in the licensing process. If people need significant dental work and can't afford to pay for it, the licensing process offers them a chance to get free services. Moreover, they are often paid for the extra time involved; it is, for them, a kind of employment.

Critics of the practice claim that no one would agree to this way of obtaining dental services unless he or she had no other option. They argue that the only reason such people are available is that the state does not provide adequate dental insurance or Medicaid support for the basic needs of the poor. If such support were available, then the supply of patients for the licensing exam would disappear. They say the licensing process merely takes advantage of the poor person's needs; it is exploitation.

Whether it counts as exploitation depends, in part, on whether those offering to pay for licensing-exam patients had within their control the possibility of helping meet these patients' needs some other way. If, for example, the licensing board could exercise influence in its state to improve the quality of dental insurance for the poor, then it should do so rather than continue to take advantage of those who need the services. If, however, there are no other options for the poor over which the licensing board could exercise any influence, then offering the opportunity may pass ethical muster.

The use of live patients thus raises a question of justice. Are the patients being taken advantage of when the society has an obligation to provide for the basic dental needs of its citizens?

Case 50: Importing Dentists for the Underserved: Two California Bills

In 2001 the California legislature passed Assembly Bill (AB) 1045, allowing a maximum of 30 dentists from Mexico, after receiving remedial instruction at a dental school, to acquire a permit to practice in an underserved area under the supervision of a licensed dentist. Presumably the practice location would be one that would serve low-income Hispanic patients. The bill was passed over the objections of the California state board and the California Dental Association.

Shortly thereafter, a second bill, AB 1116, was passed that also changed the status quo with respect to licensing dentists in California. This bill included a mechanism that would allow certain foreign graduates from any country in the world to take the licensure examination without additional education, provided that they graduated from dental schools that met certain requirements. The California state board was authorized to grant approval to schools that met the requirements of the ADA's Commission on Dental Accreditation regarding dental education.

No such legislation had ever been passed by any state. This precedent-setting situation came to pass because it was perceived that, for whatever reason, dentistry wasn't handling the problem of care for low-income people, especially Hispanic patients. The sponsors of the bills believed that by bringing more dentists into California, the problem could be better managed. Despite considerable opposition from the profession, enough votes were gathered for the bills to pass.

DISCUSSION:

The need for access to dentistry in underserved areas is severe. This case offers a strategy for addressing the problem, but, in the process, it also raises questions that have led to opposition of the plan from the dental profession. From the ethical perspective, the core problem is the injustice of having large groups of people, usually poor people with limited means and social resources, who do not have adequate access to dentistry. The response was to bring to the area a significant number of dentists who met at least a minimal standard of competency. Both bills were designed to recruit foreign dental school–graduates. According to one of the bills, they would also receive additional training and practice under supervision. The other bill permitted foreign dentists to take the licensing exam if they had graduated from an approved dental school.

The ethical assessment of the plan depends greatly on whether one assumes that these foreign dentists are equally as competent as those previously licensed in California or whether they would, on average, have lesser skills. If they are presumed equal, then there is no real problem with the plan; the protest from the profession would sound like an effort for previously licensed dentists to keep control of a tight market. If, on the other hand, one presumes that the foreign dentists have lesser skills, a presumption that may involve some stereotyping, then the moral issue is whether the patients, who are largely Hispanic, would be receiving unacceptable two-tier dental care.

Some justice theorists hold that *two-tier medicine*, in which the quality of care is dependent on one's financial and social means, is morally unacceptable. This provides a moral reason for the dental profession to protest the legislation in addition to their self-interested concerns about market influence. There is an initial problem with this basis for opposition to the schemes in that it rests on an ideal that everyone deserves the same quality of dental services. While some idealists hold to that view, it would seem to require equally vigorous protest against other arrangements whereby the poor get lesser quality dental care. Those protests have not always been forthcoming from the profession. A more general problem cuts to the heart of the claim that two-tier health care is morally unacceptable. The President's Commission, speaking about the ethics of health care, generally endorsed a moral position that everyone is entitled to a "decent minimum" of care but avoided commitment to the ideal that everyone receives the same level of services.[7] The idea here is that there is a floor below which no member of the society should fall, but that, above that floor, different levels of quality of service would be tolerable.

Other justice theorists find this ethic of a "decent minimum" unacceptable. They believe that everyone should be entitled to the same quality of care. This would imply universal insurance coverage and equal access to services in all communities. For dentistry that could mean rejecting these two bills if they are likely to provide lesser quality services for certain communities. It could also mean taking government actions that could be even more offensive to professional dental organizations: interventions into the market to pay dentists a premium for serving in underserved areas or even conscription of dentists into a public health dental service whereby they would simply be assigned to underserved areas for a period of mandatory service.

These bills begin to confront the critical problem of people not having adequate access to good-quality dentistry. If justice means arranging resources to provide more equal access, or at least to ensure fair access for the underserved, which of these strategies would best accomplish that goal?

Case 51: Pro Bono Care?

In recent years, the issue of improving access to care has become an important focus of the ADA and other organizations. For example, the ADA has launched its highly successful and award-winning "Give Kids a Smile" program, which, during National Children's Dental Health month each February, encourages willing dentists across the country to provide examinations, preventive measures, and definitive care to low-income children. Doing so emphasizes the ADA's interest in issues of access to care. Similarly, the ADA also promotes increased access to dental services by supporting the improvement of the Medicaid system. Furthermore, the ADA supports the Health Resources and Service Administration in promoting interdisciplinary partnership on this theme, and several states are holding dental access summit meetings designed to help eliminate barriers to care.

With the profession now taking a more active role in helping to promote reduced cost and pro bono care, the question arises as to how individual dentists see their responsibilities in this regard. Should all dental professionals do something for low-income or disadvantaged citizens? Should dentists participate in the Medicaid program even if they don't like it? Should the provision of care for the economically disadvantaged be part of every dentist's regular routine?

DISCUSSION:

Although individual practitioners can also play a significant role in the improvement of access, thus far they have not participated widely in the Medicaid program. Some dentists state that they would rather provide free care than treat Medicaid patients because of the low rates of reimbursement, the mounds of paperwork, and the bureaucratic delay of payment. Some practitioners, of course, already provide free or partially free care. Scarcely a week goes by that the *ADA News* does not report the activities of an individual or group providing dental services for needy people.

With these thoughts in mind, several questions arise. What should the position of the profession be about increasing access? The portion of the ADA program focusing on improving Medicaid suggests that society bears a responsibility for seeing that those without adequate means have access through Medicaid or similar government-funded programs. Thus, one option is that professional groups meet their obligations to the public in the policy-making arena by advocating the establishment and use of publicly funded programs. Another option, however, would be for professional groups to adopt the position that the improvement of access is an important consideration for everyone in the profession. Either of these would be alternatives to another interpretation of what justice (perhaps qualified by consideration of the autonomy of dentists) requires: that the provision of free care be left to those who want to do it.

The basic moral issue with respect to individual practitioners is to what extent, if any, they should provide reduced-cost or pro bono care for those who are unable to afford basic care. If dentists were to view pro bono as an important consideration, how much time should they set aside for it—a half day a week, a half day a month, one day a year? If they commit to the idea that all dental professionals owe some pro bono care to the community, they need to decide how to select the patients who will benefit. The principle of justice would urge that they concentrate on those who are worst off. The principle of social utility would support giving attention to those who can be helped the most. Sometimes these are the same people and the choice is obvious, but in other cases, it may not be. Moreover, neither principle necessarily supports merely taking the first group of patients that comes calling (up to some predetermined limit that the dentist sets). The patients who are mobile and aggressive enough to ask for help may not be the ones in greatest need or the ones who can be helped the most. Dentists also need to consider whether their contributions should be within their private offices or by donating their services in public clinics.

While the norm of every health professional providing his or her fair share of pro bono services is deeply ingrained in traditional health care ethics (even if the norm is often honored only in its breach), there are also moral arguments in support of a public program such as an adequately funded version of Medicaid or a universal dental insurance system in which all members of the community would be entitled to basic dental services funded through a public program. One of the great concerns about pro bono care as a response to the lack of adequate access for indigent patients is that it is inevitably stigmatizing; it condemns its patients to the classification of "charity cases." Not only is there a risk that the care will evolve as inferior, but there is also an insult to the dignity of the patient that comes from being so stigmatized. Medicaid in its present form could pose similar risks, but a universal insurance system would make it more difficult for the dentist to know the details of family social status. In addition, the pro bono solution leaves it up to very vulnerable people to seek out a willing provider of care. For these reasons, some would prefer a national right of access as the fair way to make basic care available to everyone rather than relying on the charity of dentists. They believe that even if every dentist did his or her share, there would still be an indignity to pro bono dentistry. It might be necessary until a fairer, more public solution is available, but its opponents think it is not ideal.

If a practitioner considers treating Medicaid patients in the office as an approach to providing equitable access, several concerns may arise. For example, one can become known as a "Medicaid dentist" and thereafter become swamped with requests for appointments. Just locating an office in a certain geographic area could expose a dentist to more than his or her fair share of cases. Then there are the practical problems of whether to "cluster" the appointments for the reduced-fee group or integrate them into the overall practice and whether to manage the problem of broken appointments by overbooking. That would reintroduce the problem of a two-tier system of care.

Microallocation: Allocating Dental Resources in the Dentist's Office

Thus far the cases in this chapter have been concerned with allocations of scarce dental resources at the societal level—how to allocate a state's dentistry funds or a county's budget. Even after these issues are resolved, however, there still remains the problem of resource allocation by the individual dentist in his or her office. The next series of cases asks how individual or small groups of dentists justly or fairly allocate resources, especially when Medicaid patients and those covered by health maintenance insurance are involved.

Case 52: Special Treatment for Medicaid Patients

Only 25% of dentists in a certain southeastern city accept children on Medicaid as patients because of the low profitability involved. Dr Dorothy Price feels that she has a responsibility to treat children from low-income families, but she also wants to minimize her financial loss.

In an effort to control office overhead, she schedules all of her Medicaid patients in roughly 2-hour blocks of time. In this way she is usually able, using two carpules of local anesthesia, nitrous oxide, and a papoose board as needed, to perform all necessary treatment.

Dr Price feels that this is a reasonable approach to the financial aspect of the problem but is troubled by other aspects. For her non-Medicaid patients, unless the amount of pathosis dictates an aggressive approach, she spaces the treatment over several visits and uses nitrous oxide and the papoose board only if necessary. For her Medicaid patients, she is concerned about the possible adverse effects of performing a large amount of treatment at one time, especially when it requires the use of the papoose board.

Is Dr Price justified in treating her Medicaid patients differently?

Case 53: Compromise Care Based on Type of Insurance

Ms Debbie Traber was a dental hygienist who worked for an agency. She received a 1-day assignment to work in an office located in an affluent suburb of Philadelphia. Her employer concisely briefed her about her responsibilities for the day. She was expected to spend an average of 45 minutes per patient. She would see three types of patients and her guidelines for approaching them were as follows:

Type 1 was a patient on Medicaid, which paid $16 per case for periodontal treatment. This patient was to be dispatched within 15 minutes. An air scaler was to be used; no hand scalers were even to appear on the tray.

Type 2 was a patient insured by a health maintenance organization (HMO). This type of patient should receive good treatment, but it should be done fairly quickly. No "frills" such as root planing should be provided. Ms Traber also should not bother with a sales pitch.

Type 3 was a patient with third-party payment insurance. This type of patient was to receive the best and most thorough treatment Ms Traber was capable of providing. Type 3 patients should also receive Ms Traber's best efforts to promote the more expensive aspects of dentistry. She should take as much time as was necessary with a Type 3 patient.

Ms Traber felt extremely uncomfortable with her instructions and found it difficult to comply. Furthermore, the dentist told her she spent too much time with her first two HMO patients. She considered what to do.

DISCUSSION:

Dr Price and Ms Traber are each confronting the demands of multiple payers willing to pay very different amounts for their patient's dental care. Ms Traber has found herself in the midst of a three-tier dental care system. We'll discuss her case first. Consider the ethics of the first and second tiers. Type 2 patients are said to be receiving "good treatment" but with no "frills." From the perspective of getting what is paid for, that sounds like what might be called a decent, acceptable level. Surely not everyone should receive the most thorough treatment Ms Traber is capable of giving. Therefore, the first problem raised by this case is whether it is ethically acceptable to provide care below this level to Medicaid (Type 1) patients, for whom reimbursement is set at $16 per case.

Continuing with the same perspective, let us assume that the Type 2 HMO patients generate a reimbursement considerably above this $16. Is it not fair to spend more time giving better care to those who pay more for their care? Would it not be unfair to give both Type 1 and Type 2 patients the same level of care even though the compensation is quite different?

Not everyone agrees that this perspective is an adequate one from which to pass judgment. When patients come to a dental office for a "cleaning" or a "prophylaxis," the common expectation is that they will receive, at the minimum, stain removal, polishing, scaling to remove calculus, and oral hygiene instructions. Every professional knows that it is impossible to do a thorough removal of calculus or anything else in 15 minutes. People who work in such an environment and who are concerned about doing good work are in the uncomfortable position of perpetual compromise. Certainly, patients should expect to receive less treatment if the reimbursement is less. But how does one handle the situation where even minimally adequate care is probably impossible to deliver? Would it be fair to all of the patients if office policy permitted employees to inform patients of their participation in a three-tier system and what it meant for them? Even if that is not office policy, should the practitioners disclose it on their own?

Dr Price in Case 52 faced a similar problem. She seemed legitimately concerned that Medicaid patients receive care and appeared to be carrying more than her share of the load. Still she has created a two-tier system of care with those at the first tier being booked in 2-hour blocks (presumably with longer waiting times) and provided large amounts of treatment (possibly requiring a papoose board) at a time. How does this treatment compare with that given to Type 1 patients by Ms Traber? Has society reached the point at which it will openly acknowledge the acceptability of two-tier care, or should we insist that all people have a right to the same level of care?

The case for single-tier care poses additional questions. Should Type 1 patients be raised to Type 2–level care, or vice versa? Should dentists be expected to absorb the loss for the low-reimbursement patients, or should they insist that the reimbursement be raised?

Ms Traber faces an additional problem with her Type 3 patients. If the "no-frills" treatment is fair and adequate, are some patients entitled to an additional level of special care? If so, the doctrine of informed consent would appear to suggest that these patients be adequately informed that they are, in effect, buying this special level of care. One might argue that the care provided to Type 3 patients constitutes deceptive overtreatment. Should the other patients also be receiving this highest level of care even though they do not have resources to pay for it? Or consider Ms Traber's problem from another point of view. She is not supposed to give the Type 2 HMO patients any sales pitch, whether they needed to be informed about expensive forms of dentistry or not. In contrast, she is instructed to give the Type 3 patients a sales pitch, perhaps whether they need it or not. The tensions between these forms of insurance coverage with respect to undertreatment and overtreatment are discussed in chapter 12.

Conclusion

The cases in this chapter press us to determine whether there is a fair and equitable distribution of care, whether the goal should be simply to maximize the good done, or whether autonomy gives people the right to choose whatever level they desire and can afford. This concludes our account of general principles in dental ethics. In the chapters in Part II, we have seen that the moral principles of autonomy, veracity, fidelity, and justice all impose potential limits on the morality of maximizing the good. We now turn to Part III for a series of case studies involving special issues in dentistry that demonstrate how these normative ethical principles are applied in some specific problem areas.

References

1. Aristotle. Nicomachean Ethics, Book 5. Ostwald M (trans). Indianapolis: Bobbs-Merrill, 1962.
2. National Institutes of Health. Consensus development conference statement: Dental sealants in the prevention of tooth decay. J Dent Educ 1984;48(suppl):12–131.
3. Daniels N. Am I My Parent's Keeper?: An Essay on Justice Between the Young and the Old. New York: Oxford University Press, 1988.
4. Callahan D. Setting Limits: Medical Goals in an Aging Society. New York: Simon and Schuster, 1987.
5. Titmuss RM. The Gift Relationship: From Human Blood to Social Policy. New York: Random House, 1971.
6. Dossetor JB, Manickkavel V. Commercialization: The buying and selling of kidneys. In: Kjellstrand CM, Dossetor JB (eds). Ethical Problems in Dialysis and Transplantation. Boston: Kluwer Academic, 1992:61–71.
7. President's Commission for the Study of Ethical Problems in Medicine and Biomedical and Behavioral Research. Securing Access to Health Care, vol 1. Washington, DC: US Government Printing Office, 1983.

Part III
Case Studies of
Special Problems

chapter 11

Ethical Concerns in Schools of Dentistry

In this chapter

- Morality in Academic Life
- Protecting the Welfare of Clinic Patients
- Ethics in Dental School Administration

Cases

- Borrowing a Friend's Laboratory Work
- Problems with Cultural Diversity?
- Friendship Versus Obligations
- Judicial Board Dilemma
- No Choice for the Patient
- When Faculty Disagree, Student Adjusts
- Advancement Committee Blues

Schools of dentistry, like other academic settings, provide a context for many ethical problems, including cheating on examinations, stealing books and school property, and straightforward physical abuses. In addition, dental schools, like medical schools, must deal with ethical situations that are peculiar to caring for patients. However, some of the ethical problems found in dental schools, especially those related to the completion of clinical requirements, are unique to the dental curriculum. In many of these problems, the ethically correct behavior is so clear that no real moral dilemma exists. Cheating on examinations is an example. Although we may not know how to avoid these ethical violations, we are at least clear that they are violations.

In the cases in this chapter, the ethical choices are somewhat less obvious. The first section focuses on cases that arise in the didactic and laboratory setting, the kinds of problems that can occur in preclinical years or, for that matter, in any academic setting. The second section presents cases where the moral conflict arises in the clinical training of dental students. Often the problem is one of conflict of interest between the education of the student and the clinical welfare of the patient.

Finally, there are problems that arise in the administration of a dental school: matters of fairness to students, conflicts among faculty, and so forth. These will be presented in the third section of the chapter.

Morality in Academic Life

The pressures of academic life for dental students are severe. Sometimes course requirements almost seem to the student to interfere with getting an education. Moreover, students increasingly come from different cultures and subcultures. Sometimes what seems clearly wrong in one culture may be acceptable practice in another. The first two cases in this section present these problems in the context of student laboratory work.

Case 54: Borrowing a Friend's Laboratory Work

Tom Novak was a freshman dental student in a southeastern dental school. Sara Simms, a good friend, was one of several students vying for part-time employment that involved laboratory work for the orthodontic department. The department had asked all applicants to submit examples of laboratory work that they had done for courses in other departments. Sara had saved most of her laboratory projects but had disposed of the wax carvings of teeth that she had made for dental anatomy.

To solve the problem, Sara asked Tom if she could borrow his wax carvings to turn in. Tom felt uncomfortable with the request. It was not that

Sara was a poor student; her carvings were as good as his. It was not even that she might beat him out of the job, because he was not interested in the position. But he was still uneasy about the request and felt that she should not have asked.

DISCUSSION:

Tom has a feeling that something is wrong here. What, specifically, is his objection? Assuming that Sara's work was as good as Tom's, this is somehow different from cheating on an examination when one is unprepared and does not know the answers. Tom's work was comparable to Sara's, but that does not seem to be sufficient. Why not? Would not Sara be put at an unfair disadvantage if she did not have work of the same quality as hers to submit?

Assuming that the work was of comparable quality, this is a moral problem related to the principle of veracity. By submitting Tom's work, although it is of comparable quality, Sara is being dishonest. The dishonesty in this case, where the result is the same as it would have been had she saved her own work to submit, may not be the same, but it is still dishonest.

Some might argue that what is wrong here is that the general practice of submitting another student's work is bound to lead to bad consequences in the long run. That could be the basis of Tom's discomfort. But others would claim that there is something intrinsically wrong with what Sara proposes.

A similar problem is presented in the following case, only here the instructor has reason to doubt whether the foreign student who makes use of another's laboratory work has the same moral understanding of the act as do the instructor and the other students.

Case 55: Problems with Cultural Diversity?

Dr Paula Stansbury has been teaching restorative dentistry for 25 years. A number of changes in dental education have occurred over the years, including—at least at her school—the enrollment of increasing numbers of foreign students. This leads to the obvious occasional challenges in communication, but Dr Stansbury has a growing feeling that there is a bigger moral challenge. She thinks that there might be differences in ideas of right and wrong between the foreign and American students.

One example involves student A, who was from a foreign country and who borrowed student B's laboratory project, saying that he wanted to learn from what B had done. Student B had already completed the project and received his grade. Student A then turned in student B's project as his own. Student

A's actions were discovered. When challenged, student A argued that he could not see what was wrong with his actions.

Dr Stansbury admits that it is hard to be sure that illustrations such as this do not stem from differences in individuals rather than in groups. In either case, she is frustrated and saddened by such examples, which seem to be on the rise, but she does not know what to do about them.

DISCUSSION:

Compare the previous case with Case 54. What are the important moral differences? Notice that in this case, the student who submits a fellow student's work is not being evaluated on work that he has demonstrated he is capable of doing, whereas in Case 54 the work submitted is known to be of comparable quality. Is that difference morally important?

There is a second difference worth noting. While Dr Stansbury and most of the other students in the class probably would have no trouble concluding that submitting another's laboratory work is unethical, there is doubt in Dr Stansbury's mind that student A is making the same ethical judgment. The student says he could not see what was wrong with his actions. Is it possible that he comes from a culture in which such behaviors are tolerated or, indeed, considered acceptable?

If so, how should Dr Stansbury take that fact into account in deciding what to do? The issue here is whether there is a "true" right or wrong answer to this problem, or whether it is merely culturally relative. One approach to this kind of problem is to try to imagine that we do not know in which culture we are. Is there something so irrational about submitting another's laboratory work, so contrary to reason, that all reasonable people, no matter what culture they are from, ought to see its wrongness? Are there grounds here for recognizing extenuating circumstances? What should Dr Stansbury do?

The problem of what a professor who finds what she considers dishonesty in student performance should do suggests other moral dilemmas arising in student-faculty interaction. The next case asks whether faculty ought to consider their personal relationships with students they find engaged in academic dishonesty.

Case 56: Friendship Versus Obligations

Dr Carolyn Pope was an instructor of removable prosthodontics. She had just seen Mary Heckman, a third-year student, forge a faculty member's signature on a patient chart. Dr Pope had been walking by the student lounge when she saw Mary with her back to her, seated at a table. Dr Pope and Mary had known each other for years, beginning as family friends, and their friendship had deepened as faculty and student. Dr Pope was going to say hello to Mary, got close enough to see the forgery, and stopped. There was always noise in the student lounge, so Mary was unaware of Dr Pope's presence.

Dr Pope was terribly upset and did not know what to do. Under the school's guidelines, she was obligated to turn Mary in to the judicial board. However, she felt such a personal bond that she did not know if she could do it. She retreated, at least temporarily, and thought about what she should do.

DISCUSSION:

Dr Pope's first problem is determining how wrong her friend's action really is. The forgery might have happened under a variety of circumstances. Mary might have been faking the completion of a certain key requirement. She might actually have done the procedure, seen that it was of poor quality, and then tried to avoid having her instructor see it. On the other hand, Mary might have been trying to avoid contact with an instructor with whom she had a personality conflict. Maybe the instructor was simply not around at the end of the clinic period when Mary needed the signature and Mary chose to forge it rather than to go to the instructor's office. Is one of these forgeries more wrong than the other? Consider who the forgery affects in these different situations and how the consequences differ. Is the act of signing the instructor's name equally wrong in all situations?

Next Dr Pope must figure out the role of her friendship with Mary in deciding what to do. Friendships, like professional relationships, are based on fidelity and loyalty. There could be a sense in which the two roles—friend and teacher—come into conflict, but it is hard to imagine that friendship could ever justify overlooking one's responsibility to the integrity of the educational process. Likewise, Dr Pope's long knowledge of her friend's moral character could play a legitimate role in tolerating Mary's indiscretion, but ignoring the forgery so threatens academic integrity and the school's obligations to future patients that it is difficult to let the coincidence of the friendship override her responsibility as a teacher. Are there times when friendship generates an obligation of loyalty that would excuse a forgery?

There are reasons for the general rule against forging signatures. It is a legitimate and important objective of dental education to have professional supervision of the adequacy of a student's skills. It is essential to the protection of future patients, who are the ones at risk if this rule is violated. That friendship should justify an exception seems odd. Are there any reasons why it would do so?

Many schools of dentistry have boards to review accusations of student misconduct. Called judicial boards or honor boards, they offer a way of adjudicating disputes about unethical conduct within the school community. Often they take on the atmosphere of a court with powers to discipline students who violate the norms of conduct. Unlike public courts, however, they may not have all of the trappings of due process, public accountability, and final authority of the more traditional public reviews. In addition, the allowable standard for conviction is almost always the "preponderance of evidence" rather than "beyond reasonable doubt." The following case demonstrates the kind of challenge faced by student members of the review board.

Case 57: Judicial Board Dilemma

In a large northeastern dental school, allegations of student misconduct are processed by a judicial board composed of both students and faculty, with cochairs from each group. The judicial board holds hearings and makes recommendations to the dean, who has the final authority to accept or change the board's recommendations.

Two problems are of interest in the collective experience of the board. The first is that accused students get harsher treatment from their peers than they do from the faculty. Punishments for convicted students, as administered by the dean, may be considerably watered down from the original recommendations. The second problem pertains to the lack of confidentiality. Although not a consistent problem, it springs forth from time to time from sources unknown. Both problems were factors in a case with which junior student Anne Muller was having to deal. As the elected vice president of her class, she sat on the judicial board and was hearing the case of Raymond Bissell, a classmate.

It was the second time that Raymond had appeared before the judicial board. Earlier that year he had been convicted of the theft of a classmate's handpiece. The board had recommended expulsion, but the final punishment administered was a 1-week suspension. Somehow the class had learned of Raymond's situation, and he was generally viewed as a disreputable person.

The current accusation was also of theft. This time, however, Raymond had been reported by a fellow student for a less serious infraction: stealing a wax carver and a plaster knife. Anne's problem was that she did not like Raymond and did not trust him. She believed that the thefts were part of a pattern of dishonesty that would make Raymond unsuitable for any health care profession. She was concerned, however, that her own biases were clouding her objectivity. Furthermore, the evidence was not conclusive. Raymond's accuser said he saw the theft committed; Raymond did not deny taking the two instruments but claimed he had intended to return them after he had finished working on a laboratory project. Anne tried to decide what was the right thing to do.

DISCUSSION:

This case reveals the moral problems encountered when a board is established to review the moral conduct of students. In this instance it poses what is essentially a due process problem. The typical procedure of a judicial board is that after an initial statement by the accused student, the student and faculty board members who question the accused, the accuser, and any witnesses brought in by either side are given an opportunity to state their positions. The board then discusses the case privately, typically with the expression of frank and open opinions from everyone. It would not be at all unexpected for Anne to be candid about her opinions of Raymond, including her distrust of him, her feeling that he was unsuitable as a health professional, and her concerns about her own objectivity. Furthermore, Anne may feel, as is sometimes expressed by both students and faculty, that ultimately the responsibility of the board is to protect the public from unscrupulous professionals.

The question is how the members of the board collectively should approach that important goal. Consider what would happen in a public court if a juror admitted that she did not like or trust a defendant. Do participants in school judicial proceedings have the same rights to due process—the right to a fair and impartial jury and the presumption of innocence until proved guilty—as do participants in a court case? In a public trial, jurors or judges who know the defendant personally would surely remove themselves from the case or would be dismissed as biased. How can similar protections be provided in school disciplinary proceedings?

Protecting the Welfare of Clinic Patients

Often the moral conflict between the interests of clinic patients and those of students is a more central ethical concern in health professional schools. A professional student has to have his or her first experience with patients in some way, yet it often is not in the patient's interest to be the student's first case. In dental school, there is a concentrated attempt to protect the patient with an extensive system of supervision. In addition, this has sometimes been dealt with by making the care available free or at a reduced fee; however, this has the effect of making low-income patients the "teaching material" for students. The cases in this section pose questions about the conflict between the important goals of training new students and the protection of clinic patients' welfare.

Sometimes the conflict between the interests of the teaching program and the patient is quite dramatic. If a totally unnecessary intervention were done on a clinic patient solely for the purpose of giving a student practice, particularly if the intervention posed real risk, pain, or inconvenience to the patient, it would clearly seem to be abuse. Often there are two or more plausible and defensible approaches to a problem in dentistry, each of which might have its defenders. Is it acceptable to insist that the patient choose one of these approaches to give a student needed practice? The following case presents such a problem.

Case 58: No Choice for the Patient

It is very important for residents in endodontics to gain sufficient experience in the management of periapical surgical problems. However, in many dental schools this type of surgery is in short supply. Sometimes there just are not enough patients who need this specific form of treatment. Dr Kevin Leppert, a new endodontic program director in a southwestern dental school, was faced with the problem of a potential patient shortage for the first time.

The previous program director dealt with this problem by having his residents choose surgery in cases where nonsurgical, more conservative treatment could have been used. Many other programs around the country did the same thing. In fact, one school did virtually all of its surgeries at a nearby prison, whereas similar cases seen at the dental school were managed conservatively.

This troubled Dr Leppert because although the cost and outcome of the two treatments were usually similar, he had no doubt that, given a choice, most patients would select the more conservative route. On the other hand, he knew he had a responsibility to his residents and to the public to ensure that his residents were adequately trained. Dr Leppert thought about what his best alternatives were.

DISCUSSION:

Dr Leppert's first task in analyzing the moral problem he faces is to identify the moral issues. Reflecting on the principles presented in Part II of this text, two issues seem relevant: respect for autonomy and how to determine whether social benefits are morally relevant in clinical decision making.

The principle of autonomy was seen as the basis for the doctrine of informed consent. According to the principle, people who are substantially autonomous have a moral right to be self-determining about their health care. Hence, they should be informed of the plausible treatment options and their risks and benefits. In this case, there seem to be plausible surgical and nonsurgical treatment options. The principle of autonomy and the related doctrine of informed consent require that Dr Leppert inform the clinic patients of both the surgical and nonsurgical treatment options and give them a choice. That, of course, is likely to lead patients in this case to elect more conservative treatment.

The doctrine of informed consent does not always require that the dentist be willing to provide all possible treatment options. Would it be sufficient for Dr Leppert to tell his clinic patients that the nonsurgical option exists and is available in private practice but that, to give students needed experience, the clinic offers only the surgical option?

The reason for this policy is clearly that, in the long run, society will benefit from having endodontists capable of performing the surgical intervention. And dental schools, in general, have long taken the view that patients who come to dental schools for treatment implicitly understand that the conditions under which treatment is provided, and indeed the treatment itself, may differ somewhat from that provided by licensed practitioners.

Hence, Dr Leppert's second problem. The traditional clinical ethic for health care professionals is that their moral duty is to do what is best for the patient. This has been modified in recent years to include the commitment to protect the rights as well as the welfare of the patient. Because of this, under the rubric of informed consent, dentists must sometimes respect the patient's informed refusal of a recommended treatment. Clinical ethics has tended to hold on to the idea of focusing only on the patient's rights and welfare, not on incorporating societal interests into their judgments. This is often seen as part of the ethics of fidelity, part of the implied promise of the clinician to the patient.

If Dr Leppert informs the patients that it is clinic policy to make available only the surgical option, is he abandoning the clinician's commitment to be patient-centered? Does an academician have moral duties to his students and to society that inevitably conflict with the rights and welfare of clinic patients?

In some educational and research settings in which an important reason exists for patients to receive an intervention that they would not otherwise elect, payment for the patient's time, inconvenience, or burden is considered. Dr Leppert could consider paying volunteers to agree to the surgery in cases in which the surgical option was clinically appropriate but unattractive to patients. If patients understood that the two treatments were equally effective and that the payment was to compensate for the patient's burden as a way of giving students needed experience, would this approach resolve the problem for Dr Leppert?

A similar moral problem can arise for dental students who examine clinic patients if instructors have different views about what is in a patient's interest. The following case finds a student trapped between the conflicting opinions of two instructors.

Case 59: When Faculty Disagree, Student Adjusts

Mrs Sara Silberman, age 70, was a patient of senior dental student David Saul. Although Mrs Silberman was in good health, other parts of her life were difficult. Her husband had entered a nursing home 6 months previously and her sister had recently died. Mr Saul worked up a patient history and, with his instructor, Dr Mill, established a treatment plan.

Phase one of the plan revolved around problems with an existing three-unit fixed partial denture that replaced the mandibular left first molar with inlays on the second premolar and second molar as retainers. The second molar needed endodontic treatment, which dictated the removal of its inlay, in turn destroying the fixed partial denture. It was thus necessary to cut off the first molar pontic at its junction with the second premolar. Once the endodontics was completed, a new fixed partial denture would be made. Phase two involved the fabrication of a maxillary removable partial denture to replace missing teeth and to establish occlusion on the left side. Mr Saul presented the treatment plan, and Mrs Silberman accepted it.

Mr Saul intended to work with Dr Mill during Mrs Silberman's treatment. However, on the day that treatment was to begin, Dr Mill was sick and was replaced by Dr Bentham. As dental students the world over rediscover daily, not all instructors think alike. Dr Bentham disagreed with Dr Mill on some fundamental ideas. First, he did not think that a maxillary removable partial denture was going to do much good. It was technically difficult, and Mrs Silberman might have trouble getting used to having teeth there because she had been without them for so long. Second, because cost was a factor, why not just leave the mandibular second premolar inlay alone? The second molar could be crowned and the space for the missing first molar could be left unrestored. This plan would be much less expensive. Furthermore, Dr Bentham thought it was unlikely that the mandibular teeth would shift without the fixed partial denture. Mrs Silberman's requirements for occlusion on the left side were minimal anyway because most of her maxillary teeth on that side were missing. Dr Bentham explained his ideas to Mrs Silberman, who seemed confused but interested.

Mr Saul listened with dismay. He had been caught in the middle before but never on such a large scale. He had to admit that Dr Bentham's views had merit. However, the plan was already established and approved by his patient. In addition, he needed the fixed partial dentures to fulfill requirements to graduate. Mr Saul was upset but did not feel that he was in a position to speak freely. He kept quiet for the moment and thought about how to handle the situation.

DISCUSSION:

As with the previous case, Mr Saul needs to identify exactly what the moral issues are. This is another case in which the interests of the patient may not be the same as those of the student or of the instructors. As in Case 58, the problem arises of whether patients of teaching clinics should have the same freedom of choice as do private patients.

One approach to this case is to, once again, look at it as a problem of autonomy and informed consent. Mrs Silberman "accepted" the treatment plan proposed by Mr Saul and Dr Mill, but it seems clear that she did not give an adequately informed consent. There are at least two possible treatment strategies for Mrs Silberman, each seen as plausible by at least one instructor. They seem to offer different risks and benefits, different costs, and possibly different outcomes. Dr Mill and Mr Saul have a moral duty to explain those options to Mrs Silberman. Dr Bentham has a similar obligation.

Mr Saul faces an additional problem; he is caught between two faculty members. It is a traditional practice in health care for a referring or consulting practitioner to avoid criticizing the primary caregiver's efforts unless they are grossly deficient. Is that an acceptable and relevant factor in this case: Should Mr Saul side with Dr Mill, the original clinician involved, or is giving priority to the original clinician morally irrelevant? Mr Saul could plead ignorance, insisting that the two clinicians resolve the dispute among themselves. Is that the student's best option? If so, he could be left with another moral problem. What should he do if the two instructors jointly agree on one strategy and Mr Saul still realizes that Mrs Silberman has not really given an informed consent after considering the treatment options?

This kind of situation occurs frequently in dental education and is probably unavoidable. Considering the questions raised here, in an ideal world, what policies and personal factors should be in place that would allow a satisfactory resolution to such problems?

Ethics in Dental School Administration

Some ethical problems in schools of dentistry arise not from the conduct of students or the conflict between the interests of dental students and their clinic patients, but from longer-term judgments about the administration of the school or the welfare of future patients. The problem can arise when graduating a student who lacks adequate skill may jeopardize the welfare of future patients, as in the following case.

Case 60: Advancement Committee Blues

The dental school's fourth-year advancement committee met in early May to determine the fate of that year's class. Most students passed without difficulty, but some had problems. Occasionally the problems were severe, like those of Charles Menefee, who was in his senior year for the second time.

The first time, he failed four of his 12 classes for a year-end grade point average of 1.50 and a cumulative grade point average of 2.07. At that time he was required to retake all of the courses that he failed plus additional requirements in most of the rest of the curriculum.

Now, a year later, he had made virtually no progress in meeting his requirements. He was not seeing patients in a timely manner and several had withdrawn from his care. Furthermore, there were reports of deceitful behavior in his relationships with both patients and faculty. For example, he had started several fixed partial dentures without having completed necessary periodontal therapy. Examples like these convinced many in the group that Mr Menefee did not belong in a professional school. Other members of the committee felt differently. They pointed out that during his first 3 years he had progressed satisfactorily, if not superbly, and that even after his terrible first senior year, he still had a cumulative grade point average greater than the minimum 2.00. His difficulties in patient care were attributed to depression, as was his unwillingness to accept help. Furthermore, the quality of his care, while not spectacular, was at least acceptable.

A motion was made to dismiss Mr Menefee. The committee continued to debate whether he deserved another chance.

DISCUSSION:

School rules permit graduation with a minimum 2.00 cumulative grade point average, but the committee also takes into account other factors, such as moral character, when deciding who will graduate. The issue is whether the school should function as society's agent for screening out potential members of the profession who are deficient in moral character or who have medical or emotional problems that may interfere with their practice of dentistry. Society could rely on graduation from dental school to be a signal of satisfactory completion of course requirements and a certification by representatives of the profession that the dentist can adequately take care of patients, or it could use the licensing procedures for that role.

If the committee has doubts that Mr Menefee can provide adequate care for patients, there are several reasons for that conclusion: Mr Menefee's poor grades, his failure to see patients in a timely manner, the reports of his deceitful behavior, and his depression. What is the moral relevance of each of these to the graduation decision? Should the depression count as an excuse for the questionable performance or as a basis for concern about future problems? Are any of these factors relevant in deciding whether Mr Menefee should graduate?

Conclusion

This chapter dealt with ethical issues pertaining to issues that arise during the formative stages of dentists' professional lives. The cases of the next chapter shift to an entirely different and more widely discussed set of problems: the ethics of third-party financing.

chapter 12

Ethical Issues in Third-Party Financing

In this chapter

- Disputes About Whether Procedures Are Beneficial
- Disputes About Marginally Beneficial but Expensive Care
- Disputes About Valued but Excluded Care

Cases

- Insurance Consultant Says No to Bioresorbable Membrane
- Obligations of an Insurance Consultant
- Insurance Coverage and Incomplete Treatment
- How Often Should Fluoride Treatments Be Given?
- Arbitrary Rejection
- A Closed Panel Dilemma

In two previous chapters we have looked systematically at the problems of balancing harms and good (chapter 6) and allocating scarce resources (chapter 10). Often the good that needs to be balanced and the resource that needs to be allocated involve money. Dentists cannot provide all of their services without compensation; they must be given some kind of payment so that they can provide for themselves and their families.

Until recently, the traditional fee-for-service method was usually used. Unlike medicine, which has long relied on insurance and publicly supported and charity care, dentistry was available, except in special cases and emergencies, primarily to those who paid directly for services rendered. This could mean that, despite a long history of dentists providing a certain amount of free care, some patients were forced by financial considerations to go without badly needed services.

The emergence of dental insurance has changed this somewhat, but it may have introduced a new set of ethical problems as well. Dental insurance is often considerably different from medical insurance, especially in its orientation toward prevention rather than treatment. The emphasis on prevention is a consequence of the fact that dental policies resemble prepaid health care more than they do true insurance. Medical insurance, like homeowners, automobile, and life insurance, exists primarily to cover unexpected and often very expensive events. When medical policies cover diagnostic or preventive services, they do so on an actuarial basis to contain costs in the long run. In contrast, dental policies are written to "prepay" predictable and affordable diagnostic and preventive services that people value. Furthermore, even when corrective dental treatment is required, the total cost is still smaller and more predictable than is most medical care, no matter how bad the problem is.

Another feature of dental insurance is that, although the terms of most policies are superficially variable, they are fundamentally similar in their structure. They all involve patient copayments for most services, and the less expensive services have the lowest copayments. Nevertheless, variability in the policies can lead to moral problems and confusion. For example, under the terms of a typical policy, it is often confusing to patients that while they pay nothing out of pocket for their examination or prophylaxis, they may be responsible for a 50% copayment for fixed partial dentures and a 20% copayment for amalgam and resin composite restorations. Thus, although total fees are usually lower in dentistry than in medicine, patient copayments are often proportionately higher. This sometimes leads to misunderstandings and conflicts between dentists and patients about the costs of treatment and the type of treatment provided.

Despite these differences between dentistry and medicine, there is a major similarity in the ethical tensions between capitation programs and traditional indemnity insurance. Capitation programs foster undertreatment and underutilization; fee-for-service programs foster overtreatment and overutilization.

The underlying ethical principles relevant to the economics of dentistry, dentists' relationships with insurers, and setting financial limits on care have been covered in Part II. Many of these cases involve disputes over whether care is really beneficial (see the cases in chapter 6) and what should be done when an intervention is marginally beneficial but very expensive or when an insurer openly declares that a procedure is not covered (see the cases in chapter 10). Many of these cases also raise problems of what patients should be told about insurance companies that impose such limits. (The issues surrounding patient autonomy and informed consent are presented in chapter 8.) In this chapter, we look at additional cases that pose these questions while focusing specifically on insurance and the relationship among insurer, dentist, and patient.

Disputes About Whether Procedures Are Beneficial

We have seen in cases in previous chapters that deciding whether an intervention will do more good than harm is itself a controversial issue. In chapter 6 we saw that competent dentists can disagree with each other and that patients may sometimes disagree with their dentists about whether an intervention is, on balance, a benefit.

Part of this problem stems from the recognition that all judgments about benefit and harm inherently contain a subjective dimension. Deciding whether a treatment is, on balance, beneficial requires that the anticipated good be compared with the potential harm. Deciding how much good is done and how bad an envisioned side effect is are both value judgments to which no amount of dental science can provide completely definitive answers. (For more discussion of this problem see the introduction to chapter 6 and the accompanying cases in that chapter.)

Because of the subjective nature of judgments about benefits and harms, it is understandable that dentists disagree about how beneficial a treatment is in comparison with alternatives or even whether the treatment is, on balance, beneficial at all. It is also understandable that laypeople might reasonably come to a different value judgment about these matters.

An understanding of the subjective nature of clinical decisions is necessary to make sense out of the increasingly complex and frustrating problems of the dentist's relationship to the insurer or to the manager of a prepaid capitation health care plan that covers dentistry. No rational subscriber would want to fund a service that was known in advance to be useless. Surely, insurers are within their rights not to cover such services. Some procedures can be demonstrated by good dental science not to produce the effects the dentist or the patient desires. For example, for many years oral surgeons often surgically managed nonpainful temporomandibular joint problems with symptoms of clicking or popping by physically repositioning the displaced meniscus. It is now clear that this treatment is completely ineffective. Eliminating such services may generate empirical disputes, but once it is agreed that the intervention will not have an effect, there is little ethical support for funding the service.

Much more commonly, there are disputes between insurers and dentists (or their patients) about whether there really is a benefit from the service. Because these are value judgment calls, it is not surprising that different people reach different conclusions even when they are acting in a disinterested, conscientious way. The following two cases involve disagreements about whether particular treatments are of any value. The cases in later sections of this chapter deal with claims against insurers in which the parties probably would agree that there is some value, but there may be disagreement about whether there is enough value for the insurer to fund the care.

Case 61: Insurance Consultant Says No to Bioresorbable Membrane

Dr Gordon Long submitted a preauthorization request to a patient's insurance company for the management of a 10- to 12-mm bony defect on the distal root of a molar using a bone graft with the barrier membrane Resolut Adapt (WL Gore and Associates, Flagstaff, AZ). This bioresorbable membrane, composed of copolymers glycolide (PGA) and trimethyene carbonate, is surgically placed to lie between the bone graft and the overlying gingival tissue. Its presence keeps the gingival epithelium from proliferating into the defect site. This barrier action is the essence of its success because it is the proliferation of gingival epithelium that confounds the regeneration of new connective tissue and is a major factor in bone graft failure. The regeneration of new connective tissue attachment has been well documented in monkeys[1] and dogs,[2] and some success has been reported in humans.[3–5] Many periodontists believe that the use of barrier membranes has radically improved the management of deep vertical periodontal pockets. Based on clinical trials, 90% success rates, as measured by evidence of tissue closure, now seem possible, compared with 20% in the more commonly used surgical debridement.

Other periodontists approach the use of barrier membrane techniques with some caution. Although it is true that connective tissue closure of the defects is well demonstrated, it is also true that the formation of new bone is unpredictable.[6] Presumably the insurance company looked to this type of evidence when it took the position that the proposed care was not of clear net benefit and notified both the patient and Dr Long of its view.

Dr Long had been turned down before on similar requests and was angry with the insurance consultant's lack of understanding of current developments in the field. The refusals also annoyed him because they tended to raise questions in the patient's mind about Dr Long's competence. It was difficult to continuously fight with insurance companies; Dr Long wondered whether he should decide on a less efficacious treatment approach.

Case 62: Obligations of an Insurance Consultant

Dr Douglas Kates is a periodontist who serves part-time as a dental consultant for a major insurance carrier. He reviews complex or controversial cases involving restorative or periodontal therapy that are submitted by dentists from around the country.

Recently Dr Kates received a request from a general practitioner for the approval of periodontal treatment for a 47-year-old man with no overriding medical complications. The treatment plan consisted of: *(1)* home care instructions, *(2)* scaling and root planing, *(3)* gingivectomy on two buccal segments, and *(4)* a bone graft (freeze-dried allograft) to replace extensive interradicular bone loss on a mandibular first permanent molar.

Dr Kates was impressed with the overall treatment plan. It showed much more knowledge of periodontics than he usually saw from a generalist. However, the bone graft troubled him because he thought it would probably fail. Freeze-dried allografts have shown greater than 50% fill in almost two thirds of the cases for intrabony defects but are only minimally effective in furcation defects.[6] Other approaches would predictably yield better results, especially the use of PGA barrier membranes with allografts. The latter method would have been Dr Kates' choice.

However, Dr Kates was glad that the dentist had not attempted to use the barrier membrane because general dentists rarely had formal training in its use. The manipulation of PGA membrane is so technique-sensitive that failures are common in untrained hands. That was probably why, at a fee of $985, it was the most expensive choice. For a fee of $765, the bone graft chosen by the dentist might have led to new bone formation, but unreliably so. Despite equivocal evidence of their success, these grafts were still regularly used in furcation defects by some periodontists. Other approaches, though less expensive, could only be expected to slow the progress of periodontal disease but could not be expected to generate new bone.

Dr Kates thought about whether to approve the overall treatment plan or to disapprove the bone graft while approving everything else. He had been so impressed by the dentist's overall approach that he wanted to encourage the dentist by approving the entire treatment plan. He also knew that in the event that he rejected the request, the dentist could resubmit it for review by a different consultant. About half of such cases under appeal were approved.

What should Dr Kates do? Do his obligations lie with a patient he does not know, with the submitting dentist he would like to encourage, or with the insurance company that pays him?

DISCUSSION:

The previous two cases are complicated. Let us first look at them from the point of view of dentists who serve as consultants to the insurance companies. What precisely is the consulting dentist's task? Is it only to determine if a procedure is covered under the terms of the policy? Is it to make sure that the clinical decision is based on acceptable scientific evidence? Is it to review and approve of the dentist's value judgment, trading off the chance of success with other treatment alternatives? Keeping in mind that the assessment of the side effects requires a completely nonscientific judgment about the trade-offs and alternatives, is the consulting dentist's task to decide whether to concur in the judgment that the side effects justify the procedure?

Let us assume that one of the operating rules for such dentists is that they are not to approve procedures that are not of known value. By definition, any procedure that is labeled "experimental" cannot be of known value.

Randomized clinical trials in which some subjects undergo experimental procedures and others do not are ethical only when it is more or less plausible that it is unknown whether the procedure is likely to be better or worse than the alternative treatment. Thus, any procedure that is still in an ethically acceptable clinical trial may be one that insurers would decide against funding.

Even procedures that are not experimental may produce real doubt about their benefit in specific patients. Presumably the consulting dentist should also disapprove of funding when it is not expected that a routine procedure of clinical practice will be of net benefit. In the case of the bone graft with a barrier membrane, presumably competent dentists disagree about whether the procedure will provide better treatment compared with its alternatives. Hence, it is important to know why these dentists disagree and what is the nature of their disagreement. They may be appealing to different facts, in which case the consultant must establish whether data support the desired outcome. Or they may value the outcomes or possible side effects differently. In the case Dr Kates is reviewing, there seems to be real doubt that the bone graft will work in that patient's particular circumstances. Moreover, there is concern about discomfort. If Dr Kates doubts the general practitioner's estimate of the likelihood of success, it is understandable that he would question funding the procedure. If he doubts whether some agreed-upon likelihood of success is worthwhile, given the discomfort and other possible side effects, we need to know why he makes the value judgment that he does.

Given the complexity of the decisions made by Dr Kates and other dentists who serve as consultants for insurance companies, it is debatable to what extent they should have a free hand to decide for or against procedures such as these bone grafts. They could be told that they should only assess the scientific data that support the clinician's recommendation. They could be given explicit rules about funding or not funding experimental procedures or other classes of treatment.

In evaluating these cases, we need to determine who else could be expected to make these value judgments. One approach is to assume that the insurer is a rational, self-interested economic agent who will have to make value judgments such that the particular insurance package he or she is selling will be marketable. Presumably patients (or the employers who choose dental insurance for them) will select the plans that, in the long run, meet their needs and desires most effectively. Furthermore, employers will match benefits and costs in order to remain within a preconceived total cost. This approach is plausible when the coverage item is one that the typical consumer can anticipate needing—routine prophylaxis, for example—but it is unlikely to work for a procedure that is sufficiently obscure that buyers of insurance are unlikely to think about it and base their insurance purchase on whether it is covered.

Another approach is to assume that the money generated by an insurance plan can be divided into two "pots." One would be the salaries of the insurance company administrators, management costs, etc. That amount could be set by free-market forces or by regulators in the way that public utility rates are set. The remaining funds could be viewed as "belonging" to the subscribers to use as they see fit. Even in this situation, however, there is a need to rationally allocate these benefits in an actuarially sound way. Logically, the managers would have no real interest in how the subscribers' pot of money was spent. Likewise, consulting dentists would have no basis for deciding which values should be served or which moral principles should be used in deciding whether to maximize efficiency or distribute benefits equitably. (This conflict between utility and justice or equity was the focus of the cases in chapter 10.)

If neither insurance company managers nor health professionals have an interest in or a basis for deciding how the subscribers' money is spent, then some have suggested that the subscribers themselves must allocate their pot of money. They could do this directly, such as in meetings of health maintenance organization (HMO) subscribers to decide what the general principles of coverage should be and which kinds of services should be given priority. They could also use indirect means—patient representative panels and labor negotiations—to further articulate which kinds of services are important. Finally, they could engage a consulting dentist to fine-tune the decisions on a case-by-case basis. This consultant, however, would be selected by the subscribers because he or she would represent the subscribers' values and be trusted as their gatekeeper. This would mean that Dr Kates or the dentist who was questioning Dr Long's treatment plan should be in tune with the subscribers as a group when it comes to making decisions about whether there is a net benefit of the treatment. The problem gets complicated, however, because even though this consultant dentist is hired by the group, he or she still has to work with rules and his or her interpretation of them. Different members of the group will have different values, and the consultant's judgment will probably always make some individuals unhappy. There is no collective unified understanding. Instead, the policy is an average of many different preferences that, when realized, will show variation. This raises a further question about the moral duty of clinicians who make themselves available as consultants for insurers or managed care plans. Traditionally, the dentist's moral commitment was to work for the welfare of the patient only. We saw in the cases in Part II that increasingly this has been expanded to include working for the rights as well as the welfare of the patient. Now, however, people are suggesting that dentists might legitimately work for public agencies or private insurers in roles that conflict with the welfare of individual patients. In these cases, if dentists are hired to make judgments on behalf of the insurer, they appear to end up with divided loyalties.

The moral principle of fidelity (discussed in chapter 7) plausibly would require that the consultant dentist refuse to accept any such commitments. Alternatively, a dentist might be able to engage in a division of moral labor, remaining loyal to the individual patient when in the clinical setting but shifting loyalties to an employer or a collectivity of patients when contractually committed to them. For example, a dentist could accept employment by which he or she was accountable to an HMO to see that no ineffective care was funded (even if the patient and patient's dentist think that the care is valuable).

This poses a serious problem for any dentist who accepts an assignment from a labor union or a group of insured patients to serve as their gatekeeper. Theoretically, this dentist could be informed about the preferred value judgments of the subscribers and told to try to make allocational choices based on those values. The subscribers as a group would recognize that individuals from within their group would occasionally not get the care that they desired. Increasingly, dentists are accepting such assignments. While they seem incompatible with the traditional professional obligation to remain loyal to the individual patient, dentistry practiced in a social setting must involve moral judgments based on competing interests. That will necessarily mean not giving every patient everything that he or she could conceivably want.

There is a closely related problem raised by these two cases. We have seen that there is a real dispute about whether these treatments offer more good than harm. Apparently reasonable, competent, dedicated dentists can disagree, in part because some issues are inherently subjective evaluations of the alternatives.

In these cases, the problems of informed consent discussed in the cases in chapter 8 emerge once again. If Dr Kates believes that the bone graft is not worthwhile (even though the patient's clinician does find it worthwhile), the patient would seemingly have a right to be informed of the disagreement about the treatment course. Alternatively, if Dr Kates did concur with the general practitioner, even though both knew that a significant proportion of competent dentists would not concur, the patient would plausibly have a right to know that other dentists had a differing view. This patient's treatment plan and insurance funding cannot be left to the luck of the draw as to whether the insurance company's dentist and the patient's dentist happen to be on the same side of the dispute. It would be reasonable to inform the patient of the dispute regardless of whether these two dentists happen to agree.

Disputes About Marginally Beneficial but Expensive Care

Many of these issues arise even more vividly in cases in which all parties involved acknowledge that some benefit is likely to come from the proposed procedure, but cannot agree on how much benefit or on whether the benefit merits funding. As we have seen, deciding exactly what the benefits and risks are and deciding how to quantify these benefits and risks is an inherently subjective matter that involves extensive value judgments. This next group of cases involves insurance judgments about whether to fund care that is acknowledged to be at least marginally beneficial, but is also expensive compared with the benefits.

Case 63: Insurance Coverage and Incomplete Treatment

Dr Theresa Tinsley is a general dentist who conscientiously and routinely incorporates periodontal therapy into her treatment plans. Recently her receptionist told her that an increasing number of patients had refused to come in for their periodontal treatment. At first Dr Tinsley did not understand this disturbing trend because her patients were all agreeing to her treatment plans, but she soon saw how it happened.

Dr Tinsley integrates restorative and periodontal care into her treatment plans along with her home care instructions. Often the restorative phase is finished before the periodontal phase. At some point during the treatment, the patients become fully aware that their insurance covers less than they thought it would—particularly the periodontics. Although patients see the value in the restorations, the importance of the periodontics seems less compelling, and they stop coming when they fully comprehend what their out-of-pocket costs will be. Typically, the cost of the periodontal treatment could be $780, and the major component of the care is deep scaling. With a copayment of 20%, the patient would pay $160. Dr Tinsley would have become aware of this trend sooner, but a good supply of new patients masked the patients she was losing.

Dr Tinsley wondered how she could manage the problem. There were so many different dental insurance policies with so many different approaches that she herself was not always completely aware of the details of the coverage. However, as difficult as it was for her, it was more of a problem for her patients.

Dr Tinsley considered how she could work effectively without being influenced by the insurance coverage. She also wondered how far she should go to help her patients understand their coverage.

Case 64: How Often Should Fluoride Treatments Be Given?

Dr Bernard Donaldson was a pediatric dentist who was strongly committed to applying fluoride to his patients' teeth. He routinely encouraged fluoride application for all children beginning at age 3 and continuing through adolescence.

Many insurance policies cover professional fluoride treatments only once a year. Consequently, some dentists set their office policies based on the frequency of recommended fluoride treatments to conform to the prevalent insurance coverage. This conflicts with the view, endorsed by a large segment of the dental community, that fluoride applications should be given every 6 months. A complicating factor is that the necessary frequency of fluoride application varies from patient to patient.

Billy Saunders, age 8, had received yearly fluoride treatments from Dr Donaldson for the past 5 years. For the first time Billy was beginning to develop some early caries lesions, and it was apparent to Dr Donaldson that a yearly fluoride treatment was not sufficient. He explained to Billy's mother that twice-yearly applications would be better but that the insurance company would only pay for yearly application. He told Mrs Saunders that the charge for the second application would be $45, at which point she said they would have to make do with the insured treatments.

DISCUSSION:

These two cases represent the problems created by dental insurance coverage limits. In Case 63 the patients may need additional education from Dr Tinsley to understand the importance of continuing their therapy. However, because the patients stop coming only when the insurance coverage ceases, it seems likely that they see some of the value but do not consider the care important enough to pay for the remaining services entirely out of pocket.

If that is true, then everyone involved in both of these cases would appear to see that the net effect of the services is beneficial. They do not receive the additional services because the insurance will not pay for an admittedly beneficial intervention—the periodontal treatments or fluoride application—and because they are unwilling or unable to pay for their own needed treatment.

The issue is whether rational people who were planning a dental insurance system would insist that all possible beneficial services be covered by the insurance. There are a number of reasons why they would not. In certain instances, for example, some services are so marginally beneficial in comparison to costs that subscribers to an insurance plan would reasonably insist that it is not in their best interest to have those services covered; they would prefer the cash.

In the real world of insurance, subscribers are not often given the chance to cast such votes. If the market is competitive, however, those selling insurance know that if they guess wrong about what patients would like covered, patients will vote with their dollars in favor of some other provider. So the issue is whether rational subscribers would support coverage for the periodontal and fluoride treatments in these two cases.

Consider Billy Saunders and his parents in Case 64. One could imagine a hypothetical meeting of subscribers trying to decide whether to include fluoride treatments for children in their insurance coverage. They would plausibly vote to include the service but then would have to face the question of how often to provide it. Surely they would favor once a year, but then they would face the question of whether to provide it twice a year. (If they favored twice a year, they would face the question of whether to provide it three times a year, and so forth.) If they understood the effects, they would realize that the second application of the year would not benefit most people at all. Some with higher caries rates, like Billy, would be helped even though the benefit of the second application would be less. Thus, as the frequency of fluoride applications increases, the clinical effects decline, even though the costs for each treatment are about the same. The subscribers could keep funding applications up to the point that no further treatments did any good whatsoever, but that may not be reasonable. For most, there would come a frequency such that the benefit would be so small in proportion to the costs that it would not be worthwhile to fund the additional treatment.

Dr Donaldson realizes that there is an additional problem. Not all patients need fluoride applied at the same frequency. Thus, even if once a year is perfectly reasonable for many patients, it may not be reasonable for some patients for reasons related to pathology, diet, hygiene habits, or even tooth morphology. The completely rational and fair insurance plan would probably try to give each patient the same fraction of their maximum possible benefit. That could mean different frequencies of fluoride treatment for different patients with no patient getting treatment at a frequency that would give absolutely maximum benefit. Unless there were an easy and objective way to measure need for fluoride, perhaps the best an insurer can do is to state a crude limit, such as one treatment per year. Does that justify imposing such a limit even on patients like Billy Saunders who have unusual needs? If not, once we realize that there is decreasing marginal benefit from increasing frequency so that no one should be funded to get every last bit of benefit, how do we set such limits?

Thus far in the discussion, we have dealt with issues primarily related to some problems created by insurance and whether rational people ought to expect that dental insurance policies should cover all possible beneficial services. Now let us turn our attention to the problem from the standpoint of what the dentist might do about it. Can Dr Tinsley, for example, improve her patients' acceptance of the periodontal treatment that they need? Apparently, her patients see the value in it, but not enough to pay after the insurance benefits run out. How should Dr Tinsley approach her patients in this regard? What kinds of issues should she address with them? Can you picture how a conversation between Dr Tinsley and a patient might go?

Disputes About Valued but Excluded Care

The previous cases involved care that was excluded from dental insurance even though it was desired by the patient (or surrogate for the patient) and would plausibly be called good dentistry. Those cases, however, all involved treatments that offered benefits that were admittedly marginal compared with the costs. Some dental insurance exclusions are different in that the service is an expensive and highly valued intervention. For example, an insurance program might simply not cover fixed partial dentures, no matter how clear the need. The following case presents such an exclusion and forces us to examine its morality.

Case 65: Arbitrary Rejection

Mr Ben Roberts was a new patient of Dr Richard Stroh. Having previously lost a mandibular first permanent molar, he both needed and wanted a fixed partial denture to replace the missing tooth. The adjacent teeth also had problems. The second molar required endodontic treatment and a crown; the second premolar had moderately deep distal caries.

Mr Roberts had insurance that he and the dentist thought would provide coverage for the fixed partial denture. Dr Stroh's interpretation of the policy was that it would pay for the endodontics and the two crowns but would not cover the pontic to replace the first molar. Mr Roberts agreed to pay for the pontic. Dr Stroh sent in the necessary forms and radiographs for pre-authorization.

The insurance company refused his plan, saying that it would not pay for any of the crowns if the final outcome was to be a fixed partial denture. Furthermore, if Dr Stroh received payment from the patient for the pontic, he would be guilty of insurance fraud. Although Dr Stroh investigated the matter at different levels of the company, the response was the same. Mr Roberts refused or could not afford to pay for the fixed partial denture himself.

Dr Stroh was disturbed by the insurance company's policy and wondered what he should do.

DISCUSSION:

The insurance company's position sounds truly arbitrary. To pay for the crowns if a fixed partial denture is not attached, but not if it is, seems to serve no purpose except to save the insurer some money. Apparently the insurer claims that the wording of the policy excludes any support of pontics. Assuming that that is their interpretation, is such a policy ethically justified?

We have seen in previous cases in this chapter that all insurance policies must have exclusion clauses and that, after excluding services that are truly useless, they will also exclude some procedures that are at least somewhat beneficial. Several criteria have been put forward as the basis for exclusions. Some services are excluded because they offer very low benefit-cost ratios. We saw in chapter 10 that one of the ethical problems with allocating on the basis of efficiency (the principle underlying appeals to benefits and costs) is that such allocations can be unfair to people who are hard to treat. Another basis for excluding services is equity. Under that consideration, those who are well off would have less claim to benefits. Still another basis, especially in dental insurance, is the belief that the purpose of insurance is not to cover all beneficial services but to spread out unexpected major costs. Finally, some exclusions might be utterly arbitrary, as the exclusion in this case seems to be.

Sometimes procedures are covered or not covered for no good reason. Many people, including employers and insurers, look upon such policies simply as mutually agreed-upon contracts with no moral implications. No one forces employers to buy the plan, and nothing prevents them from renegotiating the terms of the plan if they are unhappy with it. Insurers feel that if the plans were not meeting the needs of the employees and employers, the market would adjust and alternative plans would be offered. Here, however, it may not be enough to attempt to justify the exclusion on the grounds that insurance just can't cover everything. An appeal to fairness suggests that if the crowns are covered for someone who would need them without the pontic, then they ought to be covered even if the pontic is needed. Fairness suggests that people with similar needs should be treated similarly.

The problem of developing insurance policies that exclude some expensive, beneficial services was faced in this case by a dentist providing clinical care for a patient. The same problem can arise for dentists employed by insurers or capitated prepaid dental plans.

Case 66: A Closed-Panel Dilemma

Dr Daniel Shaum was interviewing for a job running a closed-panel dental facility. It was a substantial operation that involved the supervision of 60 dentists at two different sites. The salary and benefits were very good. With his master's degree in business administration and past experience, Dr Shaum considered himself the ideal candidate, a judgment that he thought the president of the company shared.

The president spelled out Dr Shaum's prospective responsibilities. Dr Shaum was to emphasize to the dentists he supervised that they should gear their actions to maximize the profits of the company. Under the terms of the company's contracts, profits would be maximized, for example, if they did relatively few crowns and more amalgam restorations. Similarly, they should do fewer fixed partial dentures and more uncomplicated removable partial dentures.

The president also pointed out that the nature of the dental insurance business was such that it was difficult for insurance companies to get long-term contracts. Two-year contracts were the average because employers attempted to cut costs by negotiating better deals with new insurance companies after short contract periods. Therefore, Dr Shaum needed to make it clear to the dentists under his supervision that they also must think in that short-term framework: Do what will last for 2 years. Along the same line, optional surgical procedures should be kept to a minimum because of their cost. For example, if a dentist were treating an 18-year-old whose third molars were clearly impacted but who predictably would be symptom-free during the next 2 years, the dentist should not recommend their removal, even though the timing for the surgical procedure might be ideal.

Dr Shaum was quite concerned about the constraints that would be placed on him in his management of the dentists. Most of the company's policies were in conflict with his instinct to act in the interests of the patient. Yet the job had such great financial benefits that he wondered if he could afford to turn it down if it were offered, as it probably would be. Dr Shaum considered what he should do.

DISCUSSION:

Compare this case with Case 65. Both cases involve funders of care that, by setting limits on care, eliminate some services that seem clearly desirable. In both cases it could be argued that the plan managers should have the right to exclude some services, even some that are expensive but beneficial. One controversial issue is whether the managers are obliged to provide a group of services or are only obliged to make their exclusions clear. Is the real problem with the company president's instructions to Dr Shaum the exclusion of services that will provide only long-term benefits, or is the problem not making this policy clear to members? One principle of ethics, sometimes referred to as the principle of publicity, holds that a test of the ethics of a policy is whether the policyholder would be willing to announce publicly what is being done. Would this company's policy pass this test? Would the policy be acceptable if the company and its dentists were willing to make the policy clear?

Conclusion

The cases of this chapter frequently found dentists in situations where the interests of patients conflicted with those of insurers or prepaid plans. The next chapter shifts to a clinical problem with ethical concerns that span the entire scope of dentistry: HIV and other bloodborne diseases.

References

1. Nyman S, Gottlow J, Karring T, Lindhe J. The regenerative potential of the periodontal ligament. An experimental study in the monkey. J Clin Periodontol 1982;9:257–265.

2. Aukhil I, Pettersson E, Suggs C. Guided tissue regeneration. An experimental procedure in beagle dogs. J Periodontol 1986;57:727–734.

3. Becker W, Becker BE, Berg L, Prichard J, Caffesse R, Rosenberg E. New attachment after treatment with root isolation procedures: Report for treated Class III and Class II furcations and vertical osseous defects. Int J Periodontics Restorative Dent 1988;8:8–23.

4. Pontoriero R, Nyman S, Lindhe J, Rosenberg E, Sanavi F. Guided tissue regeneration in the treatment of furcation defects in man. J Clin Periodontol 1987;14:618–620.

5. Pontoriero R, Lindhe J, Nyman J, Karring T, Rosenberg E, Sanavi T. Guided tissue regeneration in degree II furcation-involved mandibular molars. A clinical study. J Clin Periodontol 1988;15: 247–254.

6. Hancock E. Regeneration procedures. In: Nevins M, Becker W, Kornman K (eds). Proceedings of the World Workshop in Clinical Periodontics. Chicago: The American Academy of Periodontology, 1989; Section VI:1–25.

chapter 13

Ethical Issues Involving HIV and Other Bloodborne Diseases

In this chapter

- The Duty to Treat
- Disclosure of Patients' HIV Status
- HIV-Infected Dental Health Care Providers

- Clinical Decisions Involving HIV-Infected Patients
- Ethics of the Cost of Care in HIV-Infected Patients

Cases

- HIV Issues for a Periodontist
- Who Should Treat HIV-Infected Patients?
- Lied to Again
- Dentist and Physician Differ About an HIV Test
- The HIV-Positive Dental Student

- Should the Dentist Be Tested?
- Should a Biopsy Be Performed Despite an Extremely Low Platelet Count?
- Periodontal Therapy in a Patient with Idiopathic Thrombocytopenia?
- Informed Consent with No Options

The AIDS epidemic has posed so many controversial ethical issues for dentistry that virtually all of the important problems of this book could be addressed in the context of bloodborne diseases—especially AIDS; its precursor infection, HIV; and hepatitis. In this chapter a number of cases focusing on ethical issues involving these diseases are gathered for a cohesive look at their complex problems. The issues exist in the context of compelling epidemiological data. By the early 21st century, an excess of 500,000 Americans—possibly as many as 200,000 more—were infected with HIV. Worldwide, the number is an overwhelming 40 million. In the United States, 20,000 people die from AIDS each year. Worldwide, the annual number is more than 3 million.

Although bloodborne pathogens can be transmitted between dental professionals and patients in either direction and even between patients, it is clear that these incidents are rare. When transmission does occur, it is more likely to be from patient to dental professional than the reverse. The number of HIV infections transmitted from patient to dentist is not precisely known. However, in a study involving more than 4,000 dental personnel, many of whom were either treating patients with AIDS or who were at risk for AIDS, only two dentists without risk behaviors were HIV positive.[1] Since the beginning of the AIDS crisis, only five instances of possible transmission from dentist to patient have been reported, all from the same dentist.[2] According to a 2003 report from the Centers for Disease Control and Prevention (CDC), there have been no reported cases of HIV transmission from dental professionals to patients since 1992 and no reported cases of hepatitis B virus (HBV) transmission since 1987.[3] In addition, no cases of dental professionals transmitting hepatitis C virus (HCV) to patients have ever been reported. The risk of transmission in either direction exists when an exposure, defined as contact of blood or other body fluids with a nonintact skin or mucous membrane surface, occurs. A 2002 CDC study showed that of 208 participants in a surveillance system who reported a percutaneous exposure, none experienced a subsequent HIV infection, even though almost half of the exposures produced blood and 13 percent of the patients were known to be HIV positive.[4] In addition, a decade-long review of percutaneous exposures reported that dental workers experienced an average of approximately three exposures per year, the number having steadily declined over the 10-year period.[4]

Despite these reassuring statistics, the fatal nature of HIV and other bloodborne infections raises so many ethical issues that such patients present what amounts to a review of the range of ethical issues of dentistry itself. This chapter includes cases on the duty of the dental professional to treat patients with bloodborne diseases, the duty of patients to disclose their status, the duty of the dental professional not only to disclose his or her infection status but also to be tested for infection, the problems of assessing risks and benefits in the context of bloodborne infections and the related consent issues, and finally, the issues raised by the economics of treating seriously ill patients with short life expectancies. Sometimes all of these issues converge in a single case, as in the following introductory example.

Case 67: HIV Issues for a Periodontist

Ms Roberta Krebs, age 32, had been referred by a general dentist to Dr James Freeland, a periodontist, for the management of mild-to-moderate periodontitis. Ms Krebs was HIV positive and stated as much in her medical history.

Dr Freeland agreed to treat Ms Krebs but told her that there would be some additional costs because of increased infection control precautions. Ms Krebs expressed concern that the extra fees were discriminatory toward HIV-infected patients but said she accepted Dr Freeland's views about the necessity for the increased costs.

Ms Krebs suggested that Dr Freeland submit all costs, including those for the infection control procedures, to her insurance company. This could be done under an "extenuating circumstances" category. Dr Freeland pointed out that the use of that category might jeopardize Ms Krebs's confidentiality and lead to problems later. They therefore decided to submit the costs as a maintenance procedure. Dr Freeland felt uncomfortable with this submission and told Ms Krebs that in the event of any inquiry from the insurance carrier, he would have to disclose the facts of the situation to them. If the claim were denied, it would be handled out of pocket by Ms Krebs.

Dr Freeland also informed Ms Krebs that he treated patients on a selective basis and did not have to offer treatment to everyone who requested it. He told Ms Krebs that his main concern was that he would become widely known as a referral source for HIV patients. One reason for this attitude was that Dr Freeland employed a valued hygienist with decidedly negative views about treating HIV-infected patients. He could use another hygienist for the occasional HIV patient; however, this second hygienist might object if she were the only one expected to treat HIV-infected patients. Ms Krebs said she understood Dr Freeland's position.

While discussing Ms Krebs's situation with the referring dentist, Dr Freeland discovered that the other dentist did not know that Ms Krebs was HIV positive. Ms Krebs had not actually lied to him; the dentist had simply not asked her any leading questions. Dr Freeland hoped that the other dentist would continue to treat Ms Krebs and that Ms Krebs would not find out about Dr Freeland's inadvertent breach of confidentiality.

DISCUSSION:

The first task in a case as complex as this one is to begin identifying the ethical issues and distinguishing them from nonevaluative clinical issues. What are the core issues raised by this case?

Dr Freeland's first assumption is that it is ethical for him to choose the patients he wants to treat. Is this an acceptable starting point for the discussion of HIV-infected patients in dentistry? That will be the issue in the cases of the first section of this chapter.

Ms Krebs told Dr Freeland about her HIV status while the dentist was taking her medical history. If she realized that her access to treatment might be in jeopardy with such a disclosure, would it not be in Ms Krebs's interest to withhold this information? Whether patients have the moral right to withhold such information is the focus of the cases in the second section of this chapter. The link between the patient's duty to disclose his or her HIV status and the dentist's duty to treat HIV-infected patients will become apparent.

Also linked to the question of patient disclosure is whether dentists and other dental professionals have a duty to disclose their own HIV status to their patients. Being HIV positive poses some extremely small, but real, risks to patients. Moreover, because of the case of Kimberly Bergalis, the young Florida woman who was apparently infected by her dentist, patients are aware of this risk even if they may not adequately appreciate how small it is. Depending on how one answers the question of the duty to disclose, a related problem arises: whether dentists have a moral duty to be regularly screened for their HIV status.

Other issues can be identified in Dr Freeland's relationship with Ms Krebs. Special treatment decisions will have to be faced. Dr Freeland says that there will be some additional costs because of increased infection control precautions. However, it is common practice to take universal precautions to control not only HIV but other possible infections as well. If the precautions are universal, is it not morally wrong of Dr Freeland to use special precautions in Ms Krebs's case? Special calculations of risks and benefits will arise in such cases, issues that will be examined in the fourth section of this chapter.

Assuming that some special treatment costs are generated by the special precautions, Dr Freeland and Ms Krebs face the question of whether Ms Krebs's insurer will cover the added procedures. The patient will absorb the risk of having to pay for these added costs, apparently to avoid telling the insurer about her HIV status. This raises some interesting consent issues. Is it up to the dentist or the patient to decide whether the protection of confidentiality is worth the risk of generating these extra costs? What does the patient have to be told as part of the consent process? The question of the possible allocation of the scarce pool of resources that could otherwise be used for other patients makes clear that this case also poses social ethical questions that deal with the principles of beneficence and social justice in allocating resources. Does Ms Krebs have a claim to additional resources for the special precautions? If so, should they be paid for out of the pooled insurance funds that would otherwise be available to benefit other patients? These social ethical issues are discussed in the final section of the chapter.

The Duty to Treat

Dentists, like surgeons, are among the health professionals most exposed to blood and other bodily fluids that potentially could transmit HIV or other bloodborne diseases. When patients such as Ms Krebs in Case 67 make their status known to a dentist, it is natural to consider that one would prefer to treat other patients with whom the risk is less. Since the plagues of the Middle Ages, health professionals have faced the question of whether there is a duty to treat a patient in need when to do so would not be in the professional's interest. Dentists, like other health professionals, face this issue with renewed urgency in the era of AIDS. The next case asks whether there is a moral duty for each dentist to treat his or her share of these high-risk patients.

Case 68: Who Should Treat HIV-Infected Patients?

Dr Morton Cross, the director of a large midwestern city dental health department, faced a chronic problem in getting dentists to treat HIV-infected patients. Some cities set up special clinics to handle the situation, but his city had no funds for that kind of solution. Instead he obtained support for an HIV ombudsperson, who took calls from HIV-infected prospective patients and tried to arrange treatment using a list of dentists known to be willing to treat such patients.

The system worked reasonably well, but it disturbed the city dental health director that such a system was necessary. He believed that, in most cases, treatment could and should be given in the private dental office; the risks of treatment should be more evenly distributed.

DISCUSSION:

The American Dental Association's (ADA's) Council on Ethics, Bylaws and Judicial Affairs has held that "[a] decision not to provide treatment to an individual because the individual has AIDS or is HIV seropositive, based solely on that fact, is unethical."[5] If the ADA's position is morally correct and if the dentists in Dr Cross's community abided by it, his problem would apparently be solved.

It is not clear what this duty means, especially in a context in which one's colleagues are not carrying their fair share of HIV-infected patients. At its worst this could mean that the most conscientious dentist would take the most high-risk patients. If the risk of infection were greater than it is in the case of HIV, this could even mean that the most morally committed, conscientious dentists would be exposing themselves to significant risks and would, in extreme cases, eliminate themselves from the possibility of helping other patients.

In Dr Cross's case, there are apparently enough dentists willing to treat HIV-infected patients that the burden is distributed sufficiently; no one dentist is completely overwhelmed. Nevertheless, fairness as well as good dentistry suggest that this is not the best arrangement. Is Dr Cross correct in assuming that, in most cases, treatment should be given in the private dental office? If so, then should he not be dissatisfied with the easier, if more unfair, efforts of the ombudsperson?

If Dr Cross intervened more aggressively, to the point that each dentist in the community agreed to treat his or her own HIV-infected patients and further agreed to take a fair share of the new patients, would that solve the problem? Would not certain dentists, because of their clientele and geographic location, still carry more than their share of HIV-infected patients? What plan should Dr Cross pursue?

Disclosure of Patients' HIV Status

One reason why it is claimed that dentists have a duty to treat HIV-infected patients is to prevent patients from withholding their HIV status. Case 43 in chapter 9 described a patient who withheld his HIV status. The following case presents a similar problem.

Case 69: Lied to Again

Mr Ted Fisher, aged 35, came to Dr Marilyn Wistar for treatment. His medical history was unremarkable, including his negative response to questions about bloodborne diseases, but his dental needs were considerable. Two carious teeth needed extraction and many restorations were indicated.

The first extraction was technically uneventful, but the socket did not heal properly. Dr Wistar requested a blood workup and a consultation from a physician, Dr Samuel Sharrington, who said that the reason the patient did not heal was his longstanding HIV infection.

This was not the first time that Dr Wistar had been lied to by an HIV-infected patient. It seemed to her that such patients felt their responsibilities regarding disclosure were different for dentists than for physicians.

DISCUSSION:

Current standards of practice require that universal precautions be taken against transmission of infection during dental care. Mr Fisher's withholding his HIV status from Dr Wistar then poses an interesting problem: If Dr Wistar is already using the precautions thought necessary to prevent HIV transmission, is there any use she could make of the information? If the information is not of any use, there is no reason why Mr Fisher should be expected to disclose his HIV status. On the other hand, controversy remains over the question of whether it is really true that the information is of no use. For example, in this case, if the HIV status changed the way the socket would heal, it could lead the dentist to make different clinical choices. What is appropriate care for the person without known HIV could in some cases be the wrong care for someone with different immune conditions or a different capacity to heal.

Dr Wistar discovered that her patient was HIV positive from the physician, Dr Sharrington. This raises the question of whether Dr Sharrington's disclosure constituted a breach of confidentiality. Assuming that Mr Fisher did not want Dr Wistar to know his HIV status, we can presume that he would not have consented to the disclosure. Reflecting on the principles of fidelity and the promises made to patients about keeping information confidential, Dr Sharrington may have had a duty to not disclose his discovery. If Dr Sharrington is concerned about the risk to a colleague, this could be a case of a serious threat of bodily harm to a third party (the dentist) that would justify breaking confidence without the patient's permission. On the other hand, if Dr Wistar is using universal precautions, it is hard to classify the risk as a "serious threat." If Dr Sharrington wants to transfer the information to Dr Wistar in order to enable better clinical decisions, it is a potential disclosure for the benefit of the patient, in which case, based on the discussion in chapter 8, the patient's permission would be necessary. Disclosure of patient information between colleagues is generally routine if the disclosure is needed to further patient care. However, the reason is that normally we can presume that the patient would consent to the disclosure. In this case, there is good reason to suspect that Mr Fisher would not have consented. This same reasoning would apply if Dr Wistar received a request from another dentist for a transfer of records so that Mr Fisher could receive further dental care.

The question of fidelity in the relationship between dentist and patient introduces another issue in this case. If the dentist-patient relationship is to be one based on fidelity, the obligation is not solely that of the health care professional; the patient also bears responsibility. The patient should disclose to the health care provider all information that he or she would reasonably need to know to provide care. There is every reason for Mr Fisher to realize that this information is potentially important, if not for the dentist's self-protection, then at least to be taken into account in making clinical decisions about what constitutes appropriate care. If the patient fails to share such information, there is a breach of trust, just as there would be if the dentist broke the implied promise of confidentiality.

Some dentists may develop their own concern for knowing the HIV status of certain patients. In the following case a dentist wants this information but attempts to rely on a physician to obtain it. The physician is unwilling to cooperate.

Case 70: Dentist and Physician Differ About an HIV Test

Ms Alice Ford, age 55, was examined in a dental school clinic by Dr Lena Giordano, who saw that she had oral candidiasis. Ms Ford was a diabetic, which possibly could account for the candidiasis; however, she had also had a blood transfusion around 1983. Because of Ms Ford's history, Dr Giordano decided to request a consultation and a blood workup from her physician. The request included an HIV test, to which Ms Ford agreed.

The consultation came back with the suggestion that the candidiasis must be explained by the diabetes because this patient gave the physician no reason to suspect that HIV infection might be a problem. The physician refused to perform the HIV test.

DISCUSSION:

It is striking in this case that the conflict about whether to perform the test seems to be between the dentist and physician. When there is a dispute between two health care professionals, it is sometimes presumed that one of them is the "gatekeeper"—the one with the authority to make the choice. Here there may be moral reasons to refrain from performing the test. Should it come back positive, Ms Ford's life will change radically. She may face discrimination in employment and insurance. Because of this, some providers refrain from performing HIV testing. On the other hand, there are good reasons why both professional and patient would want to know. Is there any reason why a physician should act as a gatekeeper and decide whether to perform a test that the dentist desires for clinical care?

On the other hand, neither health professional seems to have considered the patient's role in this decision. Is it the patient who wants to prevent the test from being done? Ms Ford "authorized" the test, but it is not clear whether she was actively eager to have it done or was merely agreeing to the dentist's plan. If Ms Ford is interested in having the test performed, perhaps even in sharing the results with Dr Giordano, there is no reason for the physician to oppose it. The dentist could use the information in the treatment of the candidiasis.

HIV-Infected Dental Health Care Providers

If controversy exists about the right of patients to withhold their HIV status, similar controversy surrounds the right of dental professionals to hide or refuse to learn about their status. For obvious reasons, many dentists are reluctant to disclose to patients if they test positive for HIV. The following case sets the problem in the context of dental students, while Case 72 involves a practicing dentist.

Case 71: The HIV-Positive Dental Student

In the late 1990s, dental schools began to face ethical dilemmas pertaining to HIV-positive dental students. The first case was that of a third-year dental student at the Washington University School of Dentistry in St Louis who was dismissed from the school after it became known that he had tested positive for HIV antibodies. University officials said that the school acted out of its responsibility to protect patients who were receiving treatment at the school's clinic.[6]

Shortly thereafter, at the Medical College of Georgia, a somewhat different approach was formulated for a dental student who was also in his clinical years and had tested positive for HIV. The student was prohibited from engaging in further patient care in the regular clinic but was allowed to fulfill his requirements by treating HIV-positive patients.[7]

DISCUSSION:

Since those early cases, much has been learned about HIV infection, but a uniform policy for all dental schools has not been formulated. In all probability, some schools find ways to exclude HIV-infected students under criteria that invoke concerns about physical fitness for practice but avoid direct reference to HIV. Many schools have a policy of no discrimination against HIV-infected students at the time of admission, providing they are not so ill that they cannot function well enough to fulfill the academic and clinical requirements. For students who disclose their HIV status, either before or after admission, some schools have pre-appointed expert panels that can convene to recommend how to manage the students in everything from counseling to restricting their activities.

Despite all of the concerns about HIV, dental schools may face more problems in what their policies are with respect to students with hepatitis. Some, perhaps most, dental schools have policies that deny admission to known carriers of hepatitis B. This position has attracted some criticism and a few lawsuits, forcing the re-evaluation of these policies. In addition, some dental schools deny admission to students who are positive for hepatitis C. Others, however, reject that position, saying that evidence indicates that they are not dangerous to patients.

The current positions of dental schools on the admission of students with bloodborne diseases will affect dental students, practitioners, and the public for years to come. Considering the interests of all parties, what should the policies be for the admission and retention of students who are infected with HIV or are carriers of hepatitis B or C?

The treatment of these students raises a number of questions. Is there any ethical difference in the way in which the dental students were treated by the two universities?

First, questions arise about whether there are good reasons to let the students continue to see patients. Do the potential risks to patients ethically justify the universities' actions? Is there any reason why the students should not be permitted to treat HIV-positive patients? What about HIV-negative patients? The CDC has a policy on health care workers infected with HIV and hepatitis B. Its policy does not address hepatitis C because the cases have arisen since the CDC statement was written, but the policy would appear equally applicable. That policy reads:

> HCWs [health care workers] who are infected with HIV or HBV (and are HBeAg positive) should not perform exposure-prone procedures unless they have sought counsel from an expert review panel and been advised under what circumstances, if any, they may continue to perform these procedures. Such circumstances would include notifying prospective patients of the HCW's seropositivity before they undergo exposure-prone invasive procedures.[8]

The CDC includes as "exposure-prone" procedures those interventions that have a plausible risk of transmitting blood or body fluids from the health professional to the patient. Examples include surgeons whose procedures require placing fingers and sharp instruments in close proximity when the visual field is impaired. Dentistry is also given as an example of the CDC's definition of a profession at risk for exposure-prone procedures.

This suggests that if students are to have continuing contact with patients, a group of dental professionals (such as a faculty committee) would have to determine that the risk is acceptable. Moreover, the students would be ethically obligated to disclose their HIV status to their patients. Presumably, that means that the patients would be given the option to refuse to receive care from these students and still have access to other students in the clinic. If, however, the patient contact included elements that did not meet the criteria for being exposure-prone, the students could continue those functions without specific committee approval and without disclosure to patients. That is the policy currently in effect for physicians not engaged in high-risk procedures.

The second question raised by this case is whether there are reasons why the students might be permitted to continue in school without fulfilling their clinical requirements. If there are dental careers that would be suitable for individuals who agreed not to see patients, then that is an option the schools should consider.

Third, should there be an effort to ensure confidentiality of the infected dental students, and how would that be compatible with the apparent CDC consent requirement? While dental students, like all patients, deserve to have their medical information kept confidential, as we have seen in chapter 8, disclosure is required when it is necessary to protect third parties from serious threats of harm. That could plausibly justify the requirement of disclosure to patients, but it is hard to imagine how that could be accomplished without risking disclosure to fellow students and supervising faculty.

In the previous case, the issue was whether an infected dental caregiver was obligated to disclose his HIV status. In the following case, a dentist does not know if he has been infected. One way to avoid having to disclose one's HIV status is to refuse the tests necessary to determine it.

Case 72: Should the Dentist Be Tested?

Dr Kevin Pryor was 38 years old and had been in general practice for 5 years. Dentistry was a second career for him; he had spent several years as a high school biology teacher. He was married and had two young children, a new house, and more debt than most of his contemporaries because of his late start in the profession.

One day, while treating a young male patient, Dr Pryor stuck himself with an explorer. Blood entered his glove, but he saw none seep out. He was sure that the patient did not see it. Dr Pryor was alarmed by what had happened because he knew the patient was in a high-risk category for HIV infection. He continued to treat the patient while he thought about what to do. It was clear that under federal regulations he was required to record the injury and was encouraged to be tested for HIV. However, he was greatly concerned about what would happen to his practice and his young family if he were to test positive and have to consider the possibility of giving up his practice. Dr Pryor thought that maybe it was better not to know.

DISCUSSION:

Dr Pryor is reluctant to find out his HIV status. He is worried that he might lose his practice and his ability to support his family if he tests positive. This implies that if he is tested, he has an obligation to report an HIV-positive result to his patients, an implication supported by the CDC policy quoted in the discussion of the previous case. It also implies that his patients would not continue in his care if they knew that he was HIV positive.

Does it make sense for a patient to want to know his or her dentist's HIV status? Because the risk of transmission is very small, many people, including those in the dental profession, have maintained that it would be irrational for the patient to do anything with such information and that it would therefore be unnecessary for the dentist to disclose his or her HIV status. This in turn raises two separate questions: *(1)* Is it irrational to want to know something if one can do nothing about it, and *(2)* is there really nothing that a rational patient would do with such information?

Choosing a dentist is a complex process for most people. Often, if not always, there are several dentists from whom to choose and assessing competency is difficult. Two or more dentists in a community may be equally competent (or believed to be so by the layperson who is choosing a dentist). Patients also take into account many other factors, such as convenience, personality, and cost. If the patient is at a point of approximate indifference between two or more available dentists and then is told, "By the way, one of these dentists has tested HIV positive," would it be irrational for the patient to take that into account when choosing between the dentists who were, prior to this disclosure, more or less equal?

On the other hand, a dentist may rightly feel that this is unfair. He or she might argue as follows:

"Thinking of the clinical process, I cannot understand how Kimberly Bergalis (the Florida woman apparently infected by her dentist) could have been infected by dental procedures as I visualize them. Two of the most common ways that dentists bleed are *(1)* through needle sticks, which occur either while giving an injection (rare) or by capping the needle afterward (more often) or *(2)* by penetration of a bur during cavity preparation. The needle stick produces one or two drops of blood that, because it occurs extraorally, rarely enter the patient's oral cavity. I do not think that I have ever bled onto a patient from any of the sticks that I have experienced. The bleed from a bur wound does occur intraorally. However, the event is rather startling and the hand exits the mouth immediately. Even if blood is introduced during the withdrawal, dilution by saliva occurs, which would lessen the chances of the dentist's blood entering the patient's bloodstream.

"Having said all this, I recognize that parts of it might be wishful thinking rather than statements of fact. Furthermore, if a dentist is careless or ill, it is easy to imagine the comingling of fluids. This would be especially true if the dentist has symptoms of HIV because the risks of sticks and of contamination are higher because of potential diminution of physical and/or psychological powers."

The issue may ultimately rest on whether patients would rationally take HIV status into account when deciding between two more or less equal dentists. If they would, then perhaps Dr Pryor's fear is not simply that patients will react with irrational hysteria but that they will have reasons, at least in marginal cases, to avoid a dentist who is known to be HIV positive.

On January 16, 1991, the ADA released an interim policy (not since revised) on HIV-infected dentists. The key sentence is: "Thus, until the uncertainty about transmission is resolved, the ADA believes that HIV-infected dentists should refrain from performing invasive procedures or should disclose their seropositive status."[9] Thus, this policy is consistent with the CDC's position. If a dentist believes that he or she must disclose such status if it is known, is it acceptable for the dentist to avoid this significant problem by refusing to be tested?

Clinical Decisions Involving HIV-Infected Patients

Thus far, the cases in this chapter have dealt with the duty to treat HIV-infected patients and with disclosure by patient or dentist of HIV status. There are additional ethical issues posed by the patient whose treatment must take place in the context of his or her HIV-positive status. New kinds of risks and benefits must be considered. New information must be incorporated into the consent for it to be adequately informed. The first case in this section poses problems of calculating risks and benefits for the HIV-positive patient.

Case 73: Should a Biopsy Be Performed Despite an Extremely Low Platelet Count?

Jeffrey Perry, a 37-year-old man with AIDS, had previously experienced a severe necrotizing vasculitis of the palatal gingiva, thigh, and esophagus simultaneously. It took a month-long administration of high doses of intravenous steroids before the vasculitis was stabilized and discharge was possible. One week later, Mr Perry returned with an extremely painful, rapidly growing tongue mass. In addition, his platelets had dropped precipitously from $330,000/cm^3$ to $6,000/cm^3$. Mr Perry was bleeding heavily from the previously affected gingival tissues, necessitating transfusions. He was admitted to the intensive care unit. Dr Kenneth Vaughn, the attending dentist, was asked to see Mr Perry.

Dr Vaughn arranged for an oral surgeon to aspirate the tongue lesion and the oral surgeon determined that the lesion was not hemorrhagic. Its true nature, however, was not known. The medical team wanted to perform a biopsy of the tongue lesion to plan appropriate treatment that would include the elimination of the pain. However, the oral surgeon was reluctant to comply because he thought it was too risky in the face of a critical hematologic deficiency. He preferred to wait until the coagulation profiles improved.

Mr Perry's pain was intractable despite intravenous morphine. Mr Perry desperately wanted immediate treatment. There was no guarantee that a biopsy would prove to be a key factor in deciding treatment. Dr Vaughn considered whether to perform the biopsy himself.

DISCUSSION:

Mr Perry's treatment raises a number of important clinical ethical issues that draw on the principles of Part II of this book. If all else is equal, the goal of treatment is to produce the best balance of projected benefits and harms. In chapter 6, we saw that these assessments often involve complex, subjective value judgments. In this case there are significant risks in doing the biopsy immediately, but there are also reasons, including the patient's desire to expedite treatment, to do the biopsy at once. Is this a situation in which reasonable people might make different choices, so that the rational thing to do is to explain the options to Mr Perry and to let him choose, or is there some reason why dental expertise can provide the correct answer?

Consider the claim that Mr Perry was in intractable pain in spite of intravenous morphine. How does this compare with reports from skilled clinical pharmacologists that virtually all pain can be controlled, especially if one is willing to tolerate some diminution in alertness, with the use of sufficient analgesia?[10] This may be another aspect of the benefit-harm calculation. Perhaps the dentist was unwilling to take the risks of respiratory depression and even death to control the pain. Is this the sort of problem in which the patient or his surrogate should be asked whether the risk is worthwhile? How does the fact that the patient has an advanced case of a fatal illness influence the judgment about giving narcotic analgesia?

Cases 74 and 75 also bring up the questions of calculating risks and benefits along with the ethics of consent. In an era of cost containment, are these the types of situations where nearly useless medical and dental procedures can be eliminated, thus providing significant savings while losing little, if any, net benefit?

Ethics of the Cost of Care in HIV-Infected Patients

In the cases in chapters 6 and 10, there were times when the classical ethic of doing what was best for the patient may not have been the morally right thing to do. Other patients may have had stronger claims to the resources because more good would be done or because fairness required giving more equal access to care. This issue arises with particular drama in the case of critically and terminally ill patients. For these patients, the benefits of dental treatment are constrained by the brevity of the benefit. Sometimes, as when a patient is in great pain, the intervention may be justified; in other cases, the use of the resources causes more doubt. The following two cases pose issues of efficiency and equity in the treatment of HIV-infected patients. Is there good reason to limit care in each case?

Case 74: Periodontal Therapy in a Patient with Idiopathic Thrombocytopenia?

Michael Hurt, a 43-year-old man with AIDS, was admitted to a veterans hospital with cryptococcal meningitis, hearing loss, severe tinnitus, and oral bleeding. Dr Jay Branoff, a dentist on the hospital staff, examined Mr Hurt's mouth and found spontaneous, copious bleeding from the gingival tissues. Oral hygiene was very poor, and there was severe gingivitis. Mr Hurt said that he had not seen a dentist in many years. The oral bleeding was primarily related to a blood dyscrasia, idiopathic thrombocytopenia, but it was greatly complicated by the extent of the gingivitis.

Mr Hurt was aggressively treated for the meningitis and the thrombocytopenia. However, his platelets did not rise significantly and his oral bleeding persisted. The bleeding was so severe that it required many transfusions over a period of more than 2 months. He responded to treatment for the meningitis and his auditory symptoms gradually disappeared.

Dr Branoff knew from previous experience that the oral bleeding would continue despite the transfusions as long as the severe gingival inflammation persisted. Although the treatment of choice was thorough scaling and root planing, there were arguments against this plan. Mr Hurt had been in the hospital for a very long time and was in a debilitated condition. It was unclear whether the medical team would be able to improve his clotting ability enough to successfully withstand the additional bleeding caused by the procedure. Preparatory treatment for the scaling and root planing would also be very expensive, and the efficacy was uncertain. Dr Branoff and the medical team considered what to do.

Case 75: Informed Consent with No Options

Dr Joan Dwyer maintained a general practice in a low-income area of a large city. One of her patients was a 33-year-old man with AIDS who had a toothache in a maxillary first premolar. The tooth showed deep occlusal caries and a 3-mm apical radiolucency was seen radiographically. The tooth was a good candidate for endodontic treatment and a crown, but Dr Dwyer intended to extract it. The patient was still in reasonably good physical condition and could be expected to live for several years; however, he had long since exhausted his financial reserves and was receiving medical assistance from the state. For adults, the state provided funds only for emergency procedures. The extractions would not be a problem, but the likelihood of getting approval for endodontics was very low and it would be impossible to get authorization for the crown.

Dr Dwyer hated to extract the tooth but saw no other real option. She felt that the patient assumed that the tooth needed to be removed. Still, she was concerned about what to tell her patient. In a situation like this, what was the point of talking about all the options? Not doing so bothered her, but she thought it might only make him feel worse if he was again reminded of the consequences of his illness.

DISCUSSION:

Cases 74 and 75 pose different problems of justice in the context of HIV infection. Dr Branoff in Case 74 appears to be unsure whether the scaling and root planing would be worthwhile from the patient's point of view. Mr Hurt may not be able to tolerate the bleeding. There is also some question of whether he will consent to the treatment. Would a reasonable patient in Mr Hurt's position agree to the periodontal therapy being considered?

Dr Branoff is also worried that the treatment is very expensive. What role does expense play in this case? The Veterans Health Administration is paying for the care. If the funder has not objected, it is hard to imagine why Dr Branoff should worry about it. At least in the traditional ethics of the profession, the clinical dentist's responsibility is to take care of the patient, not to worry about the cost of such care to society, the insurer, and the patient.

Suppose that the insurer, after careful consideration, decides that scaling and root planing is too expensive to be justified in cases like this. Similarly, this may be the circumstance in Case 75. For adults the state provides only emergency care; that excludes the endodontics and the crown. The patient in Case 75 is being treated the same way that other adults are. Some interpretations of the principle of justice would say he is being treated equally. They claim it is not unethical to exclude endodontics and crowns if the state does so for all patients it is funding. Only if he is worse off than other citizens or if the state owes him something more would he have a special claim. Would it be any different if the restriction applied only to patients with a life expectancy of less than 6 months? The state is not expected to provide all the beneficial care that any private, self-paying patient could get. It is the state's obligation to limit care to a decent minimum. Are the endodontic therapy in Case 75 and the periodontal therapy in Case 74 above or below that decent minimum?

Now think for a moment about Case 75 from a different standpoint. Given the dim prospects for any other option than extraction, how should Dr Dwyer approach the part of informed consent that deals with treatment options? Considering her sensitivity to the psychological implications of AIDS for her patient, should she merely confirm what she believes his expectations to be—that extraction is the only option—or should she find a way to discuss all of the possibilities? What should Dr Dwyer tell her patient?

Conclusion

The cases in this chapter cover a variety of issues, including the duty to treat, the professional's obligation to disclose personal HIV status, confidentiality, clinical decision making, and ethical issues in the cost of care. The final chapter switches to an entirely different problem for dentistry: how to deal with colleagues who are incompetent, dishonest, or impaired.

References

1. Cottone J, Terezhalmy G, Molinari J. HIV infection and AIDS. In: Practical Infection Control in Dentistry. Philadelphia: Lea and Febiger, 1991:67–68.

2. Update: Transmission of HIV infection during invasive dental procedures—Florida. MMWR Morb Mortal Wkly Rep 1991;40:377–381.

3. Kohn WG, Collins AS, Cleveland JL, Harte JA, Eklund KJ, Malvitz DM; Centers for Disease Control and Prevention. Guidelines for infection control in dental health-care settings—2003. MMWR Recomm Rep 2003;52(RR-17):1–61.

4. Cleveland JL, Gooch BF, Lockwood SA. Occupational blood exposures in dentistry: A decade in review. Infect Control Hosp Epidemiol 1997;18:717–721.

5. American Dental Association Council on Ethics, Bylaws and Judicial Affairs. Principles of Ethics and Code of Professional Conduct, with official advisory opinions revised to January 2004. Chicago: American Dental Association, 2004.

6. Strom T. HIV infection spurs student dismissal, suit. ADA News 1989; Jan 2:1,8.

7. Comer RW, Myers DR, Steadman CD, Carter MJ, Rissing JP, Tedesco RJ. Management considerations for an HIV positive dental student. J Dent Educ 1991;55:187–191.

8. Recommendations for preventing transmission of human immunodeficiency virus and hepatitis B virus to patients during exposure-prone invasive procedures. MMWR Recomm Rep 1991; 40(RR08):1–9.

9. American Dental Association. Interim policy on HIV-infected dentists. Chicago: American Dental Association, 1991.

10. Twycross RG. Ethical and clinical aspects of pain treatment in cancer patients. Acta Anaesthesiol Scand 1982;26(suppl 74):83–90.

chapter 14

Incompetent, Dishonest, and Impaired Professionals

In this chapter

- Incompetent Dental Practice
- Fraudulent, Dishonest, and Illegal Practice
- Impaired Dentists

Cases

This book has covered a wide range of ethical principles and case problems. One major problem area remains to be addressed: colleagues who are significantly deficient in professional practice. In some cases, dentists simply practice dentistry incompetently. Their intentions may be good. Perhaps at one time these dentists had good skills, but time has passed them by. In some cases they may never have been practicing up to standard, but they somehow graduated from dental school and became licensed to practice. Virtually all codes of professional ethics call for dentists to maintain their professional competence. The American Dental Association (ADA) says that all dentists "have the obligation of keeping their knowledge and skill current."[1]

In rare cases dentists may not lack competence but nevertheless may engage in fraudulent, dishonest, or illegal practices. These could range from filing fraudulent insurance claims to lying to patients to prescribing illegal drugs. While these actions are quite rare, they are clearly unacceptable. They pose difficult problems for colleagues committed to protecting the integrity of the profession.

The dentist who observes an incompetent, dishonest, or impaired colleague has an obligation, often expressed by the professional codes as a duty—at least in cases of serious and continuing concern—to report a colleague or to take other action to see that patients are adequately protected. The ADA holds that "[d]entists shall be obliged to report to the appropriate reviewing agency as determined by the local component or constituent society instances of gross or continual faulty treatment by other dentists."[1]

The issues raised by such problems are more complex and controversial than they may first appear. In the cases in this chapter, dentists who suspect colleagues of substandard practice must make difficult decisions about whether the practices are truly unacceptable and, if so, whether some purpose will be served by taking action. If the decision is made to act, a number of options are open, all of which are likely to be unpleasant and controversial. While the ADA views the professional society as the appropriate place to initiate action, other possibilities come to mind, including making reports to licensing boards or legal authorities and informing present or future patients. The ADA seems to recognize the legitimacy of informing patients in some cases but warns that the dentist should do so in a way that is not critical of a colleague's practice: "Patients should be informed of their present oral health status without disparaging comment about prior services."[1] This might be a formidable task if the dentist feels morally obliged to convey that a prior dentist's work was truly unacceptable.

Although the problem of substandard practice by colleagues is difficult no matter what its explanation, not all reasons for such inadequate practice raise the same moral issues. The cases in this chapter are divided into three topics: incompetent practice, fraudulence and dishonesty, and impairment by mental illness or substance abuse. The focus is not on whether practicing dentistry under these conditions is acceptable—clearly it is not—but on the responsibility of colleagues who observe such problems.

Incompetent Dental Practice

Significant Incompetence by Colleagues

From time to time, a dentist unfortunately sees a colleague's work and finds it to be substandard. Sometimes the dentist is honestly unsure just how substandard the colleague's practice is; there is legitimate room for professional disagreement about treatment strategies and the standard of adequate skill. Other times it is clear that a colleague's practice is grossly inadequate. Before discussing the morally difficult cases of borderline or questionable incompetence, we first discuss cases where there seems to be no room to dispute the inadequacy of the performance. We shall assume, in these cases, that the incompetence is beyond dispute.

Case 76: Crowns and Posts, but No Endodontics

Dr Stanley Kilgore was a general dentist in a town of nearly 5,000 people. Mr Alan Fiorio, age 70, came to see him at the suggestion of Dr Kilgore's assistant, a friend of Mr Fiorio. Mr Fiorio had previously been treated by Dr Jones and was now in pain. Because he lived in a small town, Dr Kilgore had seen other patients who had been to Dr Jones and had not been favorably impressed. However, this was by far the worst treatment that he had seen.

The overall quality of the treatment was poor, but the main problem was with the maxillary incisors, all of which had been crowned. Two of the crowns also had posts extending into the root canal. This was fine except that no endodontic treatment had been done. These particular teeth had large abscesses. They were so mobile that Dr Jones had attempted to ligate them together by wire. Even so, Mr Fiorio would soon lose one of them. Mr Fiorio told him that he had paid Dr Jones almost $3,000 for the treatment.

Dr Kilgore became very angry at what he saw and felt sorry for Mr Fiorio. He was convinced that Dr Jones was regularly practicing seriously incompetent dentistry. He considered what to do.

Case 77: The Broken File

Mr George Sakonis was referred to Dr Marvin Goldberg, an endodontist, for treatment of a mandibular first molar. The referring dentist had been treating the tooth unsuccessfully for several weeks using both instrumentation and the prescription of two or three different antibiotics.

Dr Goldberg examined Mr Sakonis and found that a broken file had been left in one of the canals. The referring dentist had not told him about it and probably had not told the patient either. Although in this case the broken file was probably not the source of the pain, its presence was disturbing nonetheless.

Dr Goldberg's plan was to inform Mr Sakonis of his findings, to open the canal to begin treatment, and to begin antibiotic therapy with a different agent. When he told Mr Sakonis about the file, Mr Sakonis became extremely agitated. He could not understand why he had not been referred to the specialist earlier. He said he was going to demand that the referring dentist pay for his treatment and also for the work time that he had lost during his course of treatment.

Dr Goldberg had often been put in the position of being expected to answer why a previous dentist had underfilled a root canal, perforated a root, or left a broken file. However, Mr Sakonis's situation was more troublesome than most. Dr Goldberg considered what his ethical position was in relation both to Mr Sakonis and to the referring dentist.

Case 78: Problems with an Orthodontic Transfer Patient

Nan Keating was a 13-year-old girl who had been undergoing orthodontic treatment for 18 months and had just moved into the city. She had been referred to Dr Jack Testa for the completion of her treatment. The referring orthodontist said that the case could be finished within 3 to 4 months. Nan was a delightful girl, and her parents, both of whom came for the first visit, were friendly and concerned for her welfare.

Dr Testa examined Nan and discovered to his dismay that there were significant problems. First, the maxillary right second molar had caries that probably extended into the pulp. Obviously this had not happened overnight. Second, although the left side had been treated to a Class 1 occlusion, the right buccal segment was still Class 2. This would require far more than 3 or 4 months of treatment—perhaps a year.

Dr Testa had two problems on his hands: breaking the news to the parents and determining how to treat the patient. The clinical problem was difficult, but not as difficult as telling the parents.

Clinically Dr Testa thought that because the maxillary right second molar was compromised and because the third molar was developing nicely, he could remove the second molar, use that space to correct the Class 2 molar position, and later make sure that the third molar erupted into the former position of the second molar. Nan's parents, though quite upset, seemed to agree with his plan.

Dr Testa sent Nan to a general dentist for the extraction but later learned that a temporary restoration had been placed instead. Silence prevailed until 9 months later, when Mrs Keating returned for Nan's records and said good-bye.

DISCUSSION:

For purposes of this discussion, we can assume that the judgment of the dentists in these three cases is beyond controversy. Dr Kilgore, Dr Goldberg, and Dr Testa all have concluded that a colleague's work is significantly substandard. Dr Kilgore considered his colleague's work the worst that he had ever seen. While Dr Goldberg would acknowledge that breaking a file is something that even a competent dentist can do, failing to recognize the broken file, to inform the patient, and to treat the problem is a significant error. Dr Testa's colleague either purposely misled the patient or seriously underestimated the complexity of the problem. Who is at risk here and what are the dentists' options?

Consider first what is owed to the immediate patient. Both Dr Goldberg and Dr Testa were reasonably frank in describing the current clinical situation to their patients. The effect of their disclosures was predictably upsetting and, in Dr Testa's case, resulted in the loss of the patient. They might, in retrospect, have considered not fully disclosing what they saw. That would have made their lives easier, but it hardly agrees with the principle of veracity. It also means that any treatment of these problems would have been without an informed consent because the patients would not have known the true nature of their treatment. Dr Testa could have been content with dealing only with the caries lesion and leaving the right buccal segment in its Class 2 position, but that would have meant failing to practice the best-quality dentistry. The patient and her family deserve to know the treatment alternatives if their consent is to be adequately informed. A more complex problem emerges if, after explaining the options, Nan's parents insist on what Dr Testa considers the inferior option.

Additional questions arise concerning whether a dentist who discovers a colleague's poor work should speak directly with the offending dentist and, if so, should attempt to get the patient's payment refunded. For example, Dr Kilgore could try to get Mr Fiorio's payment refunded and could make clear to the colleague whose work was unacceptable that he feels that the dentistry is incompetent. Whether Dr Kilgore, Dr Goldberg, and Dr Testa should approach the offending dentists may turn out to depend on the circumstances. If the colleagues are believed to be naïve about their incompetencies, diplomatic communication might be productive, but if these dentists have histories of grossly inadequate work, then a more aggressive response may be called for—for example, reporting them to a licensing board.

Protecting the patients could well involve making clear to them why the current dentists are approaching the original dentists and warning the patient of the colleague's incompetence so that the patient will not return for further inferior dentistry. However, this raises the question of whether this can be done without violating the ADA Code, which requires that a dentist not speak disparagingly about a colleague.

Considering the risk for future patients, these dentists seem to have a moral duty to go beyond discussion with the offending colleague to ensure their practice improves. If increasing the dentist's awareness of his or her inadequacies is unlikely to bring about change, there may well be a duty to report him or her, depending on the circumstances, to the local dental society or the state licensing board. These options are explored further in cases later in this chapter.

Suppose that none of these agencies takes action and the offending dentists continue their incompetent practice. Is there more that Dr Kilgore, Dr Goldberg, and Dr Testa can or should do? They might criticize the colleague publicly, talk to the press, or warn other patients. These are all radical actions not normally contemplated in traditional professional ethics, but sometimes they may be necessary to fulfill one's duty to protect the welfare of patients. In considering whether to take such actions, these dentists might want to take into account whether they had had previous negative experiences with the offending colleagues. Dr Kilgore has seen other problems from Dr Jones, whereas Dr Testa is seeing a patient who has just moved into the city. Dr Testa might have to consider whether he has a duty to contact a dentist in a strange city or report him to that area's professional society or licensing board.

The dentists' general obligation seems quite clear: Whether they approach the offending dentist, take action through professional channels, or "go public," they have a moral duty to do something to ensure that these and future patients are protected from grossly inadequate practices.

Cases 76 through 78 involved substantial incompetence that one dentist discovered while treating a patient who was initially treated by another dentist with more or less the same level of competence. Sometimes, however, a specialist has an opportunity to view the work of a generalist who cannot be expected to manifest the same level of competence in the field of a dentist who is a specialist in some other aspect of dentistry. In these cases the specialist faces similar moral questions about how to protect the patient and others but now must factor in an adjustment so that the dentist who has not specialized in the area will not be held to unrealistically high standards. The following case presents such a choice.

Case 79: The Crispy Tissue

Dr Morton Kleeman, an oral pathologist at a dental school, received a biopsy specimen for histopathologic diagnosis from a well-known oral surgeon who frequently sent him inadequate specimens. This particular one was worse than most. It was a tiny piece of charred tissue that had been removed by electrocautery and was impossible to read. Full of pique, Dr Kleeman signed it out as "second-degree burn." Fifteen years passed before the oral surgeon sent Dr Kleeman another biopsy specimen.

DISCUSSION:

For oral pathologists to properly diagnose tissues, the specimen must meet certain standards of size and handling technique. Most specimens that they receive are adequate, but some are not. Furthermore, inadequate specimens tend to be sent repeatedly by the same individuals.

The collective experience of pathologists is that nothing will change the behavior of the referring dentist who submits poor specimens. If suggestions are made, the referring dentist sometimes gets angry and refuses to send more specimens. Because the pathologist relies on referrals for income, he is reluctant to unnecessarily antagonize those who send him tissue.

The problem for the pathologist is how to handle these poor specimens. What should be said to the referring dentist? What are his obligations to the patient, to future patients, to the referring dentist, and to himself?

Marginal Incompetence

The previous cases involved substantial incompetency in which the dentist's judgment of his or her colleague's or a referring dentist's work was not in dispute. Often, however, the colleague's work presents a more borderline problem. For instance, a clinician's work is routinely slightly substandard or reflects slightly out-of-date technique, or the colleague is generally known to do excellent work but has made a significant mistake in a single patient. The following case presents a version of this problem.

Case 80: A Periodontist Sees Another Periodontist's Patient

Mr Robert Stilwell, age 56, had been under the care of a periodontist, Dr Theodore Petrovich. Recently Dr Petrovich had told Mr Stilwell that his disease had progressed to the point where his teeth should be extracted and dentures made. Mr Stilwell was desperate to save his teeth and asked his general dentist if something could be done. His dentist referred him to Dr Joseph Donofrio, another periodontist, for consultation and treatment.

Dr Donorio agreed that Mr Stilwell's condition looked bad. Despite the possibility that Mr Stilwell's home care may have been questionable, Dr Donofrio thought that Mr Stilwell probably had been mistreated by Dr Petrovich. In Dr Donofrio's opinion, Dr Petrovich's diagnosis had been incomplete and his treatment had been ineffective.

Although a case could be made for complete dentures, Dr Donofrio could see that with selective extractions and the use of implants, followed by fixed partial denture treatment, it might be possible to save Mr Stilwell's dentition. It was a costly and lengthy treatment, but it could be done.

Dr Donofrio's problem at this point was what to tell Mr Stilwell. He did not want to create unnecessary problems with Dr Petrovich, whom he viewed as a colleague, but he felt that he had to be honest with Mr Stilwell about his condition.

DISCUSSION:

As with most cases in the real world of dentistry, this case raises a number of ethical issues. The ethics of truth-telling discussed in chapter 9 is the point at which Dr Donofrio appears to feel that he must start. The patient, Mr Stilwell, did not specifically ask Dr Donofrio whether he would recommend the original treatment plan; Mr Stilwell wanted only to keep his teeth. Dr Donofrio could try to finesse the problem by claiming that if he did not say anything he would not be lying, only withholding the full truth. While in some relationships, one need not say everything one knows, in the fiduciary relationship between dentist and patient, the professional is in a position in which he or she knows things that the layperson could not be expected to know. There is a trust that requires that the professional communicate openly.

The principle of fidelity, discussed in chapter 7, is also relevant here. Dr Donofrio is committed to tell Mr Stilwell what he would reasonably want to know as part of the consent process. Dr Donofrio may also have professional bonds with his colleagues. There was a time when that may have implied that one did not say disparaging things about a colleague's work—even when they were true. A professional, however, cannot have an obligation never to contradict a colleague's judgment. He cannot feel obliged to refrain from speaking critically of a colleague's work if he is convinced that it is substandard. Even if he believes that a case can be made for complete dentures, that cannot mean that he should refrain from presenting other options. The alternative needs to be presented, especially because Mr Stilwell wants to save his teeth.

Incompetent Friends and Partners

Dealing with an incompetent fellow dentist who is a stranger or at least a distant acquaintance is hard enough. In the next case the issue is compounded with an additional complication: a partner begins to realize that her colleague is perhaps not performing to expected standards.

Case 81: Two Views of a Cracked Tooth

Dr Jill Porteus and Dr Shelly Thomas worked together as partners, which is to say that they shared building space and expenses. However, Dr Porteus felt that they often did not share the same values and perhaps the same ability.

Recently, their dental hygienist asked Dr Thomas to examine her husband, who had a toothache. The pain was in a maxillary premolar and had begun when he bit down on a hard object. The tooth was sensitive to percussion and Dr Thomas thought that she saw a vertical crack. The hygienist also casually asked Dr Porteus to take a look. Dr Porteus agreed with Dr Thomas and in fact could see a slight separation of the tooth at the crack during clenching.

Dr Thomas told the patient that a crown was needed. Dr Porteus thought that this was a poor solution because it seemed likely that the crack extended into the root. If so, it would only be a matter of time before the pulp became abscessed.

Dr Porteus debated what to say. In her view, bad judgment was no stranger to Dr Thomas. Previously when Dr Porteus had made suggestions, Dr Thomas only became irritated. In addition, the hygienist liked Dr Thomas and respected her ability. Dr Porteus decided not to say anything.

DISCUSSION

Is Dr Porteus justified in not saying anything? She has obligations to the patient, the hygienist, and Dr Thomas. The principle of fidelity that creates duties of loyalty to one's patient also creates other kinds of loyalties—in this case, loyalty to a partner.

Dr Porteus has an interest in making sure that her partner does not practice incompetently. That is one reason she might feel compelled to speak to Dr Thomas. If that were her concern, this problem would be solved by severing the partnership. But Dr Thomas's patients would still be exposed to the risk of incompetent practice. If Dr Porteus has duties beyond protecting her own interest (if she has duties to the patients), then severing the partnership will not solve the problem. As a dental professional, she must do something to see that the patients are protected. That probably means confronting Dr Thomas.

A Hygienist's Awareness of Inadequate Dental Practice

Previous cases have dealt with incompetent and inadequate dental practice as perceived by colleagues, consulting specialists, friends, and partners. There is one other group of people with ample opportunity to observe a dentist's practice: the dentist's office staff. In the following case a hygienist recognizes significant inadequacies in her employer's practice.

Case 82: Skip the Home Care Instructions

Ms Lorna Pleasant was newly employed in Dr Louis Diamond's practice, which consisted largely of prosthodontics. Mrs Sally Merit was a patient in the practice and a heavy calculus former. Ms Pleasant completed a partial scaling and then instructed Mrs Merit on home care procedures.

While at the reception desk to make an appointment to have the scaling completed, Mrs Merit complimented Ms Pleasant on her thoroughness and especially her excellent home care instructions.

As soon as Mrs Merit left, Dr Diamond reprimanded Ms Pleasant for taking too much time with the patient. He said that complete scaling should always be done in one visit and that Ms Pleasant should not bother with home care instructions.

Ms Pleasant was very disturbed by Dr Diamond's actions. Many patients required more than one visit, and Ms Pleasant felt that home care instructions were part of her obligations as a hygienist. She wondered what she should do.

DISCUSSION:

The problem of conflicting loyalties that was discussed in the previous cases also arises here. Hygienists, dental assistants, and other professional office staff have obligations of loyalty to serve the interests of their patients just as dentists do. Ms Pleasant was certainly concerned about the dental health of Mrs Merit and her other patients. Yet she also had obligations of loyalty to her employer, Dr Diamond. Moreover, the fear of losing one's job is always a factor in a hygienist's decision in situations like this. Does Ms Pleasant also have to take into account obligations to herself and her family?

Is there any justification for a policy of omitting home care instructions in this situation? If not, what are Ms Pleasant's options? How would you evaluate each of the following?

1. Asking Dr Diamond to defend his policy
2. Consulting with other staff to see if they concur that the practice is unacceptable and jointly asking Dr Diamond to permit the home care instructions
3. Reporting the case to the dental society
4. Resigning in protest

What other options are available for Ms Pleasant?

Fraudulent, Dishonest, and Illegal Practice

Thus far in this chapter we have examined cases of dentists engaged in what appears to be incompetent practice. Generally, these cases have involved dentists who simply have lost the skill or judgment necessary to practice up to standard (or perhaps have never had that skill in the first place). However, it is clear that some dentists practice substandard dentistry solely for their personal gain in ways that are dishonest, illegal, or both. The following cases look at such practices. In the first case it is not clear whether a dishonest or illegal practice is taking place. Later cases pose more obvious examples of such practices.

Case 83: Should the Surgeon Suggest an Implant?

Mr Walter Baron was a businessman in his early forties who lived in a small university town in the northeastern United States. His dentist referred him to Dr Allan Wagner, an oral surgeon, for the removal of a mandibular premolar.

The tooth was painful and had a history of unsuccessful treatments. Dr Wagner agreed that extraction was necessary. Before extracting the tooth, he asked Mr Baron what the subsequent treatment was going to be. Mr Baron replied that a three-unit fixed partial denture was planned. Dr Wagner saw that neither of the abutment teeth was compromised with caries or restorations. Because of these facts, it appeared to him that an implant would be a good alternative for Mr Baron.

Dr Wagner had placed many implants with good success, but he knew the referring dentist had never done implant therapy and in fact knew very little about it. Recommending an implant to Mr Baron almost certainly would irritate the referring dentist. Dr Wagner might also be accused of conflict of interest because he was the only local oral surgeon who performed implant therapy. Yet he thought that it would be a good treatment and seriously considered discussing the implant with Mr Baron.

DISCUSSION:

The key questions here are why the referring dentist recommended the three-unit fixed partial denture and why Dr Wagner prefers the implant. The referring dentist might believe that the fixed partial denture is the only option available, in which case there is a competency issue. On the other hand, he might realize that an implant is possible but wants to keep Mr Baron as his own patient to gain the income from providing the fixed partial denture. If that is the case, the issue is not competency, it is honesty.

Likewise, Dr Wagner might favor the implant because he really believes it is the best option, but he might merely want to perform the treatment to gain the income. If either dentist is pressing his choice to keep the patient for himself, it seems clear that self-interest has overpowered concern for patient welfare.

One option would be for Dr Wagner to present the options to Mr Baron and then to let him choose. That would seem to be consistent with the principle of autonomy and informed consent. What would be the advantages and disadvantages of this option? How should Dr Wagner's behavior differ depending on whether he believes the referring dentist is simply lacking in knowledge or is purposely trying to hold on to the patient?

Grossly Dishonest Behavior

In the previous case it was not clear whether the referring dentist was simply incompetent (lacking in knowledge) or was motivated by self-interest. The following two cases, however, involve clearly and conspicuously dishonest practices that raise the question of how a colleague should respond.

Case 84: Competition for an Extraction Case

Billy Baum, age 12, was referred by his grandfather, a dentist, to Dr Gary Broyles, an orthodontist, for the management of a severe malocclusion. Dr Broyles's examination showed the presence of significant protrusion and severe crowding. Although Dr Broyles usually did not like to extract teeth, the crowding was so severe that extractions were clearly indicated. He told Billy's parents his opinion.

Billy's grandfather was unhappy with Dr Broyles's opinion and contacted a former orthodontic chairman at the nearby dental school. Now retired, the former chairman suggested that Billy be seen by his son, Dr John Caplan, who was also an orthodontist. Dr Caplan examined Billy, agreed with his father that extractions were not necessary, and accepted Billy as a patient.

Dr Broyles later saw Dr Caplan at a dental meeting and asked him how he could treat Billy without extractions. Dr Caplan responded, "Oh, I will extract the teeth all right—when I'm ready." To Dr Broyles's protests, Dr Caplan said, "You might feel that you are right, but I have the patient."

Dr Broyles was upset, having previously thought of Dr Caplan as a friend.

Case 85: Fraudulent Orthodontics

Dr Philip Pressley is a general practitioner who is known as a family dentist. However, much of his practice involves orthodontics. His typical strategy for obtaining consent for orthodontic treatment (at least for patients with insurance) is to tell the parents that the child needs braces and that treatment should be started right away. He suggests that he could undertake preliminary treatment immediately—that day, if the parents so desire. They can discuss the details of the case and the fees later.

With even a tentative agreement from the parents, Dr Pressley takes preliminary measures such as making impressions or cementing brackets. If the parents refuse, he does not charge them for any appliances but he does bill the insurance company. If the parents agree, he proceeds with treatment and bills the insurance company. Then when the insurance benefits are depleted, he tells the parents that treatment is not working and refers the patient to an orthodontist, usually Dr Philip Leighton.

Dr Leighton is tired of protecting Dr Pressley and angry about his dishonesty, but he does not want to instigate trouble.

DISCUSSION:

The practices of the dentists in these two cases raise ethical and legal questions. Both seem to be engaging in dishonest or deceptive practices for the purposes of gaining new patients. They may believe that their behavior is legal even if it is not ethical. However, each dentist is clearly not providing all of the information that the reasonable patient would want to know prior to giving consent for treatment; they are treating without an adequate consent. Thus the practices seem unethical and illegal as well.

The real issue is not the assessment of Dr Caplan or Dr Pressley. These deceptions are severe enough that we can assume that they are at least unethical. The real issue is how the colleagues who become aware of these practices should respond. Dr Broyles and Dr Leighton could confront the offending dentists directly. They could report them to the local dental society or state licensing boards. There are also steps beyond this that could be taken, such as directly alerting patients and the local press. Should Dr Broyles and Dr Leighton pursue these options or work strictly within professional channels?

Clearly Illegal Behavior

Although the dentists in the previous cases seemed to be engaged in clearly deceptive, unethical behavior, there was room for debate about whether the behavior was illegal. In the following case, however, the offending professional's behavior is clearly illegal. A dentist asks his hygienist to assist in an insurance fraud. Because we can presume there is no moral defense of the dentist's request, the focus of the discussion is on what, ethically, the hygienist should do.

Case 86: A Request to Participate in a Fraud

Ms Sandra Gonce, a dental hygienist, had been working for a dentist, Dr Jeffry Holmes, for almost a year. One Saturday afternoon, shortly after the staff had left, a fire started in a small laboratory used mainly for radiograph processing and storage space for dental casts of current and former patients.

The fire was put out promptly and was contained entirely within the laboratory. Ms Gonce was the first to hear about the fire and notified Dr Holmes. He suggested that they clean it up early on Monday.

By Monday morning, he had called his insurance company and received instructions to document all lost partial denture frameworks of ongoing cases, as well as any equipment destroyed by the fire. Dr Holmes instructed Ms Gonce to list everything, even cases that had long since been delivered to the patient. She was also expected to list equipment that had been broken before the fire. He intended to submit all of it to the insurance company.

Ms Gonce thought that the total claims, most of them fraudulent, might amount to as much as $10,000. She considered what to do.

DISCUSSION:

Assuming that there is no disagreement that the dentist's request was unethical, is there any possible ethical defense that would support Ms Gonce's cooperation in the request? She might consider that she is merely an employee and that she would be doing nothing more than following orders were she to do as she was told. The "just following orders" defense, however, has never been adequate to defend participation in a fraud. She might consider that she has a duty of loyalty to her employer, but that defense does not seem to carry any more weight. She might consider that, if she protests, she will lose her job and jeopardize the welfare of her family, but that does not seem to support her cooperation either. Her options seem to be to confront the dentist, to report him to various authorities, if necessary, and finally, to contemplate resignation.

If there is any defense for her to do nothing, it rests in her claim of "necessity"; that is, that the consequences to her of refusing to cooperate (including the risk of losing her job) would be so horrendous that she has, in effect, no other option. What do you believe would be the consequences of refusing to cooperate? Is there any point at which such an impact on the hygienist would morally justify her cooperation in a fraud? Are there any other reasons that would justify her collaboration, such as a sense that the insurance company has treated her or her employer unfairly in the past or that without the fraud the practice would be lost and patients would suffer? Would any of these purported extenuating circumstances or risks to the hygienist herself ever justify cooperating in insurance fraud?

Impaired Dentists

Thus far we have looked at incompetent and dishonest dentists. Both incompetence and dishonesty carry with them an implied degree of culpability; the straightforwardly dishonest dentist surely knows what he or she is doing, and the incompetent dentist often bears at least some responsibility for failing to maintain his or her skills or at least recognize his or her incompetence and withdraw from the area of practice.

Some dentists, however, are impaired by a mental handicap that may be beyond their awareness. The two cases that follow deal with a dentist with a possible mental illness and another who suffers from drug dependency. One of the issues in these cases is the extent to which the impairment excuses the behavior and whether dentists with such impairments should be held responsible. Whether they are or not, their colleagues face important ethical questions.

Case 87: Should Referrals Stop?

Dr Henry Wolfe has been referring patients to Dr Keith Johnson for many years. Dr Johnson is an oral surgeon and is generally well respected throughout the professional community. Dr Wolfe personally has seen no reason to be concerned about the quality of Dr Johnson's professional care. However, over the last few years, Dr Wolfe has been made aware of some disturbing stories about Dr Johnson. For example, he has heard that Dr Johnson recently had a series of emotional outbursts in his office. Also, reports have been circulating that Dr Johnson's fees have become disproportionately high. Recently a patient told Dr Wolfe that he did not like the lack of cleanliness of Dr Johnson's office. It was a vague complaint, not related to personal hygiene, but a complaint nevertheless. Finally, a personal friend, also a dentist, recently told Dr Wolfe that he thinks Dr Johnson's professional care is slipping.

Dr Wolfe's own observations are that Dr Johnson's care of Dr Wolfe's patients is still very good, but he is disturbed about the things that he is hearing. He is also aware that his office staff hears the same things and is concerned about the possible damage to Dr Johnson's reputation if these remarks are repeated. He wonders if he should stop referring patients to Dr Johnson. He feels that there is no objective reason to do so but worries about the significance of these disturbing pieces of information in terms of Dr Johnson's future ability to manage patients adequately.

DISCUSSION:

Dr Wolfe is beginning to suspect that Dr Johnson has developed problems, perhaps mental problems, that have the potential of compromising the quality of the care that he is giving; however, the evidence is admittedly weak. Dr Wolfe may also be worried that his own image will be tarnished if he continues to refer his patients to a dentist with a suspect reputation. What is Dr Wolfe's real worry?

Assuming first that Dr Wolfe is really concerned about the quality of Dr Johnson's practice, one option would be to stop making referrals. Would it be ethical to stop referring patients to Dr Johnson based on this flimsy evidence? If Dr Wolfe is worried about Dr Johnson's patient care in general (and not just his own referrals to Dr Johnson), he has a duty to go beyond changing his personal referrals and determine whether other patients are being jeopardized.

To the extent that Dr Johnson has a mental problem of which he is not aware, we would normally exonerate him from personal responsibility for his actions. Other unusual behavior patterns, however, may not as easily exempt one from culpability. Erratic behavior related to alcoholism and drug abuse pose such questions, as in the following case.

Case 88: Dentist on Valium

Dr James Carter and Dr Scott Seaborg were friends and partners in a general practice that they had started about 25 years earlier. Both men enjoyed their profession and their patients, but Dr Seaborg was experiencing more frustration and less satisfaction. The practice was successful, but Dr Seaborg increasingly felt that he was working more for other people than he was for himself. Taxes and the costs of accountants and lawyers were draining him emotionally as well as financially. Even though he prided himself on providing his employees with an outstanding benefits package, these benefits were an additional expense.

To alleviate these tensions, about 10 years ago Dr Seaborg began taking one 5-mg tablet of Valium a day. After several months the effect of the Valium seemed less, and he increased the dosage. After 5 years he was taking 15 tablets a day.

While he was taking the Valium, most of the time Dr Seaborg was convinced that his patient care had actually improved because he perceived himself to be calmer and less hyper. There were times, however, when he acknowledged that he cared less about the consequences of his actions. He also worried about his decreased energy levels. Lunchtime naps became part of his routine, and by the end of the day, he had no energy for any activities with his family. Sometimes he felt like a walking zombie. That sort of self-appraisal was infrequent, however. For the most part he viewed himself as a person who was doing what it took to cope with life. During this period, Dr Carter was essentially unaware of what was going on in his partner's life. He was concerned about the naps and sometimes felt that his partner was not very happy, but it never went beyond that.

After 5 years of taking Valium, Dr Seaborg abruptly stopped his habit. His mother had died 2 years previously, and he was still dealing with that loss. He saw his uncle and another family member affected by alcohol and drug abuse. In his practice, he was surrounded by frustrations. There were too many patients who had unrealistic expectations or were in pain and wanted immediate relief but at the same time complained about the cost. Altogether, Dr Seaborg felt himself sinking and believed that the Valium was a contributing factor. At the same time, he did not view himself as a Valium addict, and he wanted to prove to himself that he could stop.

Dr Seaborg had intended for his withdrawal, like his habit, to be accomplished in secrecy. However, the daily 75-mg dose had taken its toll. His wife found him unconscious and convulsing and took him to the hospital. His recovery was slow, and he experienced hand tremors that persisted for months. In addition to finally telling his wife about his habit, he decided to also tell his partner. Dr Carter was moved by Dr Seaborg's experiences and was extremely sympathetic and supportive.

For about 6 months, Dr Seaborg's life improved dramatically. He abruptly stopped smoking and began exercising regularly and vigorously. He had never felt better, but after that 6-month period he began taking Valium again. Although his exercise program and smoking cessation were liberating, they created their own pressures, and after he returned to his practice, he was faced again with work-related frustrations. This time he planned to control his Valium use by having his wife give him only one tablet a day. After a year of Valium he switched to Xanax to avoid the risks of addiction. He started with one tablet; 2 years later, he was taking 12 tablets a day.

Dr Carter had been genuinely concerned about his partner, but when he began to see the signs of his old lethargy return, he became suspicious. He also began to get angry. He felt that Dr Seaborg's previous bout with Valium addiction had put their practice at risk, and he did not want it to happen again. Then the business manager came to him with the finding that cash was systematically being removed from the practice's deposits and that the deposit slips were being altered. The business manager thought that Dr Seaborg was the one stealing the money. He was not sure how much was missing or when the thefts had begun.

Dr Carter could not imagine what his partner needed the money for, and at this point, he did not care. He was furious with Dr Seaborg and arranged for an audit. Altogether about $10,000 was missing. Dr Carter went through some of Dr Seaborg's patient records in an attempt to assess the medical and legal risks and was somewhat reassured. Other than some overhanging margins that should not have been there, Dr Seaborg's treatment did not look too bad. Dr Carter tried to figure out what to do.

DISCUSSION:

Dr Carter's response to his partner's condition began with sympathy and later turned to anger. Sympathy is appropriate for someone who has a condition that is beyond his control. One of the sociological functions of the sick role is to remove responsibility for one's behavior. Hence, a claim that alcoholism or drug dependence is a sickness is a claim for exemption from responsibility.

On the other hand, anger and blame are more appropriate responses to behavior that is within one's control. If the behavior is undertaken through free choice, then one is deemed responsible for it. The issue raised by this case is whether Dr Seaborg was repsonsible for his drug use at various times throughout this sequence of events.

Consider Dr Seaborg's initial Valium use. From the account in Case 88, there is no reason to believe Dr Seaborg was mentally disturbed or in any other way out of control when he decided to take the first tablet; many would say he was ethically responsible for that choice. If so, at some point he seems to have lost control. At what point was it? Was he responsible for making choices that led him on a course he eventually could not control?

The next issue is whether there are any significant differences between the drug abuse and stealing funds from the practice. If Dr Seaborg was out of control in doing one of these activities, was he also out of control in doing the other? Is Dr Carter's response more appropriately sympathy or anger?

Regardless, Dr Carter must consider his options. The initial issue is whether, given their more than 25-year friendship and partnership, Dr Seaborg deserves any special consideration. Dr Carter is within his rights to sever the partnership, but that would only protect Dr Carter's interests, not Dr Seaborg's patients. Dr Carter could bring suit against Dr Seaborg to recover the stolen money. Does he have any obligation to consider possible adverse effects on Dr Seaborg?

Does Dr Carter bear any ethical responsibility for Dr Seaborg's patients? One possibility would be for him to inform Dr Seaborg's patients of the nature of the problem. Would it be unethical to offer to provide care for Dr Seaborg's patients? Is that stealing patients or offering benefit to a group of patients in need—or both?

Another issue is whether, aside from the patients, anyone else should know about Dr Seaborg's problem—the dental society, the licensing board, or the press. Professional societies often have impairment programs that can render assistance. That would be one reason to contact the dental society. Even if

Dr Seaborg has a "disease" for which he is not presently responsible, does that make any difference when it comes to Dr Carter's responsibility to see that patients are protected?

Conclusion

More than most issues in dentistry, concerns about incompetent, dishonest, and impaired professionals invoke a broad range of ethical considerations. Every case in this chapter touches in some way on patients' autonomy and their right to be kept fully informed about the status of their oral health. Most of the cases involve considerations about acts of beneficence that affect one's own patients or the patients of others. The potential for doing harm to colleagues, to patients, or to ourselves is a central theme of these cases. Virtually every case raises issues of justice: What do patients deserve? What is fair to a colleague? Finally, the cases in this chapter serve as reminders of the principle of fidelity; they raise questions about the nature of commitments to patients and profession.

Reference

1. American Dental Association Council on Ethics, Bylaws and Judicial Affairs. Principles of Ethics and Code of Professional Conduct, with official advisory opinions revised to January 2004. Chicago: American Dental Association, 2004.

Appendix 1
Codes of
Medical Ethics

Hippocratic Oath[1]

I swear by Apollo Physician and Asclepius and Hygieia and Panaceia and all the gods and goddesses, making them my witness, that I will fulfil according to my ability and judgment this oath and this covenant:

To hold him who has taught me this art as equal to my parents and to live my life in partnership with him, and if he is in need of money to give him a share of mine, and to regard his offspring as equal to my brothers in male lineage and to teach them this art—if they desire to learn it—without fee and covenant; to give a share of precepts and oral instruction and all the other learning to my sons and to the sons of him who has instructed me and to pupils who have signed the covenant and have taken an oath according to the medical law, but to no one else.

I will apply dietetic measures for the benefit of the sick according to my ability and judgment, I will keep them from harm and injustice.

I will neither give a deadly drug to anybody if asked for it, nor will I make a suggestion to this effect. Similarly I will not give to a woman an abortive remedy. In purity and holiness I will guard my life and my art.

I will not use the knife, not even on sufferers from stone, but will withdraw in favor of such men as are engaged in this work.

Whatever houses I may visit, I will come for the benefit of the sick, remaining free of all intentional injustice, of all mischief and in particular of sexual relations with both female and male persons, be they free or slaves.

What I may see or hear in the course of the treatment or even outside of the treatment in regard to the life of men, which on no account one must spread abroad, I will keep to myself holding such things shameful to be spoken about.

If I fulfil this oath and do not violate it, may it be granted to me to enjoy life and art, being honored with fame among all men for all time to come; if I transgress it and swear falsely, may the opposite of all this be my lot.

Edelstein, Ludwig. Edited by Owsei Temkin and C. Lillian Temkin. Ancient Medicine: Selected Papers of Ludwig Edelstein. pp. 6. ©1967 [Copyright Holder]. Reprinted with permission of The Johns Hopkins University Press.

American Medical Association Principles of Medical Ethics[2]

Preamble:

The medical profession has long subscribed to a body of ethical statements developed primarily for the benefit of the patient. As a member of this profession, a physician must recognize responsibility not only to patients, but also to society, to other health professionals, and to self. The following Principles adopted by the American Medical Association are not laws, but standards of conduct which define the essentials of honorable behavior for the physician.

I. A physician shall be dedicated to providing competent medical service with compassion and respect for human dignity and rights.

II. A physician shall uphold the standards of professionalism, be honest in all professional interactions, and strive to report physicians deficient in character or competence, or engaging in fraud or deception, to appropriate entities.

III. A physician shall respect the law and also recognize a responsibility to seek changes in those requirements which are contrary to the best interests of the patient.

IV. A physician shall respect the rights of patients, of colleagues, and of other health professionals, and shall safeguard patient confidences within the constraints of the law.

V. A physician shall continue to study, apply and advance scientific knowledge, maintain a commitment to medical education, make relevant information available to patients, colleagues, and the public, obtain consultation, and use the talents of other health professionals when indicated.

VI. A physician shall, in the provision of appropriate patient care, except in emergencies, be free to choose whom to serve, with whom to associate, and the environment in which to provide medical services.

VII. A physician shall recognize a responsibility to participate in activities contributing to the improvement of the community and the betterment of public health.

Source: Code of Medical Ethics. ©2002, American Medical Association.

American Dental Association Principles of Ethics and Code of Professional Conduct[3]

I. INTRODUCTION

The dental profession holds a special position of trust within society. As a consequence, society affords the profession certain privileges that are not available to members of the public-at-large. In return, the profession makes a commitment to society that its members will adhere to high ethical standards of conduct. These standards are embodied in the *ADA Principles of Ethics and Code of Professional Conduct (ADA Code).* The *ADA Code* is, in effect, a written expression of the obligations arising from the implied contract between the dental profession and society.

Members of the ADA voluntarily agree to abide by the *ADA Code* as a condition of membership in the Association. They recognize that continued public trust in the dental profession is based on the commitment of individual dentists to high ethical standards of conduct.

The *ADA Code* has three main components: The Principles of Ethics, the Code of Professional Conduct and the Advisory Opinions.

The *Principles of Ethics* are the aspirational goals of the profession. They provide guidance and offer justification for the *Code of Professional Conduct* and *the Advisory Opinions*. There are five fundamental principles that form the foundation of *the ADA Code:* patient autonomy, nonmaleficence, beneficence, justice and veracity. Principles can overlap each other as well as compete with each other for priority. More than one principle can justify a given element of the *Code of Professional Conduct*. Principles may at times need to be balanced against each other, but, otherwise, they are the profession's firm guideposts.

The *Code of Professional Conduct* is an expression of specific types of conduct that are either required or prohibited. The *Code of Professional Conduct* is a product of the ADA's legislative system. All elements of the *Code of Professional Conduct* result from resolutions that are adopted by the ADA's House of Delegates. *The Code of Professional Conduct* is binding on members of the ADA, and violations may result in disciplinary action.

The *Advisory Opinions* are interpretations that apply the *Code of Professional Conduct* to specific fact situations. They are adopted by the ADA's Council on Ethics, Bylaws and Judicial Affairs to provide guidance to the membership on how the Council might interpret the *Code of Professional Conduct* in a disciplinary proceeding.

The *ADA Code* is an evolving document and by its very nature cannot be a complete articulation of all ethical obligations. The *ADA Code* is the result of an on-going dialogue between the dental profession and society, and as such, is subject to continuous review.

Although ethics and the law are closely related, they are not the same. Ethical obligations may–and often do–exceed legal duties. In resolving any ethical problem not explicitly covered by the *ADA Code*, dentists should consider the ethical principles, the patient's needs and interests, and any applicable laws.

II. PREAMBLE

The American Dental Association calls upon dentists to follow high ethical standards which have the benefit of the patient as their primary goal. Recognition of this goal, and of the education and training of a dentist, has resulted in society affording to the profession the privilege and obligation of self-government.

The Association believes that dentists should possess not only knowledge, skill and technical competence but also those traits of character that foster adherence to ethical principles. Qualities of compassion, kindness, integrity, fairness and charity complement the ethical practice of dentistry and help to define the true professional.

The ethical dentist strives to do that which is right and good. The *ADA Code* is an instrument to help the dentist in this quest.

III. PRINCIPLES, CODE OF PROFESSIONAL CONDUCT AND ADVISORY OPINIONS

Section 1 PRINCIPLE: PATIENT AUTONOMY ("self-governance").
The dentist has a duty to respect the patient's rights to self-determination and confidentiality.

This principle expresses the concept that professionals have a duty to treat the patient according to the patient's desires, within the bounds of accepted treatment, and to protect the patient's confidentiality. Under this principle, the dentist's primary obligations include involving patients in treatment decisions in a meaningful way, with due consideration being given to the patient's needs, desires and abilities, and safeguarding the patient's privacy.

CODE OF PROFESSIONAL CONDUCT

1.A. PATIENT INVOLVEMENT.

The dentist should inform the patient of the proposed treatment, and any reasonable alternatives, in a manner that allows the patient to become involved in treatment decisions.

1.B. PATIENT RECORDS.

Dentists are obliged to safeguard the confidentiality of patient records. Dentists shall maintain patient records in a manner consistent with the protection of the welfare of the patient. Upon request of a patient or another dental practitioner, dentists shall provide any information in accordance with applicable law that will be beneficial for the future treatment of that patient.

ADVISORY OPINIONS

1.B.1. FURNISHING COPIES OF RECORDS.

A dentist has the ethical obligation on request of either the patient or the patient's new dentist to furnish in accordance with applicable law, either gratuitously or for nominal cost, such dental records or copies or summaries of them, including dental X-rays or copies of them, as will be beneficial for the future treatment of that patient. This obligation exists whether or not the patient's account is paid in full.

1.B.2. CONFIDENTIALITY OF PATIENT RECORDS.

The dominant theme in Code Section 1.B is the protection of the confidentiality of a patient's records. The statement in this section that relevant information in the records should be released to another dental practitioner assumes that the dentist requesting the information is the patient's present dentist. There may be circumstances where the former dentist has an ethical obligation to inform the present dentist of certain facts. Code Section 1.B assumes that the dentist releasing relevant information is acting in accordance with applicable law. Dentists should be aware that the laws of the various jurisdictions in the United States are not uniform, and some confidentiality laws appear to prohibit the transfer of pertinent information, such as HIV seropositivity. Absent certain knowledge that the laws of the dentist's jurisdiction permit the forwarding of this information, a dentist should obtain the patient's written permission before forwarding health records which contain information of a sensitive nature, such as HIV seropositivity, chemical dependency or sexual preference. If it is necessary for a treating dentist to consult with another dentist or physician with respect to the patient, and the circumstances do not permit the patient to remain anonymous, the treating dentist should seek the permission of the patient prior to the release of data from the patient's records to the consulting practitioner. If the patient refuses, the treating dentist should then contemplate obtaining legal advice regarding the termination of the dentist/patient relationship.

Section 2 PRINCIPLE: NONMALEFICENCE ("do no harm"). The
dentist has a duty to refrain from harming the patient.

This principle expresses the concept that professionals have a duty to protect the patient from harm. Under this principle, the dentist's primary obligations include keeping knowledge and skills current, knowing one's own limitations and when to refer to a specialist or other professional, and knowing when and under what circumstances delegation of patient care to auxiliaries is appropriate.

CODE OF PROFESSIONAL CONDUCT

2.A. EDUCATION.

The privilege of dentists to be accorded professional status rests primarily in the knowledge, skill and experience with which they serve their patients and society. All dentists, therefore, have the obligation of keeping their knowledge and skill current.

2.B. CONSULTATION AND REFERRAL.

Dentists shall be obliged to seek consultation, if possible, whenever the welfare of patients will be safeguarded or advanced by utilizing those who have special skills, knowledge, and experience. When patients visit or are referred to specialists or consulting dentists for consultation:

1. The specialists or consulting dentists upon completion of their care shall return the patient, unless the patient expressly reveals a different preference, to the referring dentist, or, if none, to the dentist of record for future care.
2. The specialists shall be obliged when there is no referring dentist and upon a completion of their treatment to inform patients when there is a need for further dental care.

ADVISORY OPINION

2.B.1. SECOND OPINIONS.

A dentist who has a patient referred by a third party* for a "second opinion" regarding a diagnosis or treatment plan recommended by the patient's treating dentist should render the requested second opinion in accordance with this *Code of Ethics*. In the interest of the patient being afforded quality care, the dentist rendering the second opinion should not have a vested interest in the ensuing recommendation.

2.C. USE OF AUXILIARY PERSONNEL.

Dentists shall be obliged to protect the health of their patients by only assigning to qualified auxiliaries those duties which can be legally delegated. Dentists shall be further obliged to prescribe and supervise the patient care provided by all auxiliary personnel working under their direction.

2.D. PERSONAL IMPAIRMENT.

It is unethical for a dentist to practice while abusing controlled substances, alcohol or other chemical agents which impair the ability to practice. All dentists have an ethical obligation to urge chemically impaired colleagues to seek treatment. Dentists with first-hand knowledge that a colleague is practicing dentistry when so impaired have an ethical responsibility to report such evidence to the professional assistance committee of a dental society.

ADVISORY OPINION

2.D.1. ABILITY TO PRACTICE.

A dentist who contracts any disease or becomes impaired in any way that might endanger patients or dental staff shall, with consultation and advice from a qualified physician or other authority, limit the activities of practice to those areas that do not endanger patients or dental staff. A dentist who has been advised to limit the activities of his or her practice should monitor the aforementioned disease or impairment and make additional limitations to the activities of the dentist's practice, as indicated.

---

*A third party is any party to a dental prepayment contract that may collect premiums, assume financial risks, pay claims, and/or provide administrative services.

2.E. POSTEXPOSURE, BLOODBORNE PATHOGENS.

All dentists, regardless of their bloodborne pathogen status, have an ethical obligation to immediately inform any patient who may have been exposed to blood or other potentially infectious material in the dental office of the need for postexposure evaluation and follow-up and to immediately refer the patient to a qualified health care practitioner who can provide postexposure services. The dentist's ethical obligation in the event of an exposure incident extends to providing information concerning the dentist's own bloodborne pathogen status to the evaluating health care practitioner, if the dentist is the source individual, and to submitting to testing that will assist in the evaluation of the patient. If a staff member or other third person is the source individual, the dentist should encourage that person to cooperate as needed for the patient's evaluation.

2.F. PATIENT ABANDONMENT.

Once a dentist has undertaken a course of treatment, the dentist should not discontinue that treatment without giving the patient adequate notice and the opportunity to obtain the services of another dentist. Care should be taken that the patient's oral health is not jeopardized in the process.

2.G. PERSONAL RELATIONSHIPS WITH PATIENTS.

Dentists should avoid interpersonal relationships that could impair their professional judgment or risk the possibility of exploiting the confidence placed in them by a patient.

Section 3 PRINCIPLE: BENEFICENCE ("do good"). The dentist has a duty to promote the patient's welfare.

This principle expresses the concept that professionals have a duty to act for the benefit of others. Under this principle, the dentist's primary obligation is service to the patient and the public-at-large. The most important aspect of this obligation is the competent and timely delivery of dental care within the bounds of clinical circumstances presented by the patient, with due consideration being given to the needs, desires and values of the patient. The same ethical considerations apply whether the dentist engages in fee-for-service, managed care or some other practice arrangement. Dentists may choose to enter into contracts governing the provision of care to a group of patients; however, contract obligations do not excuse dentists from their ethical duty to put the patient's welfare first.

CODE OF PROFESSIONAL CONDUCT

3.A. COMMUNITY SERVICE.

Since dentists have an obligation to use their skills, knowledge and experience for the improvement of the dental health of the public and are encouraged to be leaders in their community, dentists in such service shall conduct themselves in such a manner as to maintain or elevate the esteem of the profession.

3.B. GOVERNMENT OF A PROFESSION.

Every profession owes society the responsibility to regulate itself. Such regulation is achieved largely through the influence of the professional societies. All dentists, therefore, have the dual obligation of making themselves a part of a professional society and of observing its rules of ethics.

3.C. RESEARCH AND DEVELOPMENT.

Dentists have the obligation of making the results and benefits of their investigative efforts available to all when they are useful in safeguarding or promoting the health of the public.

3.D. PATENTS AND COPYRIGHTS.

Patents and copyrights may be secured by dentists provided that such patents and copyrights shall not be used to restrict research or practice.

3.E. ABUSE AND NEGLECT.

Dentists shall be obliged to become familiar with the signs of abuse and neglect and to report suspected cases to the proper authorities, consistent with state laws.

ADVISORY OPINION

3.E.1. REPORTING ABUSE AND NEGLECT.

The public and the profession are best served by dentists who are familiar with identifying the signs of abuse and neglect and knowledgeable about the appropriate intervention resources for all populations.

A dentist's ethical obligation to identify and report the signs of abuse and neglect is, at a minimum, to be consistent with a dentist's legal obligation in the jurisdiction where the dentist practices. Dentists, therefore, are ethically obliged to identify and report suspected cases of abuse and neglect to the same extent as they are legally obliged to do so in the jurisdiction where they practice. Dentists have a concurrent ethical obligation to respect an adult patient's right to self-determination and confidentiality and to promote the welfare of all patients. Care should be exercised to respect the wishes of an adult patient who asks that a suspected case of abuse and/or neglect not be reported, where such a report is not mandated by law. With the patient's permission, other possible solutions may be sought.

Dentists should be aware that jurisdictional laws vary in their definitions of abuse and neglect, in their reporting requirements and the extent to which immunity is granted to good faith reporters. The variances may raise potential legal and other risks that should be considered, while keeping in mind the duty to put the welfare of the patient first. Therefore a dentist's ethical obligation to identify and report suspected cases of abuse and neglect can vary from one jurisdiction to another.

Dentists are ethically obligated to keep current their knowledge of both identifying abuse and neglect and reporting it in the jurisdiction(s) where they practice.

Section 4 PRINCIPLE: JUSTICE ("fairness"). The dentist has a duty to treat people fairly.

This principle expresses the concept that professionals have a duty to be fair in their dealings with patients, colleagues and society. Under this principle, the dentist's primary obligations include dealing with people justly and delivering dental care without prejudice. In its broadest sense, this principle expresses the concept that the dental profession should actively seek allies throughout society on specific activities that will help improve access to care for all.

CODE OF PROFESSIONAL CONDUCT

4.A. PATIENT SELECTION.

While dentists, in serving the public, may exercise reasonable discretion in selecting patients for their practices, dentists shall not refuse to accept patients into their practice or deny dental service to patients because of the patient's race, creed, color, sex or national origin.

ADVISORY OPINION

4.A.1. HIV POSITIVE PATIENTS.

A dentist has the general obligation to provide care to those in need. A decision not to provide treatment to an individual because the individual has AIDS or is HIV seropositive, based solely on that fact, is unethical. Decisions with regard to the type of dental treatment provided or referrals made or suggested, in such instances should be made on the same basis as they are made with other patients, that is, whether the individual dentist believes he or she has need of another's skills, knowledge, equipment or experience and whether the dentist believes, after consultation with the patient's physician if appropriate, the patient's health status would be significantly compromised by the provision of dental treatment.

4.B. EMERGENCY SERVICE.

Dentists shall be obliged to make reasonable arrangements for the emergency care of their patients of record. Dentists shall be obliged when consulted in an emergency by patients not of record to make reasonable arrangements for emergency care. If treatment is provided, the dentist, upon completion of treatment, is obliged to return the patient to his or her regular dentist unless the patient expressly reveals a different preference.

4.C. JUSTIFIABLE CRITICISM.

Dentists shall be obliged to report to the appropriate reviewing agency as determined by the local component or constituent society instances of gross or continual faulty treatment by other dentists. Patients should be informed of their present oral health status without disparaging comment about prior services. Dentists issuing a public statement with respect to the profession shall have a reasonable basis to believe that the comments made are true.

ADVISORY OPINION

4.C.1. MEANING OF "JUSTIFIABLE."

A dentist's duty to the public imposes a responsibility to report instances of gross or continual faulty treatment. However, the heading of this section is "Justifiable Criticism." Therefore, when informing a patient of the status of his or her oral health, the dentist should exercise care that the comments made are justifiable. For example, a difference of opinion as to preferred treatment should not be communicated to the patient in a manner which would imply mistreatment. There will necessarily be cases where it will be difficult to determine whether the comments made are justifiable. Therefore, this section is phrased to address the discretion of dentists and advises against disparaging statements against another dentist. However, it should be noted that, where comments are made which are obviously not supportable and therefore unjustified, such comments can be the basis for the institution of a disciplinary proceeding against the dentist making such statements.

4.D. EXPERT TESTIMONY.

Dentists may provide expert testimony when that testimony is essential to a just and fair disposition of a judicial or administrative action.

ADVISORY OPINION

4.D.1. CONTINGENT FEES.

It is unethical for a dentist to agree to a fee contingent upon the favorable outcome of the litigation in exchange for testifying as a dental expert.

4.E. REBATES AND SPLIT FEES.

Dentists shall not accept or tender "rebates" or "split fees."

Section 5 PRINCIPLE: VERACITY ("truthfulness"). The dentist has a duty to communicate truthfully.

This principle expresses the concept that professionals have a duty to be honest and trustworthy in their dealings with people. Under this principle, the dentist's primary obligations include respecting the position of trust inherent in the dentist-patient relationship, communicating truthfully and without deception, and maintaining intellectual integrity.

CODE OF PROFESSIONAL CONDUCT

5.A. REPRESENTATION OF CARE.

Dentists shall not represent the care being rendered to their patients in a false or misleading manner.

ADVISORY OPINIONS

5.A.1. DENTAL AMALGAM AND OTHER RESTORATIVE MATERIALS.

Based on current scientific data, the ADA has determined that the removal of amalgam restorations from the non-allergic patient for the alleged purpose of removing toxic substances from the body, when such treatment is performed solely at the recommendation or suggestion of the dentist, is improper and unethical. The same principle of veracity applies to the dentist's recommendation concerning the removal of any dental restorative material.

5.A.2. UNSUBSTANTIATED REPRESENTATIONS.

A dentist who represents that dental treatment or diagnostic techniques recommended or performed by the dentist has the capacity to diagnose, cure or alleviate diseases, infections or other conditions, when such representations are not based upon accepted scientific knowledge or research, is acting unethically.

5.B. REPRESENTATION OF FEES.

Dentists shall not represent the fees being charged for providing care in a false or misleading manner.

ADVISORY OPINIONS

5.B.1. WAIVER OF COPAYMENT.

A dentist who accepts a third party* payment under a copayment plan as payment in full without disclosing to the third party* that the patient's payment portion will not be collected, is engaged in overbilling. The essence of this ethical impropriety is deception and misrepresentation; an overbilling dentist makes it appear to the third party* that the charge to the patient for services rendered is higher than it actually is.

5.B.2. OVERBILLING.

It is unethical for a dentist to increase a fee to a patient solely because the patient is covered under a dental benefits plan.

5.B.3. FEE DIFFERENTIAL.

Payments accepted by a dentist under a governmentally funded program, a component or constituent dental society sponsored access program, or a participating agreement entered into under a program of a third party* shall not be considered as evidence of overbilling in determining whether a charge to a patient, or to another third party* in behalf of a patient not covered under any of the aforecited programs constitutes overbilling under this section of the Code.

---

*A third party is any party to a dental prepayment contract that may collect premiums, assume financial risks, pay claims, and/or provide administrative services.

5.B.4. TREATMENT DATES.

A dentist who submits a claim form to a third party* reporting incorrect treatment dates for the purpose of assisting a patient in obtaining benefits under a dental plan, which benefits would otherwise be disallowed, is engaged in making an unethical, false or misleading representation to such third party.*

5.B.5. DENTAL PROCEDURES.

A dentist who incorrectly describes on a third party* claim form a dental procedure in order to receive a greater payment or reimbursement or incorrectly makes a non-covered procedure appear to be a covered procedure on such a claim form is engaged in making an unethical, false or misleading representation to such third party.*

5.B.6. UNNECESSARY SERVICES.
A dentist who recommends and performs unnecessary dental services or procedures is engaged in unethical conduct.

5.C. DISCLOSURE OF CONFLICT OF INTEREST.

A dentist who presents educational or scientific information in an article, seminar or other program shall disclose to the readers or participants any monetary or other special interest the dentist may have with a company whose products are promoted or endorsed in the presentation. Disclosure shall be made in any promotional material and in the presentation itself.

5.D. DEVICES AND THERAPEUTIC METHODS.

Except for formal investigative studies, dentists shall be obliged to prescribe, dispense, or promote only those devices, drugs and other agents whose complete formulae are available to the dental profession. Dentists shall have the further obligation of not holding out as exclusive any device, agent, method or technique if that representation would be false or misleading in any material respect.

ADVISORY OPINIONS

5.D.1. REPORTING ADVERSE REACTIONS.

A dentist who suspects the occurrence of an adverse reaction to a drug or dental device has an obligation to communicate that information to the broader medical

---

*A third party is any party to a dental prepayment contract that may collect premiums, assume financial risks, pay claims, and/or provide administrative services.

and dental community, including, in the case of a serious adverse event, the Food and Drug Administration (FDA).

5.D.2. MARKETING OR SALE OF PRODUCTS OR PROCEDURES.

Dentists who, in the regular conduct of their practices, engage in or employ auxiliaries in the marketing or sale of products or procedures to their patients must take care not to exploit the trust inherent in the dentist-patient relationship for their own financial gain. Dentists should not induce their patients to purchase products or undergo procedures by misrepresenting the product's value, the necessity of the procedure or the dentist's professional expertise in recommending the product or procedure.

In the case of a health-related product, it is not enough for the dentist to rely on the manufacturer's or distributor's representations about the product's safety and efficacy. The dentist has an independent obligation to inquire into the truth and accuracy of such claims and verify that they are founded on accepted scientific knowledge or research.

Dentists should disclose to their patients all relevant information the patient needs to make an informed purchase decision, including whether the product is available elsewhere and whether there are any financial incentives for the dentist to recommend the product that would not be evident to the patient.

5.E. PROFESSIONAL ANNOUNCEMENT.

In order to properly serve the public, dentists should represent themselves in a manner that contributes to the esteem of the profession. Dentists should not misrepresent their training and competence in any way that would be false or misleading in any material respect.*

5.F. ADVERTISING.

Although any dentist may advertise, no dentist shall advertise or solicit patients in any form of communication in a manner that is false or misleading in any material respect.*

---

*Advertising, solicitation of patients or business or other promotional activities by dentists or dental care delivery organizations shall not be considered unethical or improper, except for those promotional activities which are false or misleading in any material respect. Notwithstanding any *ADA Principles of Ethics and Code of Professional Conduct* or other standards of dentist conduct which may be differently worded, this shall be the sole standard for determining the ethical propriety of such promotional activities. Any provision of an ADA constituent or component society's code of ethics or other standard of dentist conduct relating to dentists' or dental care delivery organizations' advertising, solicitation, or other promotional activities which is worded differently from the above standard shall be deemed to be in conflict with the *ADA Principles of Ethics and Code of Professional Conduct.*

ADVISORY OPINIONS

5.F.1. ARTICLES AND NEWSLETTERS.

If a dental health article, message or newsletter is published under a dentist's byline to the public without making truthful disclosure of the source and authorship or is designed to give rise to questionable expectations for the purpose of inducing the public to utilize the services of the sponsoring dentist, the dentist is engaged in making a false or misleading representation to the public in a material respect.

5.F.2. EXAMPLES OF "FALSE OR MISLEADING."

The following examples are set forth to provide insight into the meaning of the term "false or misleading in a material respect." These examples are not meant to be all-inclusive. Rather, by restating the concept in alternative language and giving general examples, it is hoped that the membership will gain a better understanding of the term. With this in mind, statements shall be avoided which would: a) contain a material misrepresentation of fact, b) omit a fact necessary to make the statement considered as a whole not materially misleading, c) be intended or be likely to create an unjustified expectation about results the dentist can achieve, and d) contain a material, objective representation, whether express or implied, that the advertised services are superior in quality to those of other dentists, if that representation is not subject to reasonable substantiation.

Subjective statements about the quality of dental services can also raise ethical concerns. In particular, statements of opinion may be misleading if they are not honestly held, if they misrepresent the qualifications of the holder, or the basis of the opinion, or if the patient reasonably interprets them as implied statements of fact. Such statements will be evaluated on a case by case basis, considering how patients are likely to respond to the impression made by the advertisement as a whole. The fundamental issue is whether the advertisement, taken as a whole, is false or misleading in a material respect.

5.F.3. UNEARNED, NONHEALTH DEGREES.

A dentist may use the title Doctor or Dentist, DDS, DMD or any additional earned, advanced academic degrees in health service areas in an announcement to the public. The announcement of an unearned academic degree may be misleading because of the likelihood that it will indicate to the public the attainment of specialty or diplomate status.

For purposes of this advisory opinion, an unearned academic degree is one which is awarded by an educational institution not accredited by a generally recognized accrediting body or is an honorary degree.

The use of a nonhealth degree in an announcement to the public may be a representation which is misleading because the public is likely to assume that any degree announced is related to the qualifications of the dentist as a practitioner.

Some organizations grant dentists fellowship status as a token of membership in the organization or some other form of voluntary association. The use of such fellowships in advertising to the general public may be misleading because of the likelihood that it will indicate to the public attainment of education or skill in the field of dentistry.

Generally, unearned or nonhealth degrees and fellowships that designate association, rather than attainment, should be limited to scientific papers and curriculum vitae. In all instances, state law should be consulted. In any review by the council of the use of designations in advertising to the public, the council will apply the standard of whether the use of such is false or misleading in a material respect.

5.F.4. REFERRAL SERVICES.

There are two basic types of referral services for dental care: not-for-profit and the commercial. The not-for-profit is commonly organized by dental societies or community services. It is open to all qualified practitioners in the area served. A fee is sometimes charged the practitioner to be listed with the service. A fee for such referral services is for the purpose of covering the expenses of the service and has no relation to the number of patients referred. In contrast, some commercial referral services restrict access to the referral service to a limited number of dentists in a particular geographic area. Prospective patients calling the service may be referred to a single subscribing dentist in the geographic area and the respective dentist billed for each patient referred. Commercial referral services often advertise to the public stressing that there is no charge for use of the service and the patient may not be informed of the referral fee paid by the dentist. There is a connotation to such advertisements that the referral that is being made is in the nature of a public service. A dentist is allowed to pay for any advertising permitted by the *Code*, but is generally not permitted to make payments to another person or entity for the referral of a patient for professional services. While the particular facts and circumstances relating to an individual commercial referral service will vary, the council believes that the aspects outlined above for commercial referral services violate the *Code* in that it constitutes advertising which is false or misleading in a material respect and violates the prohibitions in the *Code* against fee splitting.

5.F.5. INFECTIOUS DISEASE TEST RESULTS.

An advertisement or other communication intended to solicit patients which omits a material fact or facts necessary to put the information conveyed in the advertisement in a proper context can be misleading in a material respect. A dental practice should not seek to attract patients on the basis of partial truths which create a false impression.

For example, an advertisement to the public of HIV negative test results, without conveying additional information that will clarify the scientific significance of this fact, contains a misleading omission. A dentist could satisfy his or her obligation under this advisory opinion to convey additional information by clearly stating in the advertisement or other communication: "This negative HIV test cannot guarantee that I am currently free of HIV."

5.G. NAME OF PRACTICE.

Since the name under which a dentist conducts his or her practice may be a factor in the selection process of the patient, the use of a trade name or an assumed name that is false or misleading in any material respect is unethical. Use of the name of a dentist no longer actively associated with the practice may be continued for a period not to exceed one year.*

ADVISORY OPINION

5.G.1. DENTIST LEAVING PRACTICE.

Dentists leaving a practice who authorize continued use of their names should receive competent advice on the legal implications of this action. With permission of a departing dentist, his or her name may be used for more than one year, if, after the one year grace period has expired, prominent notice is provided to the public through such mediums as a sign at the office and a short statement on stationery and business cards that the departing dentist has retired from the practice.

5.H. ANNOUNCEMENT OF SPECIALIZATION AND LIMITATION OF PRACTICE.

This section and Section 5.I are designed to help the public make an informed selection between the practitioner who has completed an accredited program beyond the dental degree and a practitioner who has not completed such a program. The special areas of dental practice approved by the American Dental Association and the designation for ethical specialty announcement and limitation of practice are: dental public health, endodontics, oral and maxillofacial pathology, oral and maxillofacial radiology, oral and maxillofacial surgery, orthodontics and dentofacial orthopedics, pediatric dentistry, periodontics and prosthodontics.

---

*Advertising, solicitation of patients or business or other promotional activities by dentists or dental care delivery organizations shall not be considered unethical or improper, except for those promotional activities which are false or misleading in any material respect. Notwithstanding any *ADA Principles of Ethics and Code of Professional Conduct* or other standards of dentist conduct which may be differently worded, this shall be the sole standard for determining the ethical propriety of such promotional activities. Any provision of an ADA constituent or component society's code of ethics or other standard of dentist conduct relating to dentists' or dental care delivery organizations' advertising, solicitation, or other promotional activities which is worded differently from the above standard shall be deemed to be in conflict with the *ADA Principles of Ethics and Code of Professional Conduct*.

Dentists who choose to announce specialization should use "specialist in" or "practice limited to" and shall limit their practice exclusively to the announced special area(s) of dental practice, provided at the time of the announcement such dentists have met in each approved specialty for which they announce the existing educational requirements and standards set forth by the American Dental Association. Dentists who use their eligibility to announce as specialists to make the public believe that specialty services rendered in the dental office are being rendered by qualified specialists when such is not the case are engaged in unethical conduct. The burden of responsibility is on specialists to avoid any inference that general practitioners who are associated with specialists are qualified to announce themselves as specialists.

GENERAL STANDARDS.

The following are included within the standards of the American Dental Association for determining the education, experience and other appropriate requirements for announcing specialization and limitation of practice:

1. The special area(s) of dental practice and an appropriate certifying board must be approved by the American Dental Association.
2. Dentists who announce as specialists must have successfully completed an educational program accredited by the Commission on Dental Accreditation, two or more years in length, as specified by the Council on Dental Education and Licensure, or be diplomates of an American Dental Association recognized certifying board. The scope of the individual specialist's practice shall be governed by the educational standards for the specialty in which the specialist is announcing.
3. The practice carried on by dentists who announce as specialists shall be limited exclusively to the special area(s) of dental practice announced by the dentist.

STANDARDS FOR MULTIPLE-SPECIALTY ANNOUNCEMENTS.

The educational criterion for announcement of limitation of practice in additional specialty areas is the successful completion of an advanced educational program accredited by the Commission on Dental Accreditation (or its equivalent if completed prior to 1967)* in each area for which the dentist wishes to announce. Dentists who are presently ethically announcing limitation of practice in a specialty area and who wish to announce in an additional specialty area must submit to the appropriate constituent society documentation of successful completion of the requisite education in specialty programs listed by the Council on Dental Education and Licensure or certification as a diplomate in each area for which they wish to announce.

---

*Completion of three years of advanced training in oral and maxillofacial surgery or two years of advanced training in one of the other recognized dental specialties prior to 1967.

ADVISORY OPINIONS

5.H.1. DUAL DEGREED DENTISTS.

Nothing in Section 5.H shall be interpreted to prohibit a dual degreed dentist who practices medicine or osteopathy under a valid state license from announcing to the public as a dental specialist provided the dentist meets the educational, experience and other standards set forth in the *Code* for specialty announcement and further providing that the announcement is truthful and not materially misleading.

5.H.2. SPECIALIST ANNOUNCEMENT OF CREDENTIALS IN NON-SPECIALTY INTEREST AREAS.

A dentist who is qualified to announce specialization under this section may not announce to the public that he or she is certified or a diplomate or otherwise similarly credentialed in an area of dentistry not recognized as a specialty area by the American Dental Association unless:

1. The organization granting the credential grants certification or diplomate status based on the following: a) the dentist's successful completion of a formal, full-time advanced education program (graduate or postgraduate level) of at least 12 months' duration; and b) the dentist's training and experience; and c) successful completion of an oral and written examination based on psychometric principles; and
2. The announcement includes the following language: [Name of announced area of dental practice] is not recognized as a specialty area by the American Dental Association.

Nothing in this advisory opinion affects the right of a properly qualified dentist to announce specialization in an ADA-recognized specialty area(s) as provided for under Section 5.H of this *Code* or the responsibility of such dentist to limit his or her practice exclusively to the special area(s) of dental practice announced. Specialists shall not announce their credentials in a manner that implies specialization in a non-specialty interest area.

5.I. GENERAL PRACTITIONER ANNOUNCEMENT OF SERVICES.

General dentists who wish to announce the services available in their practices are permitted to announce the availability of those services so long as they avoid any communications that express or imply specialization. General dentists shall also state that the services are being provided by general dentists. No dentist shall announce available services in any way that would be false or misleading in any material respect.*

ADVISORY OPINIONS

5.I.1. GENERAL PRACTITIONER ANNOUNCEMENT OF CREDENTIALS IN NON-SPECIALTY INTEREST AREAS.

A general dentist may not announce to the public that he or she is certified or a diplomate or otherwise similarly credentialed in an area of dentistry not recognized as a specialty area by the American Dental Association unless:

1. The organization granting the credential grants certification or diplomate status based on the following: a) the dentist's successful completion of a formal, full-time advanced education program (graduate or postgraduate level) of at least 12 months' duration; and b) the dentist's training and experience; and c) successful completion of an oral and written examination based on psychometric principles;
2. The dentist discloses that he or she is a general dentist; and
3. The announcement includes the following language: [Name of announced area of dental practice] is not recognized as a specialty area by the American Dental Association.

5.I.2. CREDENTIALS IN GENERAL DENTISTRY.

General dentists may announce fellowships or other credentials earned in the area of general dentistry so long as they avoid any communications that express or imply specialization and the announcement includes the disclaimer that the dentist is a general dentist. The use of abbreviations to designate credentials shall be avoided when such use would lead the reasonable person to believe that the designation represents an academic degree, when such is not the case.

---

*Advertising, solicitation of patients or business or other promotional activities by dentists or dental care delivery organizations shall not be considered unethical or improper, except for those promotional activities which are false or misleading in any material respect. Notwithstanding any *ADA Principles of Ethics and Code of Professional Conduct* or other standards of dentist conduct which may be differently worded, this shall be the sole standard for determining the ethical propriety of such promotional activities. Any provision of an ADA constituent or component society's code of ethics or other standard of dentist conduct relating to dentists' or dental care delivery organizations' advertising, solicitation, or other promotional activities which is worded differently from the above standard shall be deemed to be in conflict with the *ADA Principles of Ethics and Code of Professional Conduct.*

IV. INTERPRETATION AND APPLICATION OF PRINCIPLES OF ETHICS AND CODE OF PROFESSIONAL CONDUCT.

The foregoing *ADA Principles of Ethics and Code of Professional Conduct* set forth the ethical duties that are binding on members of the American Dental Association. The component and constituent societies may adopt additional requirements or interpretations not in conflict with the *ADA Code*.

Anyone who believes that a member-dentist has acted unethically may bring the matter to the attention of the appropriate constituent (state) or component (local) dental society. Whenever possible, problems involving questions of ethics should be resolved at the state or local level. If a satisfactory resolution cannot be reached, the dental society may decide, after proper investigation, that the matter warrants issuing formal charges and conducting a disciplinary hearing pursuant to the procedures set forth in the ADA *Bylaws*, Chapter XII. PRINCIPLES OF ETHICS AND CODE OF PROFESSIONAL CONDUCT AND JUDICIAL PROCEDURE. The Council on Ethics, Bylaws and Judicial Affairs reminds constituent and component societies that before a dentist can be found to have breached any ethical obligation the dentist is entitled to a fair hearing.

A member who is found guilty of unethical conduct proscribed by the *ADA Code* or code of ethics of the constituent or component society, may be placed under a sentence of censure or suspension or may be expelled from membership in the Association. A member under a sentence of censure, suspension or expulsion has the right to appeal the decision to his or her constituent society and the ADA Council on Ethics, Bylaws and Judicial Affairs, as provided in Chapter XII of the ADA *Bylaws*.

References

1. Edelstein L. The Hippocratic Oath: Text, translation and interpretation. In: Temkin O, Temkin CL (eds). Ancient Medicine: Selected Papers of Ludwig Edelstein. Baltimore: Johns Hopkins University Press, 1967:6.
2. American Medical Association. Code of Medical Ethics. Chicago: American Medical Association, 2002.
3. American Dental Association Council of Ethics, Bylaws and Judicial Affairs. Principles of Ethics and Code of Professional Conduct, with official advisory opinions revised to January 2004. Chicago: American Dental Association, 2004.

Appendix 2
Informed Consent

This appendix presents a legal perspective of informed consent—something that every state in the United States has dealt with. Our intent is to provide a complementary frame of reference for discussions of the ethical issues associated with autonomy and informed consent that appear in chapter 8 of this book.

The legal requirements presented here are taken from Maryland statutes and are specific for that state. Like the requirements of most states, they conform to the reasonable person standard. The guidelines of other states, though similar in most respects, may vary somewhat from those of Maryland. Therefore, in order to ensure one's legal compliance in a given state, it is necessary to be familiar with that state's specificities.

Requirements of an Adequate Informed Consent*†

The practitioner must advise the patient of:

- The nature of the ailment.
- The nature of the proposed treatment.
- The probability of success of the contemplated therapy and its alternatives.
- The material risk(s) of unfortunate consequences associated with such treatment measured by the materiality of the information to the reasonably prudent patient.
- The consequences of no therapy.[1–3]

The scope of the information disclosure is measured by the patient's needs.

- Must include all information that is material to the decision.
- Information is material if the reasonably prudent patient, under the circumstances, would consider it and possibly change her treatment decision based upon that information.
- All risks potentially affecting the patient's decision must be divulged.[2,3]

---

*Courtesy of Roger L. Eldridge, DDS, JD, Director, Special Patient Clinic; Associate Professor, Department of Comprehensive Care and Therapeutics, University of Maryland Dental School.
†The requirements stated here in general terms are spelled out further in chapter 8, in which five specific examples of elements of an adequately informed consent are presented. These include the treatment alternatives and their risks and benefits, who will perform the treatment and what the charges will be, differing views of treatment options held by other dentists, special interests of the provider or other parties, and what procedures, if any, are for research purposes. In that chapter, it is also pointed out that the standard of a reasonable person (what is in this appendix is referred to as a *reasonably prudent patient*) must sometimes be supplemented if the dentist knows or has reason to know that the patient has unique interests that would make additional information necessary to a truly autonomous consent. In chapter 8, this is referred to as the adding the *subjective standard*.

References

1. *Sard v Hardy*, 281 Md 432, 379, A2d 1014 (1977).
2. Furrow BR, Greaney TL, Johnson SH, Jost TS, Schwartz RL. The professional-patient relationship. In: Furrow BR, Greaney TL, Johnson SH, Jost TS, Schwartz RL. Health Law: Cases, Materials, and Problems, ed 3. St Paul: West Publishing, 1997:358–452.
3. Furrow BR, Greaney TL, Johnson SH, Jost TS, Schwartz RL. Life and death decisions. In: Furrow BR, Greaney TL, Johnson SH, Jost TS, Schwartz RL. Health Law: Cases, Materials, and Problems, ed 3. St Paul: West Publishing, 1997:1059–1152.

Glossary

A priori. Derived from self-evident proposition.

Act-based theory. A kind of action theory in which principles are applied directly to individual actions.

Action theory. A theory of right action in which general principles are articulated, sometimes through the use of rules, to make moral evaluations of actions (rather than the character of the actors); *cf*, virtue theory.

Altruism. The moral position that, when pursuing good outcomes, one has a duty to strive to do good for others; contrasted with *egoism*, which focuses on the actor's own good, and *neutralism*, which pursues good without regard to whether the benefit accrues to oneself or another.

Antinomianism. The position that ethical actions must be evaluated in each situation without the use of any rules or guidelines; *cf*, legalism, rules of practice, situationalism.

Autonomy. The governing of oneself according to one's own system of morals and beliefs or life plan.

Axiology. The theory of what constitutes the good. Various theories identify such features as happiness, truth, beauty, health, and morally good character as elements of goodness.

Beneficence. The state of doing or producing good; *cf*, nonmaleficence. Also the moral principle that actions are right insofar as they produce good.

Best interest standard. Judgment based on an idea of what would be most beneficial to a patient; *cf*, substituted judgment standard.

Collegiality. The quality of relationships among similarly situated individuals—in this case professionals—that may influence or reinforce their values, function, and self-regulatory discipline.

Consent. Agreement of one party, usually the patient or surrogate for the patient, to a proposed course of action, usually proposed by a health professional. Consent is *informed* if it is based on knowledge that the decision-maker would need to choose. It is *voluntary* if the decision-maker's choice is substantially autonomous.

Consequentialism. The normative theory that the rightness or wrongness of actions is determined by anticipated or known consequences; *cf*, deontologism.

Contract. A term sometimes used to describe the fiduciary relationship in professional ethics grounded in promises or pledges.

Covenant. A solemn agreement between two or more parties that, as related to health care, emphasizes the moral and social character of the bond between professional and patient.

Cultural relativism. The claim that moral judgments are grounded only in each culture's collective opinion.

De facto. In reality, actual; *cf*, de jure.

De jure. By right, by law; *cf*, de facto.

Deontologism. A theory according to which actions are judged right or wrong based upon inherent right-making characteristics or principles rather than on their consequences; *cf*, consequentialism.

Descriptive relativism. The claim that different cultures have differing views as to which matters are believed to be moral.

Distributive justice. The just allocation of society's benefits and burdens.

Double effect, the doctrine of. The theory that an evil effect is morally acceptable provided a proportional good effect will accrue, evil is not intended, the evil effect is not the means to the good, and the action is not intrinsically evil.

Due process criterion of paternalism. A criterion sometimes used to justify paternalism by which the individual who coerces paternalistically must have observed proper procedure and have proper authorization.

Durable power of attorney. An advance directive that specifies the person to serve as the writer's surrogate decision-maker in the event the writer is unable to speak for himself or herself. It is "durable" in that it continues to govern after the writer becomes mentally incompetent.

Duty proper. A duty decided after taking into account all relevant principles and applying some theory of how to reconcile conflict among principles; *cf*, prima facie duty.

Egalitarian. A social philosophy or principle that advocates human equality.

Ethical. An evaluation of actions, rules, or the character of people, especially as it refers to the examination of a systematic theory of rightness or wrongness at the ultimate level.

Fidelity. The state of being faithful, including obligations of loyalty and keeping promises and commitments. Also the principle that actions are right insofar as they demonstrate such loyalty.

Fiduciary relationship. A relationship based on trust and confidence that commitments made between parties will be honored.

Human immunodeficiency virus (HIV). A retrovirus responsible for acquired immune deficiency syndrome (AIDS).

Justice, the formal principle of. The principle that an action is morally right insofar as it treats people in similar situations equally.

Justice. A moral principle that holds that actions or rules are morally right insofar as they distribute resources according to some pattern, regardless of whether doing so produces the greatest possible balance of benefits over harms. Different theories of justice identify different patterns; for example, an egalitarian principle of justice would distribute health care on the basis of need.

Legalism. The position that ethical action consists of strict conformity to law or rules; *cf*, antinomianism, rules of practice, situationalism.

Libertarianism. The moral theory that gives exclusive or first priority to the principle of autonomy or liberty.

Liberty right. A right to be left alone or to be free from the interference of others to act autonomously. Liberty rights, sometimes called *negative rights*, are often based on the principle of autonomy.

Macroallocation. The process of allocation, with reference to issues of justice, of total societal resources to a particular area; for example, dentistry.

Metaethics. The branch of ethics having to do with the meaning, justification, or grounding of ethical claims; *cf*, normative ethics.

Microallocation. Distribution of resources on a small scale.

Moral. An evaluation of actions or the character of people, especially as it refers to ad hoc judgments by individuals or society.

Neutralism. A characteristic of moral or ethical evaluations in which there is general application not favoring one party.

Nontherapeutic. Something that does not serve the purposes of benefiting an individual patient.

Nonmaleficence. The state of not doing harm or evil; *cf*, beneficence. Also the moral principle that actions are right insofar as they avoid producing harm or evil.

Normative ethics. The branch of ethics having to do with which actions are right or wrong, which states are valuable, or which character traits of people are praiseworthy; *cf*, metaethics.

Normative relativism. The claim that there is no single universal foundation of moral judgments.

Ordering. A characteristic of moral or ethical evaluations on which a set of principles, rules, or character assessments provides a basis for ranking conflicting claims.

Paternalism. The system of action in which one person treats another the way a father treats a child, striving to promote the other's good even against the other's wishes.

Personal relativism. The claim that a behavior or character is good or right if it conforms to one's personal standard of goodness or rightness.

Prima facie duty. A duty based on consideration of a single moral dimension of an action represented by one moral principle; *cf*, duty proper.

Principle (moral). General and abstract characteristics of morally right action; *cf*, action theory.

Profession. An occupation oriented toward service to others based on a fiduciary relationship with clients; it requires extensive specialized knowledge and is self-regulating with respect to issues of entry education and collegial discipline.

Professional standard for consent. The standard that health professionals must disclose all information that their professional colleagues similarly situated would disclose about a proposed procedure; *cf*, reasonable person standard of consent, subjective standard of consent.

Publicity. A characteristic of moral or ethical evaluations in which one must be willing to state the evaluation and the basis on which it is made publicly.

Reasonable person standard of consent. The duty of health professionals to disclose all information that a reasonable person would find meaningful in making a decision about whether to consent to a proposed procedure; *cf*, professional standard for consent, subjective standard of consent.

Rule-based theory. A kind of action theory in which rules, rather than acts, are used to apply principles to individual actions.

Rules of practice. Rules that define general practices in a society; the position that ethical action must be judged by such rules rather than by direct assessment of individual cases; *cf*, antinomianism, legalism, situationalism.

Secular ethics. Theories of what is good and bad, or right or wrong, based on criteria other than religious doctrine.

Situationalism. The position that ethical action must be judged in each situation guided by, but not directly determined by, rules.

Strong paternalism. The provision of treatment for the good of an individual against the wishes of the individual who is known to be substantially autonomous.

Subjective standard of consent. The standard that health professionals must disclose the information that the individual patient would desire in order to know whether to consent to a proposed procedure; *cf*, professional standard for consent, reasonable person standard of consent.

Substituted judgment standard. Judgment based on an idea of what the patient would have wanted considering his or her beliefs and values; *cf*, best interest standard.

Two-tiered medicine. A dual-level system of health care in which tier 1 offers coverage of basic and catastrophic health needs through required societal resources, and tier 2 provides other health needs and preferences through voluntary private coverage.

Ultimacy. A characteristic of moral or ethical evaluations that they are grounded in the highest standard by which one might judge.

Universality. A characteristic of moral or ethical evaluations in which an action or character trait should be evaluated the same by all people.

Utilitarianism. The view that an action is deemed morally acceptable because it produces the greatest balance of good over evil, taking into account all individuals affected.

Utility. The state of being useful or producing good.

Value theory. A theory in which objects or states are rationally desirable; what counts as a good or a harm.

Veracity. A moral principle that holds that actions or rules are morally right insofar as they involve communicating truthfully and avoiding dishonesty.

Virtue theory. A theory that focuses on the character traits of the actor rather than the ethics of the behavior itself; *cf*, action theory.

Weak paternalism. The provision of treatment against the wishes of individuals whose autonomy is or may be compromised.

Index

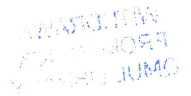